DWARFISM ~

D1274922

DWARFISM ~

MEDICAL AND PSYCHOSOCIAL ASPECTS OF PROFOUND SHORT STATURE

BETTY M. ADELSON

Foreword by Judith G. Hall, O.C., M.D.

THE JOHNS HOPKINS
UNIVERSITY PRESS
BALTIMORE AND LONDON

9 8 7 6 5 4 3 2 1

The Johns Hopkins University Press
2715 North Charles Street
Baltimore, Maryland 21218-4363
www.press.jhu.edu

Library of Congress Cataloging-in-Publication Data

Adelson, Betty M., 1935–
    Dwarfism : medical and psychosocial aspects of profound short stature /
Betty M. Adelson ; foreword by Judith G. Hall.
        p. ; cm.
    Includes bibliographical references and index.
    ISBN 0-8018-8121-8 (hardcover : alk. paper)—ISBN 0-8018-8122-6
    (pbk. : alk. paper)
    1. Dwarfism.
    [DNLM: 1. Dwarfism.   2. Health Knowledge, Attitudes, Practice.
    WE 250 A231d 2005] I. Title.
    RB140.3.A33 2005
    616.4'7—dc22   2004025487

A catalog record for this book is available from the British Library.

*In memory of Dr. Steven E. Kopits, healer of body and spirit,
and in honor of all the dedicated physicians, persons
with dwarfism, and their families, whose mutual regard and
sense of shared mission are transforming the lives of dwarfs*
∾

Contents ⌇

Foreword ～

I am honored to have been invited to write the foreword for the first book to trace broadly and insightfully the exciting developments that have taken place in the field of dwarfism treatment during the past century, particularly during the past fifty years. Betty Adelson has searched the medical literature for articles written by physicians a century ago, when confusion about the causes of dwarfism reigned, and has gone on to carefully sift through the mountain of recent entries on medical databases to garner the most valuable current information. While describing the remarkable progress that has occurred in medical research and treatment, this work also gives equal attention to the social changes that have shaped a newly emerging dwarfism community.

Dr. Adelson is a psychologist whose daughter, Anna, a nursery school teacher, was born thirty years ago with achondroplasia, the most common type of dwarfism. This combination of professional and personal experience has enabled Dr. Adelson to capture many facets of the lives of persons with dwarfism. She has skillfully blended a narrative about medical research and technological advances with more individualized descriptions of human encounters and attitudes.

When I began my career as a physician and clinical geneticist thirty-five years ago, many of the developments described in this volume were in their early stages. I had the privilege of training with Dr. Victor McKusick at a time when he was intensely involved in defining different types of disproportionate short stature. The knowledge and perspective that I acquired during those years helped me to develop effective research strategies and clinical insights. I am particularly proud of being the first author of the American Academy of Pediatrics outline for a health survey on achondroplasia, which I believe was the beginning of health surveillance for a whole variety of genetic

disorders that required understanding their natural history. That outline reveals some of the noteworthy changes that have taken place in
our approach to medical treatment since earlier eras because of our
current greater understanding of scientific method, critical periods,
and individual differences.

As a geneticist, I find it easy to say that each gene interacts with
other genes and so, although the visible difference (especially in disproportionate short stature) is the most striking feature, we now
know that every single type of short stature may affect other organ
systems besides the bones. These effects may alter life span and func-
tionality. It is remarkable that the genes have been found for more
than twenty different types of disproportionate short stature, that animal models have been developed and therapies are being tried, and
that the molecular basis of many different disorders is now much better understood. However, it remains frustrating to both researchers
and affected individuals that a great deal of that research has not yet
led to significant improvements in the lives of those affected. But we
are still in early times.

Much of what we have discovered is reported in the up-to-date references to research studies in the chapters of this volume that deal
with medical and psychosocial aspects. The later chapters, about
dwarfism organizations and the lives of individuals today, describe
some of the other great changes that have taken place. These improvements occurred because the advocacy system in the United
States led to recognition that people with disabilities should be given
the same opportunities as others: in employment, in access to care,
and through removing architectural barriers.

Thirty-five years ago, families frequently were ashamed of and hid
away affected individuals, who then never left home. Today that is un-
thinkable. Because of the advocacy and the support that have been
provided through groups such as Little People of America, families
no longer feel ashamed but rather are motivated to work toward better understanding and better accessibility. They feel pride in their accomplishments and the accomplishments of affected individuals.
This new spirit is documented in the excellent, evocative photographs

that Betty Adelson and LP graphic artist Julie Rotta have selected to accompany the text.

My association with the Little People of America and the equivalent Canadian organizations has taught me about the importance of lay parent support groups and the many roles they can play in providing information, offering social activities, and supporting research. In addition, they challenge society and professionals (both health care and other professionals) to provide the most appropriate and informed care for individuals with short stature. It would be embarrassing to enumerate the many times I have been "off base" and helped by a little person to understand a perspective on the challenges that face people with profound short stature. They have been my mentors in so many ways.

As an average-sized person, I have gained enormous respect for the accommodations that such persons must make every day. Each day is an odyssey and requires overcoming obstacles of heroic proportion that simply cannot be understood by the average-sized individual. Among the challenges that medical professionals face in treating and counseling persons with short stature is the large number of different types, each of which has different complications, different natural histories, and even different inheritance patterns (yes, almost all have a genetic basis).

Researchers and health care professionals need to understand the complexities and complications (medical, scientific, social, and psychological) that confront affected individuals and their families. There is a huge need for really good research to understand what is happening in each type. Furthermore, every family is different. A child born with dwarfism into an average-statured family, for example, encounters different circumstances from a dwarf child born into a family in which at least one parent is a little person. In addition, whatever the family composition, it has unique characteristics that medical professionals must take care to notice.

The ways in which medical and personal history are interwoven are demonstrated in several chapters of this volume. The chapter on psychosocial aspects summarizes research findings but also features the perspectives and voices of short-statured individuals and their families. The chapter addressing the birth of a child portrays the challenges that confront the average-sized parent of a child with profound short stature: the shock, the love, the need for knowledge, and the search for professionals who are most knowledgeable. The parent is often presented with a kaleidoscope of information that is confusing and continuously changing. But that is how it is!

Betty Adelson emphasizes the importance of consulting the most knowledgeable health care professionals so that an accurate diagnosis can be made and effective follow-up conducted through the years; she laments the fact that more dwarfism specialists are not available. She shares not only her own experiences, including those she encountered as a mentor to other families with dwarf children, but also those described by others in published and unpublished accounts. She explores some of the ethical conundrums that have resulted from genetic and technological progress. Her searching and balanced inquiry into a controversial issue such as limb lengthening should prove of interest to both medical professionals and families.

This book is one of the best, most thorough overviews published on dwarfism-related topics. The text is well written, but from the heart, in a way that makes it particularly useful for those who appreciate having scholarly information presented within a meaningful personal and social context. And you never stop looking for information! New findings will always lead to new questions—that is the fate of wanting to learn about a rare condition.

This is a volume that everyone dealing with short stature will want to read and then keep for future reference. Physicians, health care professionals, psychologists, family members, and affected individuals will all find it useful. It details what is known and suggests what future research is needed; it recognizes that parents and affected individuals must be part of the process. In a book that is packed with so much material, readers may choose to "jump around" in search of the answer to a specific question or turn back and read about historical approaches. The appendixes are also valuable, indicating where further resources are available.

This is an exciting time in medical history because of the major advances that are being made in molecular biology, health care, and social services. Dr. Adelson's book provides a rich background, indicating what is presently available, but it also clearly challenges the reader to think about how things will change over the next decade and the decade after that. One can anticipate that a second edition of this book will contain a great deal of new and stimulating information and many new challenges.

It is likely that further social change will occur, that more organizations will form all around the world, and that surprising new stories will appear about families and individuals. Each family is a pioneer, discovering new ways to deal with things and new approaches. What is apt to remain unchanged, however, is that the best solutions are to be found through collaboration among medical professionals, dwarfism organizations, and affected individuals.

Judith G. Hall, O.C., M.D.
Professor of Pediatrics and Medical Genetics
University of British Columbia and Children's and Women's
   Health Centre of BC
Department of Pediatrics, BC's Children's Hospital
Vancouver, British Columbia

Preface ∽

This book is a companion to my volume *The Lives of Dwarfs: Their Journey from Public Curiosity toward Social Liberation.*[1] The questions addressed in both works first surfaced thirty years ago when my daughter, Anna, was born with achondroplasia, the most common dwarfing condition, and I was thrust into bewildering new territory. As I struggled to understand and cope, I sought information in medical libraries. The first textbook entry that I read described the medical hazards of achondroplasia and then went on to say that affected persons waddled when they walked and were consigned to sedentary occupations. Accompanying photographs showed an achondroplastic female as she traveled from babyhood to maturity, naked and blindfolded, with an increasing deformity. Another medical text noted that, because of their grotesque appearance and strength, achondroplastic dwarfs were apt to be employed in circuses and were immature, with strong feelings of inferiority, often vain and fond of drink, and sometimes lascivious.[2]

My visits to physicians at several major New York medical centers did not assuage my fears about whether my daughter could ever have a fulfilling life. These professionals had little or no experience with dwarfs, made significant errors, and offered their pittance of information with considerable unease. Most of all, they communicated that they felt sorry for us. Determined to find answers, my husband, Saul, and I kept in what seemed like constant motion. Anna's average-statured brother, David, was four years old and she was just four months old when we arrived at the Moore Clinic at the Johns Hopkins Hospital. There we encountered a warm and knowledgeable team and took part in a case conference, infusing us with optimism. Subsequent friendships with other families and dwarf individuals became the next step in our pilgrims' progress, an enduring and invaluable part of our lives as parents and as people.

Because I am not a physician or a scientist (I am a psychologist), I have written a work that is not designed for specialists. Current information about specific fields of interest can be found via PubMed, the Online Mendelian Inheritance in Man (OMIM), and professional and dwarfism organizations (see Appendix 2). Space limitations preclude a comprehensive bibliography capable of accommodating the vast number of important entries now accumulating in various subspecialties. I have tried to write an overview for a variety of readers with interest in the field—physicians, nurses, genetic counselors, social workers, and medical students—and, of course, persons with dwarfism and their families.

In the fifteen years since I began my research, the world has changed greatly both for medicine and for persons with dwarfism. While I was quarrying in the past, dramatic developments were taking place in the present. For generously answering my questions and helping me to interpret those developments, I thank Drs. Francomano, Hall, Horton, McKusick, Pauli, Reid, Rimoin, and Scott. Dr. Selna Kaplan has been an excellent resource for growth hormone–related information. Most of all, I shall be forever grateful that through her good counsel I embarked early on the path that led me to Johns Hopkins and Little People of America (LPA), and ultimately to the engagement with the dwarfism community that has resulted in this book.

For the visual component of this book, I am deeply grateful to Julie Rotta, whose graphic expertise, medical knowledge, and familiarity with dwarfism and LPA proved invaluable. During the final three years of the book's preparation, she helped select the photographs, improved their quality, and undertook various related tasks. Her perspective as a person with pseudoachondroplasia enhanced my own understanding. Together, we chose images that we hoped would document the transition of persons with dwarfism from being patronized or mistreated adjuncts to the lives of others to assuming central, satisfying roles in their own lives.

Informants from the United States and abroad contributed significant information or insights. Among them are Dr. Hae-Ryong Song of Gyeong-Sang National University, Korea; Professor Tao Jie of Beijing University, China; Simon Minty, Dr. Tom Shakespeare, and Fred Short of the United Kingdom; and several correspondents from European countries. Many members of LPA have been important to chapter 5, "Lives Today," notably, Reba Hill, Paul Miller, Monica Pratt, Cara Egan Reynolds, Cathy Sarino, Angela Van Etten, and Julie Williams. I appreciate the generous responsiveness of the National Mucopolysaccharidosis Society, the Turner Foundation, Human Growth Foundation, the Osteogenesis Imperfecta Foundation, and the Magic Foundation, and individuals in those groups, notably Barbara Balaban and Lois Warshauer of Human Growth Foundation, Sally Motomura of the National Mucopolysaccharidosis Society, and Priscilla Ciccariello of the Marfan Society.

Special thanks to Joan Weiss, who offered help and encouragement at many stages; to Vita Gagne, who played a vital role in chapter 3, "The Birth of a Child," and to POLP2 members for their postings; to Gretchen Worden of the Mütter Museum for medical history; to Professor Nancy Romer for reading chapter 2, "Psychological Aspects"; to Dr. David Rimoin for reviewing an early draft of chapter 1, "Medical Aspects"; to Berna Miller Torr for helping me understand the demography of vocations; and to my daughter, Anna Adelson, for crucial help with formatting and computer emergencies.

Medical anthropologist Joan Ablon has been a major influence on me and on dwarfism research overall, demonstrating that excellent scholarship can be combined with a personal research style to ensure that the voices of persons with dwarfism are heard. My excellent agent, Sam Stoloff, urged me to divide the original tome I had written into two separate medically and culturally oriented volumes. I am very grateful to the Johns Hopkins University Press and to my sponsoring editor, Wendy Harris, for recognizing the value of this work, assisting in its development, and tending to innumerable fine points. During the final period, I benefited greatly from the perspicacity of Gretchen Primack, who deftly cut and sharpened the voluminous text. Ethan Crough also joined me then as an able, energetic research assistant.

I have written my companion works about dwarfs and dwarfism because no comprehensive chronicles existed: the need was great, and no one else was filling it. I will be very glad to cease being a walking database and to pass on to others the task of describing the next generation of noteworthy events. During this lengthy period, I have been sustained by the love and unflagging assistance of my husband, Saul, and by the pleasure of seeing my two children mature into wonderful adults—my son, David, and my daughter, Anna, who inspired my efforts.

DWARFISM ～

INTRODUCTION ～

This volume chronicles how several concurrent revolutions—medical, scientific, and social—have combined to transform the lives of persons with dwarfism. In 1900, these individuals were still seen as curiosities and were displayed as such, very much as they had been in the courts of many nations from the beginning of recorded history, both indulged and abused.[1] The mysteries of genetic mutation were as unexplored as the cosmos, and the roles of nutrition and metabolism in inhibiting growth were not recognized. Although lack of knowledge was most responsible, the attitudes of the medical establishment were also implicated in its powerlessness to be of any real assistance.

The treatment of dwarfism is now an interdisciplinary endeavor. Geneticists, biologists, chemists, anthropologists, and others are increasing the available information with dazzling speed. Although the genome has largely been unraveled and the discovery of yet another new dwarfism gene is a common event, other aspects, such as matrix biology, which will enrich our understanding of how physiological systems operate, are proving slower to yield their secrets. Generations of transgenic mice now live their lives in laboratories, as the researchers who use them try to fathom how to make short or deformed bones grow normally.

These arenas are only part of the story. What should be noted is that this progress involves a vital collaboration between physicians, both researchers and clinicians, and persons with dwarfism. At conferences of Little People of America and other organizations, doctors and members mingle comfortably. Physicians conduct clinical examinations, offer medical workshops on the latest research and clinical treatments, and distribute questionnaires for ongoing research projects. Physicians and affected individuals are ineluctably intertwined and indeed have a shared mission: improving the daily lives of persons with dwarfism. In the process, they find themselves spending a great deal of time together, coming to know one other as individuals, and sometimes forming lifelong friendships. The old authoritarian system has begun to give way, to the benefit of all. Although an enormous need remains for the volumes now appearing with "hot off the press" accounts of scientific accomplishments, an overview such as this one aims to convey more broadly the nature of this newly shared enterprise.

Dwarfism is an umbrella term that describes a vast medical universe: several hundred conditions that differ in morphology and etiology. All persons with dwarfism are short statured and often have medical problems associated with their individual types, including genetic, chromosomal, hormonal, intrauterine, nutritional, iatrogenic, and psychosocial, but at least as important are factors that transcend these. Unlike most other conditions, dwarfism has resonated in mythology, religion, and the arts throughout history. Among the daunting obstacles that all dwarfs face are omnipresent stares, comments, and often ridicule. Dwarfs tend to be viewed in relation to the single startling fact of their visible difference.

Stigma has always played a role in the lives of persons with dwarfism. The same nations that discriminate against women, blacks, and homosexuals also discriminate against dwarfs. Only recently have dwarfs become part of the movements that gathered strength in the United States in the 1960s and 1970s, in which one group after another claimed equal rights and demanded to be treated with dignity.

In February 2003, 3 foot 3 inch Monique Coneley, then editor-in-chief of the University of Wisconsin–Milwaukee *Post,* wrote an article to help educate the college community. She began:

> People do not see the real me when they look at me. The real me is a
> 23-year-old International Studies major who likes to camp, go to the
> movies, and absolutely loves to travel. This is not what people see when
> they look at me; they may see me as this poor person with dwarfism,
> a disabled person, or someone who got dealt a bad hand. Strangers see
> me not as Monique, but as a dwarf.

It's hard in today's world to be a dwarf when ridicule is condoned and when you have the medical community trying to find the gene that will eliminate dwarfism because to them it is such a horrible condition. People who are non-dwarfs have given me labels and seem to define what it is to be one.

I see my dwarfism like I see myself being Irish; it is just part of who I am and I'm proud to be both. I do not see myself as being dealt a bad hand and I do not see myself as a cripple.[2]

The simple truths embodied in Coneley's statement are central to this book's mission. The attitudes reflected by the relationships of dwarfs to their physicians, their families, and the general public help determine whether dwarfs will flourish or languish in a given society.

Even defining who is a dwarf is not a simple matter. Various height levels have been cited through the years. These days, a dwarf is commonly described as someone 4'10" or under as a result of a medical condition. However, because any cutoff must be somewhat arbitrary, persons just a bit taller whose genetic makeup, bodily characteristics, and medical problems are identical diagnostically to a given dwarfing condition are included (e.g., a 4'11" person with a gene for diastrophic dwarfism and arthritic joints).

On the other hand, individuals from short ethnic stock (Chinese or Guatemalan, for example) whose height is less than 4'10" typically do not identify as dwarfs and are generally not described as such, although they are sometimes included in studies of constitutional short stature. Very short proportionate persons whose short stature is caused by illness or nutritional circumstances may see the mythologically charged term *dwarf* as associated only with short-limbed conditions like those depicted in *Snow White*.

Labels and definitions are rarely entirely satisfying, so although in the United States, physicians and most members of dwarfism groups are comfortable with the word *dwarfs*, now viewed as a medical term, there are varied opinions about *little people*, suggestive of elves and children. The abbreviation *LP*, a neologism without much emotional baggage, is commonly used within the American dwarfism community. In much of Europe, *persons with restricted growth* or *short stature* are the preferred terms, and *short stature* also has its advocates in much of North America, Australia, and New Zealand.

A primary focus of a book about dwarfism, of course, must be the medical revolution that has played a central role in the transformation of the lives of dwarfs. The story of the remarkable developments in radiology, genetics, surgery, technology, and preventive measures that have changed the lives of dwarfs has never before been conveyed

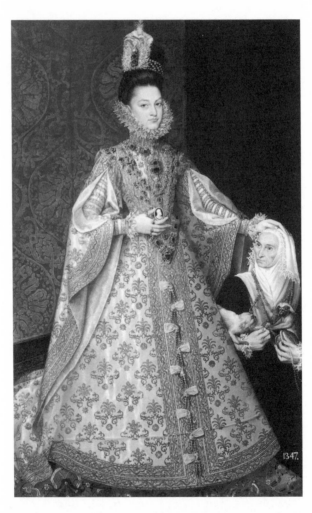

Fig. I.1. The Infanta Isabella Clara Eugenia of Spain with the court dwarf, Magdalena Ruiz (Teodoro Felipe deLiano, 1515–1590). The Prado, Spain.

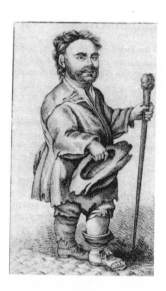

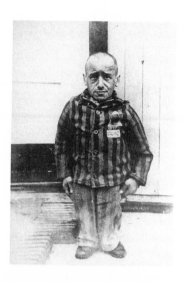

Fig. I.2. Eighteenth-century Irish exhibiting dwarf Owen Farrel. Hy Roth and Robert Cromie, *The Little People* (New York: Everest House, 1980).

Fig. I.3. Alexander Katan (1899–1943), victim of Nazi doctors in Matthausen concentration camp. U.S. Holocaust Memorial Museum.

in a single article or volume. These accomplishments are reviewed here but also located within a broader framework by featuring some of the extraordinary physicians who have starred in the drama. Their devotion to the human beings that they treat is the true raison d'être for their scientific inquiries. They are presented here as role models for the next generation of practitioners and may also help patients and families to crystallize their ideas about the kind of care they should seek. Chapter 1, "Medical Aspects," also touches on a host of ethical and personal dilemmas that have resulted from our newfound ability to diagnose in utero, lengthen limbs surgically, and attempt genetic intervention. The remaining chapters set these questions in context, by reviewing relevant scholarship and by highlighting the human consequences of these medical problems.

The progress of the past half-century does not mean that the prejudice and ridicule omnipresent in previous societies has disappeared. Heightism and beautyism, deemed by some researchers to be rooted in sociobiology (though demonstrably responsive to changes in values and mores), remain prominent. Thoughtless slights abound. During the 1998 presidential campaign, Michael Dukakis and the other Democratic candidates were referred to pejoratively as "the seven dwarfs." Woody Allen has been quoted as declaring that the words most capable of engendering humor are *feathers, herring, butter,* and *dwarf.*[3]

In January 2003, a pre–football game television show featured dwarf entertainers doing imitations of celebrities. Afterward, host Jimmy Kimmel remarked, "Aren't midgets fun? Everyone should own a midget!" Not only is *midget* now viewed as a pejorative word, but also Kimmel's dehumanizing comment recalled the days of the court era, when dwarfs could indeed be owned by the nobility; its correlate would be an appreciative remark that reminisced about slavery, proposing, "Everyone should own a nigger!" It is questionable whether most viewers registered this slur as they would have registered a racially linked insult. Consciousness about dwarfs as a beleaguered minority has surfaced only recently. However, Kimmel did receive many protests from members of Little People of America, the largest support organization for persons of short stature.

Echoes of the past when dwarfs were treated as curiosities and pets, and were exploited and ridiculed, are not apt to disappear soon. Still, encouraging laboratory research and advances in medical treatment, improved vocational opportunities, and a sense of positive identity in much of the LP community are important steps toward transformation. The first three images in this book—Magdalena Ruiz, Spanish court dwarf; Owen Farrel, Irish exhibiting dwarf; and Dutch-Jewish dwarf Alexander Katan, who was murdered in a German concentration camp—are reminders of earlier eras. The other photographs and the entire text document the monumental changes that have occurred and celebrate the new world that physicians and persons with dwarfism are creating together.

1 ～

MEDICAL ASPECTS

Before the recent genetic and technological advances, before the proliferation of new medications and surgical innovations, a doctor's presence could provide only a modicum of expertise and pain relief, along with a large dose of reassurance. These limitations were as true of the treatment of dwarfism as of the rest of medicine.

EARLY MEDICAL APPROACHES TO DWARFISM

The scholarly reader might begin by consulting J. M. Tanner for a history of early philosophical and scientific attempts to understand growth patterns.[1] But to fully appreciate the progress that has been made, one should review representative articles about dwarfism published at the beginning and the end of the twentieth century. Many articles in medical and anthropological journals in the late nineteenth and early twentieth centuries were merely descriptive case studies, with little analysis and no reference to treatment. A typical account appears in M. le Dr. Godin's 1898 article in *Société d'Anthropologie de Paris*.[2] Godin notes that 43-year-old dwarf Mlle. Agnes Sztyahaly of Budapest, whose parents and brother are of normal height, resides with Spaniards who run a circus.

Godin describes Sztyahaly's eyes, skin, and teeth, and then her fine memory, grasp of six languages, and excellent intelligence. Portraying her as courageous, lively, and witty, he remarks that she accepts her poor living quarters without self-pity. Her only weakness is that she drinks too much alcohol, but because she has seen the ravages alcohol has produced in dwarf comrades, she has resolved to stop. Godin concludes by reporting sixty measurements, including the length of her hair.

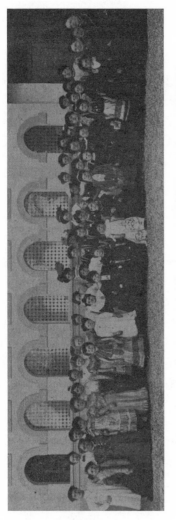
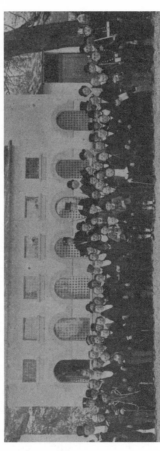

Fig. 1.1. Meeting of the dwarfs of the Jardin d'Acclimation. A. Bloch, "Observations sur les Nains du Jardin d'Acclimation," *Société d'Anthropologie de Paris Bulletins et Memoires* 10, ser. 5 (1909): 533–74. Photograph courtesy of the New York Public Library.

An article entitled "A Family of Dwarfs," published in 1891 in the respected British medical journal *Lancet,* describes a family in which the father is 5′4″ and the deceased mother is 4′10″, but all three children are much shorter.[3] Charles, "a very sharp lad," is 14 years old and 47 inches tall; he has "no hair about the pubic area and axillae, and his ideas are rather childish." Bertha is 13 years old and 44½ inches tall; Natalie is 11 years old and 36¼ inches tall. Though bright, she is puny and delicate and shows no signs of puberty. In winter she must be kept home from school.

Dr. Jacobson, the author, does not explore the reason for the children's short stature, which a modern reader might conjecture was a growth hormone deficiency. At the turn of the century, science had not yet progressed sufficiently to investigate etiology, much less treatment (which, in any event, would have been unavailable). Instead, engaged by their patients' smallness, physicians exercised their tape measures avidly and published the results. When the patients displayed any talent, their physicians would confess themselves charmed that persons so small could be capable of such feats. Some articles did endeavor to resolve scientific disputes. In 1909, an unusually large, well-publicized gathering of dwarfs (most of them entertainers) took place in France and was referred to by the name of the site where they met, "Les Nains du Jardin d'Acclimation" (fig. 1.1).[4] Members of the Paris anthropological society, in commenting on this gathering, compared their observations with previous accounts of dwarfs and pygmies. They distinguished two classes: those with no deformity and those who were termed rachitic, most often identified as achondroplasts. The proportionate dwarfs were reported to be 113.9 cm and the rachitic dwarfs were 103.6 cm. Bloch, the principal investigator, made a point of distinguishing between these pathological cases and pygmies, declaring that he did not believe (as Poncet and Leriche had)[5] in an ancient pygmy race, or that the dwarfs of Le Jardin d'Acclimation bore any connection to pygmies past or present.

Bloch, like many early investigators, distinguished only between proportionate and disproportionate, but he was perceptive enough to discriminate between sporadic and ethnic cases, a distinction that often eluded his predecessors. Still, without any evidence, he concluded that achondroplasia "was not passed on indefinitely" in the genes. Heritability was a great unknown. As late as 1977, a popular work noted, "Heredity does not seem to play an important part in dwarfism."[6]

Diagnostic categories were commonly muddled. Because of worldwide malnutrition, rickets and its resultant restricted growth were common even in advanced nations, and many bowlegged dwarfs were incorrectly labeled rachitic well into the twentieth century. Eminent geneticist Dr. Victor McKusick estimates that probably half of those early cases labeled "rachitic" were in fact not suffering from rickets, but achondroplasia.[7]

Although many "rickety dwarfs" had genetic conditions, the weak bones of others resulted from inadequate sunlight and vitamin D. Dr. James Gamble concludes that Jenny Wren, a young girl in Dickens's novel *Our Mutual Friend,* was a rickety dwarf.[8] Rickets had become endemic in major cities polluted by industrial smog. Roughly one-third of sick children under the age of two in England were suffering from rickets in 1867; in Clydeside in 1884, every child examined was found to be rachitic, whereas in rural areas, the condition was absent.

Although its origins were not understood, the disease had been known since Francis Glisson wrote his classic description in 1650, concluding, "Some Bones wax crooked. . . . Children long afflicted with this Disease become Dwarfs." True rickets has waned as environmental and dietary conditions have improved. A dramatic change occurred during World War II when, in an effort to reduce illness in children caused by poverty, vitamin D supplementation was added to milk and cod liver oil.

Rickets was hardly the only acquired condition thought to be congenital. Cretinism (dwarfism often marked by goiter and accompanied by compromised mental capacity) was described only as a glandular disorder caused by a missing or atrophied thyroid. It had not yet been recognized that this condition might also result from iodine deficiency. The decrease in cretinism is one of the more remarkable developments in the history of treatment for extreme short stature. In some parts of Switzerland, 0.5 percent of the inhabitants were cretins, almost 100 percent of schoolchildren had large goiters, and up to 30 percent of young men were rejected by the military because of a large goiter.[9] Iodization of salt was introduced in 1922, and the amount increased in 1962 and again in 1980, virtually eliminating goiter and dramatically decreasing symptoms of cretinism in areas where it was used.

Some efforts had been made in the early part of the twentieth century to establish sensible diagnostic categories.[10] In their comprehensive 1909 review of achondroplasia and other dwarfing conditions, H. Rischbieth and A. Barrington distinguished ethnic dwarfism from achondroplasia and ateliosis (proportionate short stature, referred to as "true dwarf growth"). Rischbieth and Barrington divided the categories further into six groups[11]: (1) dwarf races; (2) hypoplasia caused by syphilis, plumbism, or perhaps ateliosis; (3) intrauterine microcephaly and children born before term; (4) hydrocephaly, meningitis, and renal and intestinal conditions; (5) thyroid problems, including cretinism and infantile myxedema; and (6) rickets, which includes achondroplasia, other chondrodystrophies, and bone growth disorders. Rischbieth and Barrington offer X-rays, photographs of historical figures and patients, and an extensive catalog of dwarfs in art. This raw material makes their text, despite its errors, essential reading for those studying the history of dwarfing conditions. Early accounts of causality seem little more than a guessing game. One 1912 book about achondroplasia reports that stunting of growth is caused by amnion pressure in the womb.[12] More astonishing is Theophilis Parvin's 1893 article, "The Influence of Maternal Impressions upon the Foetus."[13] Parvin, professor of obstetrics and diseases of women and children, declares that a patient's dwarfism resulted from the mother being startled in early pregnancy by a turtle her husband had hidden in a cupboard. He includes a drawing of that patient whom his neighbors call "the turtle man" (fig. 1.2); he classifies a baby also pictured, born without most of his arms and legs, as an ectromelian, related to "the subvariety phocomelians—that is, seal-like monstrosities." Few physicians today would use the word *monstrosity*, once a standard medical term applied to physical deformities.

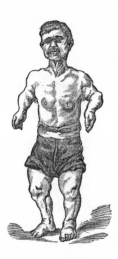

Fig. 1.2. "The turtle man," an example of early medical ignorance. Theophilis Parvin, "The Influence of Maternal Impression on the Foetus," *International Medical Magazine* 1 (1893).

Although perplexed by why some offspring of frightened mothers do not have congenital marks, while others not conceived in dread do have them, Parvin is convinced that maternal impression accounts for many, if not all, deformities, and he frames these events as designed "according to a Divine Plan." Citing Tesla's recent discoveries in electricity, he concludes that one day the mechanism governing maternal impression on the fetus will be as clear as the workings of the telephone and telegraph.

Belief in maternal impression has been pervasive in almost every culture and era.[14] Josef Warkany, in *Congenital Malformations,* mentions that ancient Greeks encouraged expectant mothers to look at beautiful statues, and sixteenth-century philosopher Montaigne used the theory to explain congenital anomalies. Warkany notes that an 1889 survey of maternal impression reported ninety cases described in medical journals. We need not feel superior to the authorities of the past because old mistakes have disappeared. Even today, Warkany suggests, people incorrectly conclude that congenital malformations are due to mutant genes, viruses, or diet. It is also still common for individuals who are uneducated about causality to declare that their dwarfism has resulted from their mothers' having seen a dwarf early in pregnancy.

Respected authorities such as George Gould and Walter Pyle offered vague and sometimes inaccurate statements in 1896: "It may be remarked that perhaps certain women are predisposed to give birth to dwarfs."[15] They distinguish two classes of dwarfs: those born healthy, who in their infancy become ill and are afflicted with arrested development, and a second group, dwarfs from birth, "conformed, robust, and intelligent." The first group is infertile; members of the second group "have more than once proved their virility." The authors note that some dwarfs who have married average-sized women have had several children, "though this is not, it is true, an indisputable proof of their generative faculties." Are the authors questioning these fathers' paternity?

Indeed they are. Respected anesthesiologist Dr. J. Mason Warren, who was also taken in by the ruse of microcephalic dwarfs exhibited in Boston as "Aztec children," believed dwarfs were incapable of reproducing, citing dwarfism authority Étienne Geoffroy St. Hilaire as well as Catherine de Medici's vain efforts to mate her dwarfs. Of court dwarf Joseph Boruwlaski, who had several children, he noted: "The paternity of Boruwlaski was not received by all without incredulity, even in his own day."[16]

Although not everyone thought all dwarfs were infertile, some adamantly opposed childbearing. After citing examples of death during childbirth, the authors of one 1878 article do not discuss ways of making childbirth safer but instead decry all marriages between a dwarf woman and a taller man. They write: "That these marriages or results of copulation in these cases, should be made a criminal offense, as much as murder, suicide, or abortion, we think no man who has studied the subject will deny."[17]

To understand these doctors' position, one needs to understand the sorry state of mid-nineteenth-century obstetrics. In 2002, Gretchen Worden, director of the Mütter Museum, a division of the College of Physicians of Philadelphia, mounted an exhibit of the skeleton of a dwarf woman who had died in childbirth. Some individuals suspected this might be a throwback to previous centuries, when physicians purchased corpses from impoverished dwarfs in return for meager payments, to display their bones at medical colleges after their deaths.

Worden's way of thinking was quite different. A knowledgeable, sensitive curator, she had done careful research to educate the public about dwarfism. She discovered that the Mütter skeleton belonged to Mary Ashberry, a 3'6" achondroplastic woman who had died in Norfolk, Virginia, after a cesarean delivery in 1856 (fig. 1.3). Ashberry had been living in a brothel, but it was unclear whether she had been employed there or had simply taken refuge. An 1879 article revealed that her childbirth had been mismanaged, resulting in death after three days of labor.[18]

Obstetrical care was inadequate for most in the mid-nineteenth century, but for dwarfs it was far worse. Of 110 cesarean surgeries in the United States, 23 had been performed on dwarf women. Only six dwarf women and twelve children survived the operations, which were often attempted very late in labor; death was commonly caused by peritonitis or exhaustion. Dr. Robert Harris, who analyzed the original description of Ashberry's labor and surgery, noted that three dwarfs had cesarean surgeries in Virginia in 1856, with the loss of two mothers and one child. The only early operation saved both mother and fetus. Harris believed that with proper, timely attention, Ashberry too might have survived. When Rischbieth and Barrington declared in 1912 that most dwarf infants with achondroplasia were born dead or died in the first year of life, they had little understanding of why, or that intervention could make a difference. They also reported (inaccurately) that there were more females than males, and that obesity was common in females but rare among males.

It is easier to forgive the errors of brave early scientists who were charting new territory with inadequate tools than it is to forgive some later authors. Here are just a few examples from a lengthy catalog. Walter Bodin in *It's a Small World* (1934) comments: "the odds against midgetism . . . are a million to one. These odds are arrived at by placing the world population at two billion. The best authorities

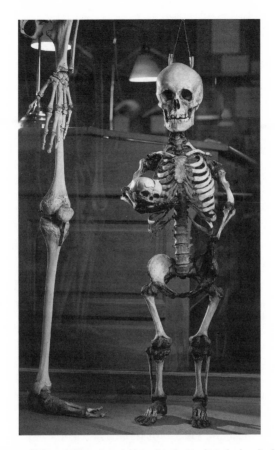

Fig. 1.3. Skeleton of Mary Ashberry, an achondroplastic dwarf who died in childbirth in 1855. Mütter Museum, The College of Physicians of Philadelphia. Photograph © 2000 Scott Lindgren.

estimate the world population of midgets at two thousand. Thus we find that of every million children brought into life one is destined for midgethood."[19]

Thirty years later, Andrew Hamilton's 1964 *Science Digest* article, "If You Were a Midget," draws on these fantastic "statistics," stating that there were "3,000 little people in the world—midgets and dwarfs—whose height is less than 4 feet six inches tall." Hamilton continues: "Because their metabolism is about one and one-half times that of an average-sized person, a 60 pound midget can stow away as much food as a 175-pound man and sometimes drink him under the table. Little people are surprisingly resistant to infectious diseases, tooth decay and baldness."[20]

One wonders whether the fact-checkers at *Science Digest* were fast asleep, but here as elsewhere writers offer "evidence" without supplying sources, as noted literary critic Leslie Fiedler did in *Freaks* in 1978: "Sexual relations are possible, at least between full sized women and male dwarfs, who are apparently as well endowed sexually as their taller peers. The evidence is more contradictory concerning the mating of Lilliputian women and normal men."[21] Fiedler goes on to state from admitted "limited personal observation" that most marriages between dwarfs and nondwarfs conceal a desire to exploit the "freak partner" either economically or sexually.

Medical authorities have also been guilty of unsupported bias. One infamous example in the 1983 edition of *Mercer's Orthopedic Surgery* describes the clinical features of achondroplasia alongside a photograph of a child who appears to have pseudoachondroplasia. Under the heading "Intellect," the author offers the following observations:

> Achondroplasts are usually of normal intelligence, and frequently they are lively and amusing. In some cases, however, the intellect is impaired and they are backward for their age.
>
> Because of their deformed bodies they have strong feelings of inferiority and are emotionally immature, and are often vain, boastful, excitable, fond of drink, and sometimes lascivious. Sexual development is usually normal, but may be retarded. Dwarfs are very muscular and excel in feats of strength; they are frequently employed in theatres and circuses, partly because of their strength and partly because of their grotesque appearance.[22]

Even in the era of the Internet, misinformation abounds. The *Encarta Encyclopedia* offers this entry under "Dwarfism":

> Dwarfism, in medicine, condition of being undersized, or less than 127 cm (50 in) in height. The term *midget* is usually applied to physically well-proportioned dwarfs. The cause of most dwarfism in Europe, Canada, and the United States is *cretinism*, which results from a

disease of the thyroid gland. Other causes of dwarfism include *Down syndrome;* achondroplasia, a disease involving short limbs resulting from improper fetal development; hypochondroplasia, a milder form of achondroplasia; and spinal tuberculosis.[23]

The unidentified perpetrator of this account manages to offend several times in a single paragraph. Dwarfs are typically defined these days as persons 4′10″ and under as a result of a medical condition. The term *midget* is considered pejorative. The cause of most dwarfism in North America and Europe is not cretinism. Achondroplasia is a genetic, not an intrauterine condition. Such gross inaccuracies make us all the more grateful for myriad discoveries now being made at a speed astonishing even to the scientists and physicians themselves.

DIAGNOSTIC CATEGORIES, ETIOLOGY, AND TREATMENT

Systematic assessment of current knowledge about dwarfism requires cognizance of both morphology and etiology (differences in appearance of individuals with dwarfism and causes of their conditions). Although full understanding requires knowledge of Mendelian and molecular genetics and radiology, it helps to begin with a simple classification system. This diagnostic outline is adapted from Linder and Cassorla's 1988 etiological arrangement of dwarfing conditions.[24]

1. *Constitutional or Familial Short Stature.* This is short stature noticeable in individuals whose parents and other relatives tend to have heights less than 4′10″. Whether from a short national stock or a taller national group whose families have nevertheless been extremely short, they usually consider themselves merely small and would not use the term dwarf, which has tended to be used more often in referring to those who have an identifiable medical condition. Nevertheless, this is the most prevalent type.

2. *Disorders of the Bone.* Also called chondrodystrophies or skeletal dysplasias, these are the more than 200 genetic conditions in which cartilage and bone have not developed normally because of a mutant gene. Persons with these conditions tend to have disproportion

of some kind in limbs or parts of limbs, between torso and limbs, or in facial features affected by cartilage growth. Often the spine and spinal nerves are involved. In some conditions there is degeneration of the hip bones.

3. *Endocrine Disorders.*

  a. Hypopituitary dwarfism. In general, proportionate dwarfism is caused either by a deficiency of human growth hormone or a problem with the receptors for that hormone. It was originally called ateliosis; persons were called midgets (now often rejected as pejorative). In childhood and young adulthood, persons with this condition tend to look much younger than their actual age and sometimes lack robustness. Sometimes, a hypothalamic rather than pituitary defect is involved; many neurotransmitters, including dopamine, can influence the hypothalamus. There are also more complex disorders that influence the secretion and function of growth hormone. The condition has proved treatable, at first with somatropin (HGH) extracted from human pituitaries and, more recently, much more widely with synthetic growth hormone.

  b. Hypothyroidism. This is a congenital or acquired problem of the thyroid that interferes with growth. Acquired hypothyroidism occurring after two to three years is often caused by autoimmune thyroiditis. Early diagnosis and treatment with thyroid replacement is very important. Hypothyroidism, formerly known as cretinism, may also be caused by iodine deficiency.

4. *Dwarfism Caused by Absent or Incomplete Chromosomes.*

  a. Turner syndrome. This syndrome, which affects only females, is caused when one of the two X chromosomes normally found in women is missing or contains certain structural defects. The condition results in short stature and nonfunctioning ovaries, with impaired pubertal development and infertility. In some patients there are additional medical concerns. Women with Turner syndrome are treated with estrogens; recently, synthetic growth hormone (rhGH) has proved useful in providing some increase in height; sometimes long-acting gonadorelin, gonadotropin-releasing hormones (GnRH), has been used to allow for a longer growth period.

b. Down syndrome. This is a genetic disorder characterized by an anomaly in cell development that results in 47 instead of the usual 46 chromosomes in every cell of the body, interfering with aspects of body and brain development. The condition is marked by a distinct physical appearance, notably broad hands and feet and slanting eyes with eyelid folds. One-fourth of individuals have extreme short stature.

5. *Intrauterine Growth Retardation.* These disorders originate while the baby is still in utero, resulting in full-term babies whose height and weight may be as much as two standard deviations below the mean. Etiology is often not identifiable, but there are probably many causes. The infants are proportionately short statured, and most have been unable to achieve average height. Recent growth hormone trials have produced some encouraging signs.

6. *Genetic Syndromes.* Bloom syndrome, Russell Silver syndrome, and Cornelia de Lange syndrome, among others, produce proportionate growth retardation and additional distinctive features.

7. *Chronic Systemic Disease or Iatrogenic Dwarfism.* Many diseases and infections such as kidney, cardiac, hepatic, and gastrointestinal can interfere with children's achieving their full growth potential. Rheumatoid arthritis in childhood has resulted in extreme short stature. Sometimes therapy for a condition (e.g., the treatment of colitis, nephrotic disease, or asthma with excessive amounts of cortisone) inhibits growth.

8. *Dwarfism Caused by Nutritional Deprivation.* Children who suffer from chronic malnutrition will not achieve their full genetic potential in height, most often because of lack of proteins. In what was once called rachitic or rickety dwarfism, the lack of vitamin D and sunlight also contributes. If a child is protein starved until the age of 5 years, full growth often cannot be recovered. Iodine deficiency has caused cretinism in many developing nations.

9. *Psychosocial Dwarfism.* A substantial literature demonstrates that when children are abused or neglected emotionally, their growth is

seriously compromised. Upon transfer to salubrious conditions, growth tends to resume. If a child experiences prolonged emotional deprivation, dwarfism can result.

A well-researched 2003 government publication offers a rare overview of many of these short-stature conditions, including chronic diseases. Aided by charts and a comprehensive bibliography, it attempts to assess conditions by disability criteria.[25]

Organizations that serve dwarfs tend to be composed mostly of persons with congenital medical conditions. In 2003, there were 8,843 members of LPA, many of them of average stature. Among 3,224 persons with dwarfism, diagnoses tended to be skewed toward bone disorders: achondroplasia, 1,995; SED (all types), 196; hypochondroplasia, 122; diastrophic dwarfism, 101; pseudoachondroplasia, 100; hypopituitary dwarfism, 73; osteogenesis imperfecta, 56; cartilage-hair hypoplasia, 40; Turner syndrome, 29; Morquio syndrome, 29; spondylometaphyseal dysplasia, 25; Kneist dysplasia, 18; metaphyseal chondrodysplasia, 14; acromesomelic dysplasia, 14; Ellis-van Creveld syndrome, 12; Russell Silver syndrome, 10; campomelic dysplasia, 10; other, 148; diagnosis unknown, 232.

Other conditions constitute a total of 143 diagnoses, many categories including just a few individuals. Although approximately half the respondents have achondroplasia, reflecting its relative frequency in the general population, one cannot assume that the incidence of other rare conditions in this database corresponds to their frequency in the general population.

The most common of these polysyllabic conditions are described briefly in Appendix 1, but comprehensive accounts can be found in Online Mendelian Inheritance in Man (OMIM), in PubMed, or in *Bone Dysplasias* by J. Spranger et al. (2002). Also useful are the LPA Medical Resource Center site on LPA Online, the Web sites of various dwarfism organizations, and the literature listed in Appendix 2.

Some of the major medical concerns of persons with chondrodystrophies (bone disorders) are spinal narrowing in the lumbar region, which may cause numbness, difficulty walking, or paralysis, and problems at the foramen magnum or upper cervical spine, which may cause muscle weakness or paralysis, breathing and swallowing problems, or even sudden infant death syndrome. Among other significant medical difficulties are joint degeneration or bone fragility, problems with hearing or vision, cleft palate or dental abnormalities, hydrocephalus, or, rarely, a heart problem. (Note: Even within a single condition, not all potential problems actually occur.)

Reading a catalog of symptoms and abnormalities is apt to be discouraging for parents and patients. Despite the daunting problems associated with dwarfing conditions, the hopeful note is that at least partial remedies now exist for most problems. Furthermore, treatment has become more sophisticated and effective with each passing year. There are continuous positive airway pressure (CPAP) and bilevel positive airway pressure (BiPAP) treatments for breathing problems, shunts to treat hydrocephalus, vents to prevent hearing loss, and surgeries for a multitude of conditions. Careful monitoring, surgical intervention, and preventive measures have become more common, thereby averting the most disastrous scenarios, such as paralysis or unremitting pain. With increased attention being given to the psychosocial aspects, a person's overall life situation can be organized in ways that minimize difficulties and maximize participation in normal activities and pleasures.

THE INCIDENCE OF DWARFING CONDITIONS

Because different definitions of dwarf have been used, and no single reference work answers the question, we are unsure how common dwarfism is. Even geneticists have hesitated to weigh in decisively. Most estimates have been based on cobbling together the results of a few of the best studies extant of incidence. Although there have been some valuable investigations, casting light on various subgroups in a number of countries, variations in methodology have made it impossible to use them to come to definitive conclusions about the incidence of dwarfism across the full etiological spectrum.[26] The absence of birth defects registries is one problem (only a few states have well-functioning registries). Those that do are required to report only cases discovered during the first year of life: growth failure discovered later often goes uncounted, because few studies of whole populations have been done. Census takers don't ring our bells and ask, "Is there a dwarf in your household?"

Consequently, there is little consensus. In 1984 Ablon noted previous estimates ranging from 20,000 to 100,000 dwarfs in the United States.[27] Many researchers have been "chondrocentric," focusing on bone dysplasias and ignoring most other conditions. Until there is serious collaboration on the problem by a demographer and a few geneticists with dwarfism expertise, we probably must content ourselves with educated guesses. However, there are ways to approach a more accurate appraisal, and in assaying them one is apt to discover that prevalence is far greater than the investigators that Ablon cited had reported.

One approach is simply to add the figures noted on various dwarfism Web sites. The incidence of achondroplasia is estimated at approximately 1 in 20,000; 1 in 20,000 for types III and IV osteogenesis imperfecta (those accompanied by dwarfism); 1 in 2,500 for Turner syndrome; 1 in 4,000 cases of Down syndrome (just those who are short statured); and 1 in 7,000 schoolchildren who have growth hormone deficiency (greater if adults are considered). Calculating the totals by using a U.S. population of 280 million, the numbers of persons with dwarfism add up to several hundred thousand. Not included here are a great many other bone dysplasias and other genetic and chromosomal anomalies, as well as other potentially dwarfing conditions such as kidney failure, juvenile arthritis, psychosocial dwarfism, and iatrogenic short stature, for which we do not have precise figures.

These figures suggest an incidence well over 200,000. That estimate is reinforced by a recent survey of Department of Motor Vehicle (DMV) statistics by Rick Spiegel—associate of the Society of Actuaries, a member of the American Academy of Actuaries, and former president of LPA.[28] To be able to get a better gauge of the incidence of very short individuals than LPA previously had available, he contacted several state DMV offices. He was not able to obtain figures from all states, but reports from a total of just seven revealed that 1 of 1,520 individuals was 4'6" or shorter, and 1 of 277 was 4'10" or shorter. Calculating only the persons who are no more than 4'6" and using a U.S. population figure of 280 million, one discovers that there are approximately 169,000 persons who are 4'6" or shorter. It is unlikely that stature like this would occur without accompanying medical etiology. Had figures been available for persons who were 4'8" or for very short individuals who were nondrivers because of their disabilities, this number would be considerably higher.

PROGRESS IN DIAGNOSTIC UNDERSTANDING OF THE SKELETAL DYSPLASIAS

When many skeletal conditions were not yet identified, or were ill understood, there was considerable disagreement on how they ought to be grouped. Physicians leaned toward being either "lumpers" or "splitters"—diagnosing through commonalities or distinctions that mark conditions. Until the mid-1960s, indiscriminate lumping often tended to be the rule: it was common for all short-limbed conditions to be referred to as achondroplasia and all short-trunk conditions to be called Morquio's by nonspecialists, despite the fact that a number of researchers had begun to assign separate names to conditions.[29] Later, individual conditions were distinguished further and regrouped into families.

By the 1960s Dr. Victor McKusick and others had noticed distinctive features in a number of disorders. When he studied the Amish in Pennsylvania, McKusick discovered two dwarfing conditions that occurred in the group with unusual frequency.[30] One turned out to be a previously unrecognized condition; because it was characterized by problems with bone growth and thin hair, McKusick termed it cartilage-hair hypoplasia; the other term for it now is metaphyseal chondrodysplasia, McKusick type. Another unusual concentration exists in Finland.[31]

Another disorder had commonly been called "six finger syndrome"; it was first identified by Ellis and van Creveld in the 1930s, and later referred to as Ellis–van Creveld syndrome. McKusick identified more cases among the Amish than had been described in all previous literature. He and his colleagues used the genealogic registry of Lancaster County, spurring later researchers to analyze genetic inheritance and inbreeding. Although cases had occurred in other groups, the concentration here was exceptional and traceable to a single founding settler. Perhaps 50 percent of those with the condition had serious heart problems, and many did not survive into adulthood. By 1972, drawing on his own work and that of American and European investigators, McKusick published his groundbreaking *Heritable Disorders of Connective Tissue,* updated in several later editions.[32]

The 1960s and 1970s were a very active period for new discoveries. Dr. David Rimoin, for example, while still a resident at Johns Hopkins, distinguished endocrine disorders in which isolated growth hormone deficiency was involved. Other physicians began to discriminate and label various conditions using precise measurements, blood samples, radiology, and attention to clinical features. McKusick organized week-long conferences on clinical delineation of birth defects at Johns Hopkins beginning in 1968, attended by international experts.

By 1985 there was a swing back in the direction of noticing significant commonalities, with Dr. Jurgen Spranger suggesting that genetically different bone dysplasias could manifest themselves in similar patterns of skeletal abnormalities. He proposed that they be grouped in "families" (e.g., the achondroplasia pattern; the SED congenita pattern; the Larsen/oto-palatal-digital [OPD] pattern, and the Stickler-Kniest pattern).[33] Later molecular work confirmed many of his clinical impressions, and refinements of classification resulting from DNA discoveries allowed the insights of molecular genetics to be combined with the knowledge already in place from radiology.

In 2002, Spranger and colleagues published *Bone Dysplasias,* a diagnostics compendium of 160 conditions that updated his 1974 seminal work produced with other collaborators.[34] In his introduction to the 2002 volume, Spranger notes that mutations of specific genes are now known to produce conditions with different phenotypes and prognoses and that the classification system of this volume represents a compromise between etiopathogenetic and clinical considerations.[35]

The old battle of the "lumpers" and "splitters" has largely been resolved. As a result of genetic mapping, some conditions formerly seen as separate are recognized as variations of a single syndrome. The latest schema of the *International Nomenclature of Constitutional Disorders of Bone* reflects the current approach, establishing thirty-three categories subdivided into more than 225 conditions. In nosology as in sociology, individuals can be discussed separately or as members of a family group. Some "unfamilied" individuals are labeled "private" conditions—diagnostic categories known to affect only a few persons in the whole world or even a single individual.

THE HISTORY OF CLASSIFICATION OF SKELETAL DYSPLASIAS

The passage of researchers toward understanding the nature of skeletal dysplasias entailed more than a century of unsteady progress. Dr. Steven Kopits's 1974 review reflects how widely spread are the dates at which the six major bone conditions he discusses were first identified.[36] Some had been noticed as early as 200 years ago, but the account had been forgotten. In one dramatic instance, Olaus Jacob Ekman, chief surgeon to the Swedish Royal Cavalry Regiment of Southern Scane, defended his thesis before the faculty of medicine in 1788. He described several cases of what he called osteomalacia and traced this hereditary bone fragility through three generations. For the most part, his work remained unrecognized until 1949, when Knud Seedorf credited him with the discovery of osteogenesis imperfecta.[37]

Achondroplasia, though described by Parrot in 1878 and Kauffman in 1892, was at first overdiagnosed and confused with other conditions. Morquio and Brailsford identified what came to be known as Morquio syndrome in independent investigations in 1929; pseudoachondroplasia was first described by Maroteaux and Lamy in 1959; they identified diastrophic dwarfism as a distinct condition in 1961.

Metaphyseal chondrodysplasia began to be discussed in 1934, but entities subsumed under it were defined only much later; Spranger and Wiedmann identified spondyloepiphyseal dysplasia in 1966. It was also not uncommon for the same conditions to have been described by different names in different decades. Horton has traced the development of approaches to bone dysplasia from the time when it relied most heavily on radiology to the present when better information about genetic mutations has become accessible.[38]

A major triumph of classification was the creation of the Paris Nomenclature for Constitutional Disorders of Bone in 1970 under the aegis of the European Society of Pediatric Radiology. It classified the skeletal dysplasias into two major groups: osteochondrodysplasias, abnormalities of cartilage and/or bone growth and development, and the dysostoses, malformation of individual bones singly or in combination. That categorization, elaborated in articles by Maroteaux in France and by Rimoin, McKusick, and Scott in the United States in the 1970s, provided a workable and much more accurate organizing system of dwarfing conditions.[39] McKusick's *Heritable Disorders of Connective Tissue* and *Mendelian Inheritance in Man* remain among the richest wellsprings of information for physicians and researchers.[40]

The impressive *International Nomenclature of Constitutional Disorders of Bone*, introduced in the 1990s, is updated biannually.[41] Divided into thirty-three categories, each containing between two and twenty-two separate diagnoses, it offers the mode of inheritance for each condition, its chromosomal locus, gene, and syndrome number in *Online Mendelian Inheritance in Man*, and presence or absence at birth. It illustrates the groups for which the gene has been discovered and the protein known—and those awaiting new information.

The approach to nosology represented by the adaptable *International Nomenclature* grid represented enormous progress. However, within the next decade, still more would be required. After the *International Classification of Disorders of Bone* was published in 1998, rapid advances in identifying molecular changes responsible for conditions caused the classification to expand to include not only thirty-three groups of osteochondrodysplasias, but also three groups of genetically determined dysostoses.[42] Spranger's 2002 *Bone Dysplasias* is a compendium representing the new integrated approach that includes emerging genetic and molecular information.

Articles such as those by Andrea Superti-Furga and his colleagues point toward the amazing reshuffling of thinking required when approaching the new information.[43] For example, phenotypically dissimilar conditions such as diastrophic dysplasia and the typically lethal achondrogenesis 1B are shown to share a common pathogenetic mechanism and are referred to as "the Achondrogenesis-Diastrophic Dysplasia family." Related mouse-model research is already in progress. The authors suggest that assessing the multitude and variety of genes by means of a molecular and pathogenetic classification that complements the existing nosology can serve as a bridge between laboratory and clinic. Resulting insights are apt to lead to new therapeutic measures. In addition, nagging questions such as the influence of paternal age as a cause of sporadic achondroplasia promised to be better understood once it was learned that there were three main classes of gene mutations causing genetic disorders.

A HISTORY OF TREATMENT ADVANCES

Thyroid Conditions

The near disappearance of rickets since World War II and the gradual reduction of cretinism have caused major changes in whole populations where the conditions were endemic. The conquest of cretinism has been a miracle of investigation and treatment. This previously common deficiency disease has been eliminated in all parts of the world where adequate nutrition and iodine supplementation are available. Nevertheless, congenital hypothyroidism still occurs and is responsible for a small percentage of instances of dwarfism; it can be treated with thyroid supplementation.

Access to knowledge and treatment limits the effect of scientific advances in most of the world. In countries such as India and Bangladesh, cretinism—now more commonly referred to as IDD, or iodine
deficiency disorder—is still a major public health problem. It is estimated that in India 270 million people are at risk for IDD; only recently has noniodized salt been banned and programs instituted
aimed at eliminating the condition by early in the twenty-first century.[44] Such surveys do not focus on stature, but it is well known that
when the deficiency is great, dwarfism is a consequence.

Congenital hypothyroidism (CH) is one of the most common preventable causes of mental retardation, occurring in 1 of 3,600–4,000
infants. Before screening became available in the 1970s, many children with this condition were moderately or profoundly retarded.
Screening for hypothyroidism is now part of the neonatal battery in
most Western nations; in the United States it is mandated in most
states.[45] Early detection and treatment is essential; studies have
shown that treatment must be provided by the third month.

Growth Hormone Deficiency, or Hypopituitary Dwarfism

The 1960s–1990s brought another major advance in therapy with
treatment for hypopituitary dwarfism, a dysfunction of the pituitary
gland in which patients are very short but proportionate. (Persons
with this condition were formerly called "midgets.") There are two
major types: in panhypopituitarism, which represents about two-
thirds of the cases, persons do not go through normal puberty and do
not reproduce; in one-third of the cases, isolated growth hormone deficiency (IGHD), patients mature sexually and can reproduce. (There
are also subgroups of IGHD.)

Through the use of human pituitary hormone, and later synthetic
growth hormone, patients have achieved average stature. Human
growth hormone (HGH) was first isolated in 1956 by Dr. Cho Hao Li
of the University of California Medical Center at San Francisco. Between 1962 and 1985 the number of patients treated with pit-hGH
increased from 150 to 3,000. In 1985, there was consternation among

physicians when it was discovered that a number of patients treated with pit-hGH had developed Creutzfeldt-Jakob disease (a condition similar to mad cow disease) and some had died as a result. Such treatment was discontinued, and the growth hormone first synthesized in 1971 by Dr. Li came into widespread use. It is estimated that more than 60,000 patients have been treated with synthetic growth hormone (rhGH).[46]

This treatment has facilitated greater height gain than before, permitting many patients to attain or exceed targeted height. The earlier treatment is started, the better the results. A French long-term study of GH-deficient children who began treatment before 1 year of age for an average of 8 years (±3.6 years) demonstrated excellent normalization of height.[47] The outlook for a child first treated at 4 years of age is much better than for one not treated until adolescence. Also, it has become clear that daily injections of small doses are more effective than larger ones administered two or three times a week.

The Kabi International Growth Study of 2,589 patients published in 1990 revealed that 85 percent of patients being treated had growth hormone deficiency, whereas 15 percent had other causes of growth failure. Most patients were three standard deviations below the mean when treatment started, and there was a preponderance of boys. The numbers of patients being treated for idiopathic and organic growth hormone deficiency seem to be steadily rising.[48]

With the advancement of molecular biological techniques, the basis for other forms of short stature has been expanded. The discovery of genes and transcription factors (PROP-1 and POU-1F1) critical for pituitary hormonal cell development has led to the identification of new forms of GH and other pituitary hormonal deficiencies.[49] One condition that has received an extraordinary amount of attention is Laron dwarfism, identified in 1966, in which growth hormone is present, but a defect in the receptor causes growth failure. Somatomedin-1 therapy is being tested to treat this recessive condition, which is particularly common in Ecuador and Israel.

There have been new approvals of GH treatment for several conditions, among them intrauterine growth retardation (IUGR), Prader-Willi syndrome, and chronic renal failure, changing the practice of endocrinology. Studies of children with IUGR indicate a significant increase in growth rate after eight years of treatment; in some instances, individuals treated for two years continued to grow normally without further treatment. In the case of Prader-Willi syndrome, beneficial effects on growth rates and metabolism have been described for most patient types, although reports of a few deaths have led to lower doses, and caution has been advised especially for obese patients with respiratory problems.

Numerous studies have been done using growth hormone to treat children with achondroplasia. It is difficult to compare results because there are many variables, but it seems that, although cartilage responds with initially increased velocity to GH therapy, the effect of GH therapy on final height seems negligible and is not predictable with the available data.[50]

Other possible uses continue to appear. For example, individuals with Crohn disease have improved significantly through the use of protein diets and growth hormone. And although studies most often report the results of treatment with adults, they suggest that the use of GH may enhance growth in children with bowel disorders.

The use of growth hormone to treat conditions that are clearly medical elicits no debate. However, in both the medical and general community, the use of growth hormone to treat persons who are merely constitutionally short has inspired ongoing controversy. On 25 July 2003 the Food and Drug Administration approved the use of Humatrope, a growth hormone treatment for persons with idiopathic short stature (of unknown origin).[51] Children more than 2.25 SD below the mean for age and sex (the shortest, 1.2%) would be eligible. This corresponds to heights of less than 5'3" in adult men and 4'11" in adult women. Multicenter trials, involving children who received doses six times weekly for about 6.5 years, indicated an increase in growth of 1½–3 inches. Although many seem to be willing to sign on for that relatively small gain, the popular press has tended to be critical or at least circumspect about "enhancement" that might cost as much as $200,000. Nevertheless, in 2004, Tercica, a newly public biotechnology company, indicated that it would seek Food and Drug Administration approval to market rh1GF-1, a new drug that they report allows patients to grow an average of one inch a year more than they would have without treatment. If approved, it is estimated that there could be a $1.6 billion market for treating 30,000 children with this first new drug in thirty years designed to increase stature.[52]

Turner Syndrome

Growth hormone has offered a height gain of several inches for girls with Turner syndrome.[53] Estrogen is often used in conjunction, both to promote development of secondary sexual characteristics and to avoid osteoporosis. It has been recommended that treatment be initiated in adolescence and be continued in subsequent decades, supplemented by calcium and exercise. Despite negative publicity about estrogen replacement therapy in postmenopausal women, a recent study has reaffirmed the importance of estrogen replacement in young women with Turner syndrome.[54] The results of ongoing research about cardiovascular disease in women with Turner syndrome have also been reported. Progress in fertility methods has enabled women with Turner syndrome to bear children using their husbands' sperm and in vitro fertilization with donor eggs.

Osteogenesis Imperfecta

The "search for a cure" often entails much trial and error and many disappointments. Persons affected by osteogenesis imperfecta (OI), a bone condition accompanied by frequent fractures and much pain, have experimented with many remedies that proved ineffective (vitamin C, synthetic calcitrol, and full-spectrum lights). The OI Foundation currently recommends against the use of Forteo (parathyroid treatment for osteoporosis) and high-dose vitamin C and takes a cautious "wait-and-see" attitude toward bone marrow transplants. Since the late 1990s, studies of the bisphosphonates have shown treatments with these medications to be promising, reducing fractures. Most notable is the drug pamidronate (administered intravenously), but similar studies of al-

endronate and other bisphosphonates (given orally) are also underway. However, controlled long-term investigations will be needed before efficacy is fully demonstrated and possible negative outcomes are
better understood. Among the other procedures currently utilized in
the management of OI are improved surgical rods that reduce bone
deformities, as well as pain relief measures, exercise, and nutrition.

Mucopolysaccharidoses and Mucolipidoses

These are a set of inherited lysosomal storage disorders caused by the
lack of enzymes that allow the body to break down and recycle cells
after the cells die. Consequently, progressive damage may occur
throughout the body, including the heart, respiratory system, bones,
joints, and central nervous system, sometimes causing early death.
Hopes for a cure have frequently been dashed, as when fetus-to-fetus
transplants proved unsuccessful.[55] However, gene mapping has led
to improved understanding, as have experiments with animal models. The potential for enzyme replacement therapy and retrovirus-
mediated gene transfer in mucopolysaccharidoses exists, and studies
with cultured fibroblasts suggest that active enzymes can be synthesized and alter abnormal cells. Some positive results have occurred,
with Dr. E. D. Kakkis and colleagues reporting success with enzyme
replacement in mucopolysaccharidosis I; Dr. S. Tomatsu, after puri-
fying a deficient enzyme and cloning the Morquio gene, is attempting to develop an effective treatment for Morquio patients.[56] Some
speculate that the most dramatic improvements may not appear until gene transplantation techniques have been perfected.

Advances in Diagnostic Tools and Surgical Procedures

General improvements in medical treatment during the 1980s and
1990s, such as sonar and magnetic resonance imaging, and the introduction of biochemical (collagen) and molecular (DNA) tests, have
been of particular importance to the treatment of dwarfism.

New procedures have been introduced to correct impairments, particularly in disorders of limbs and spine that might previously have resulted in significant disabilities and even paralysis. Orthopedic and neurological surgical techniques developed by Drs. Steven Kopits, Benjamin Carson, John Lonstein, and others have resulted in drastically improved quality of life. Joint replacement and spinal fusion are among the perfected procedures.

A particularly significant area of discovery has been problems affecting the cervical spine.[57] In early childhood, stenosis of the foramen magnum in achondroplasia is now known to have the potential to cause muscle weakness (hypotonia) or complete paralysis, apnea, swallowing problems, or sudden infant death syndrome (SIDS).[58] Techniques for delicate surgeries have improved dramatically. Breathing problems noticeable in childhood in a number of disorders, notably achondroplasia, began to be better understood in the 1980s and 1990s; they may be treated surgically or with CPAP/BiPAP devices (continuous or alternating air pressure masks to prevent apnea).

Problems of the upper two cervical vertebrae may occur in persons of all ages with a variety of conditions, including spondyloepiphyseal dysplasia and pseudoachondroplasia; abnormalities of the lower cervical spine often occur in diastrophic dysplasia, campomelic dysplasia, and Larsen syndrome. These problems may be treated with neck braces in younger children with mild deformities or with surgery, including stabilization (fusion), in later or more severe cases.

UNRESOLVED PROBLEMS: MALNUTRITION AND PSYCHOSOCIAL DWARFISM

Malnutrition remains the greatest source of growth failure worldwide and is the area where progress has been least apparent. Neither the United Nations nor individual wealthy nations have been able to address the problems of famine and poverty in more than an emergency fashion.

Psychosocial dwarfism—also known as deprivation dwarfism, the Kaspar Hauser syndrome,[59] nonorganic failure to thrive, and abuse dwarfism—is also problematic. Study after study has demonstrated that children who are rescued from an abusive or neglectful environment experience a significant growth spurt. If they are returned to their former environment, their growth is once again inhibited. Decades of research have demonstrated that growth failure was mediated by human growth hormone. Among the many interesting reviews of psychosocial dwarfism in the past several decades are one by Gardner and another by Blizzard and Bulatovic.[60]

There have been few follow-up studies of these children. One notable exception is the work of Skuse and Gilmour who discuss "hyperphagic short stature," psychosocial dwarfism involving changes in growth hormone levels.[61] They estimate that at least 2 percent of "short normal" children in England are affected by this disorder and believe that it is likely that the syndrome is genetic and that hypothalamic pathology is responsible. Unfortunately, they indicate only sketchily how they reached these conclusions. A review by Burgin in the same volume attempts to analyze the complex etiology of several kinds of psychosocial failure to thrive (PFTT).[62] It seems that psychosocial dwarfism is an area sorely in need of a careful, prospective study.

LPA has many separate diagnostic categories listed, but no subgroup of persons willing to identify themselves as psychosocial dwarfs. Are there none in the group? Are they uninformed of or ashamed of their stigmatized condition? Recent adoptions from orphanages in Russia and elsewhere have revived interest in the condition(s) and highlighted the effects of poor emotional care on physical, mental, and emotional growth.[63] Adoptive parents confronting serious physical, intellectual, and personality problems have sought help from developmental psychologists, occupational therapists, and other professionals.

THE CHANGED FOCUS OF MEDICAL LITERATURE

What a difference a century makes in the controversies addressed! Unlike a century ago, merely anecdotal case studies of individual dwarfs are rarely published. Instead, recent discoveries of genes are reported, animal model research discussed, and therapeutic and surgical outcomes evaluated. Discussions are more apt to deal with treatment: appropriate uses of human growth hormone, criteria for surgical intervention, outcomes of limb lengthening and enzyme replacement, and ethical issues such as abortion and gene replacement.

Increasingly, major genetic centers pool their resources to solve problems affecting patient populations. The aforementioned multicenter review by A. G. Hunter et al. studied 193 patients with achondroplasia, determining the rates of occurrence for each complication at various ages and also surveying patient or parent perceptions of outcomes of orthopedic surgery in chondrodysplasias.[64] Another by Mahomed, Spellmann, and Goldberg investigated the functional health status of persons with achondroplasia, finding no significant difference between their overall health and the general population's except that two-thirds had had at least one operation.[65]

Apart from the search for "miracle cures," there have been many improvements in the health of both children and adults through the application of knowledge to prevent complications and catastrophes. By determining frequency and approximate ages when a given symptom occurs, it is possible to alert patients and doctors to be vigilant and seek timely treatment. In 1984, an article appeared indicating that thirteen achondroplastic infants had died of SIDS. The collaboration of Dr. Richard Pauli and many others revealed that compression of the lower brainstem or cervical spinal cord had been responsible.[66] Unlike average-sized children who die supine, these achondroplasts had been more apt to die while in the sitting position in strollers, swings, or bouncers. Subsequently, Dr. Robert Wassman prepared an article recommending against early, unsupported sitting and against the use of such devices as doorway bouncing seats. In addition, he advised that babies be observed at specialized centers and monitored for possible neurological compression, and he suggested surgical intervention, if necessary.

Such prophylactic care has become standard practice at major dwarfism centers. Important articles about spinal problems, breathing disorders, anesthesia, and other medical questions are now available on *LPA Online.* One development resulted from collaboration between doctors and patients. It had been assumed that dwarfs, especially those with achondroplasia, "naturally" tended to be obese because of average-sized internal organs and short bones. In a 1974–75 survey of 150 members of LPA with classical achondroplasia, 75 percent said that they had problems with being overweight.[67] A study of metabolism published in 1990 revealed that obesity was twice as common in this group as in the general population. It found some high resting metabolic rates and wide variation, but no startling revelations about the relationship between achondroplasia and obesity; investigators recommended that body composition variables and caloric requirements be studied further.[68] Subsequently, Drs. Hunter, Hecht, and Scott published helpful standard weight-for-height curves for achondroplasia (fig. 1.4); Dr. Hall offered helpful recommendations about weight control.[69] Many dwarf individuals have discovered that by doubling their height in inches, they can approximate the upper limit of desirable weight in pounds (e.g., someone 36 inches tall should weigh no more than 72 pounds; a 50-inch person should be less than 100).

As a result of years of patient counseling, most young people today appear to be of moderate weight. Two generations of parents and young LPs have repeatedly been reminded by their physicians that obesity represents a danger to the skeletal and neurological structure of dwarfs, and they have taken heed. The generally good doctor-patient relationships that prevail in this community deserve much of the credit for this little publicized but remarkable success story.

Dr. Judith Hall has been particularly helpful in advising women. Little was known about the gynecological problems of female dwarfs before she and Dr. Judith Allanson conducted their survey of 163 women with chondrodystrophies in the United States and Canada. They found an increased incidence of menstrual complications. They also discovered that women with achondroplasia tended to early menopause and an increased incidence of fibroids; women with os-

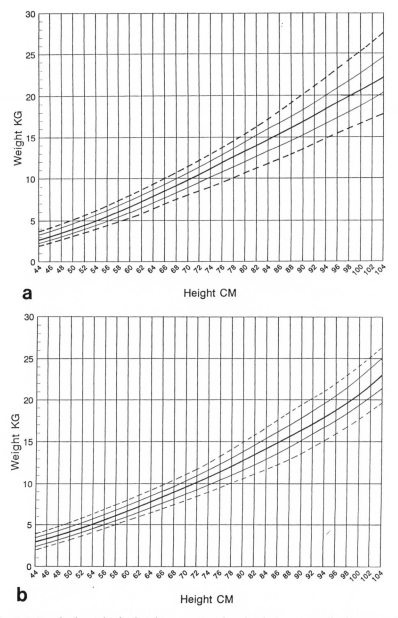

Fig. 1.4. Standard weight-for-height curves in achondroplasia. *a*, smoothed mean, +1 and 2 SD, weight/height curves to 104 cm for males with achondroplasia. *b*, smoothed mean, +1 and 2 SD, weight/height curves to 104 cm for females with achondroplasia. *American Journal of Medical Genetics* 62 (1996): 255–61.

teogenesis imperfecta were slightly older when they got their first periods; women with pseudoachondroplasia had longer menstrual cycles. Allanson and Hall recommended delivery by cesarean delivery for most chondrodystrophies and advised a general (vs. spinal) anesthetic.

Increasingly, women were eager to obtain the most recent information. In a workshop led by Dr. Judith Rossiter at the 2000 LPA conference, participants spoke freely and expressed many questions and concerns, benefiting both from Dr. Rossiter's expertise and their shared experiences. Remedies for some menstrual problems were offered; several women had found that birth control pills, particularly Alesse, reduced cramps and promoted shorter, lighter periods. Dr. Rossiter, an obstetrician/geneticist specializing in high-risk pregnancy, recommended that a pediatric speculum be used for vaginal exams and suggested ways to deal with pregnancy complications, such as problems sitting in late stages of pregnancy and possible compromised lung function for some conditions.

Unlike in previous eras, short-statured couples such as Anu Povinelli, 3′1″ tall, and her 3′3″ husband, Mark, who both have spondyloepiphyseal dysplasia, are now finding expert help that allows them to have children. Anu had previously been advised never to attempt pregnancy. However, the couple located a supportive obstetrician/geneticist specializing in high-risk pregnancy and dwarfism near their home in Phoenix, Arizona, and Anu had a successful cesarean delivery, giving birth to their daughter Priya in 2003 (see fig. 3.11).

PROTAGONISTS IN THE DWARFISM DRAMA

There are several major medical centers with expertise in dwarfism, some staffed by LPA Medical Advisory Board members. To communicate the spirited atmosphere in which progress in dwarfism research and treatment is occurring, a number of individuals who helped to shape that history will be highlighted. Many such experts have been influenced by the philosophy of geneticist and cardiologist

Dr. Victor McKusick, who has always felt that research, teaching, and the best patient care were inextricably entwined. He advises young physicians and researchers to "find work that gives you a chance to help people, that satisfies our natural curiosity about ourselves, and is intellectually challenging," thereby "finding a career that is thoroughly soul-satisfying—that's how I characterize my work, soul satisfying."[70]

McKusick has made major contributions to a number of fields. His work has been significant both for short-statured individuals and for those who are unusually tall—patients with Marfan syndrome, a heritable disorder of connective tissue whose manifestations include tall stature, heart disease, and eye problems. In a Marfan literary anthology, one poet advocate calls for a humanistic approach by the medical establishment[71]:

INVITATION
By Lucy Hook Porter

I am a person
I am not
a problem
to be solved
not an age
not a diseased body part
not a condition
not a research subject
not "Bed 1"
don't be
so slow to come in
so quick to leave
sit down if you can
look at me
listen to me
touch me
I need you to

> See me
> hear me
> know me
>
> I am not
> A problem
> To be solved
> I am a person
> To be loved

The careers of McKusick and others are testaments to their understanding of such sentiments. Although the research of these scientists is a source of fascination in itself, they never forget that it exists to serve real individuals, with whom they often enjoy lifelong personal relationships. The physicians who trained under McKusick at the Johns Hopkins Hospital are now dispersed worldwide. The influence of this Johnny Appleseed of genetics on dwarfism research and treatment cannot be overstated.

The LPA Medical Advisory Board

Just as individual dwarfs a century ago were apt to live in isolation, medical clinicians and researchers tended to work alone. There are now far more ongoing contacts and cooperative efforts. The board that serves LPA consists of physicians who have made outstanding contributions to research. It also includes a few exemplary social workers and administrators. At the annual national LPA conference, many individuals schedule clinic appointments, and still more attend the general meeting where board members present recent developments in the field and answer questions. Smaller workshops led by physicians focus on specific conditions and topics of interest. Medical Advisory Board members are also available throughout the year by phone or e-mail.

Most of the individuals discussed below have trained or worked at

Johns Hopkins during part of their careers. The list is influenced by my acquaintance with certain notable physicians; I apologize for the account's slant toward the American experience, with insufficient attention given to major figures such as Mörch, Spranger, Lamy, Maroteaux, and Wiedmann. I hope, nevertheless, to capture the flavor of how accomplishments such as theirs are revolutionizing dwarfism research and treatment.

Dr. Victor A. McKusick

It may be impossible to find a single physician who has made such monumental contributions to so many disparate fields of medicine as Victor McKusick. The recipient in 1997 of the prestigious Lasker prize, the highest honor in medicine, he has also been granted innumerable other awards and honorary degrees. Although he has done important research in cardiology, internal medicine, and heritable disorders of connective tissue, he is most famous for his preeminent role in creating the new field of genetics. His groundbreaking *Mendelian Inheritance in Man,* first published in 1966, has had numerous editions. Now available online, it is the most important reference work for physicians and researchers investigating inherited conditions.

The best description of McKusick's career trajectory appears in his illuminating 1989 *JAMA* article "Forty Years of Medical Genetics."[72] He writes about his early influences, his long association with the Jackson Laboratory for Mammalian Research in Maine, his studies of the Amish, and his biographical essays about figures important to the history of medicine. The compelling thread that reappears throughout McKusick's article is his enduring fascination with both investigative and clinical genetics.

During the 1960s and 1970s, when Dr. McKusick was conducting some of his most important research, he also maintained personal contact with patients at the Moore Clinic, often presiding at case conferences held during clinic days. Typically, patients and families met with an internist, an ENT (ear, nose, and throat) physician, an orthopedist, a social worker, and any other relevant staff members. At the end of the day's appointments, the specialists discussed each patient's condition with the family.

After experiencing the fragmented world that characterized the medical establishment elsewhere, patients usually found the Moore Clinic an oasis of calm, caring, and enlightenment. Few of the families who met with Dr. McKusick on these occasions were aware of the worldwide reputation of this courtly, quietly knowledgeable physician. Only later did some come to know that the clinic's structure and ambience had been his creation.

Although the Moore Clinic had functioned as an outpatient chronic disease center since 1914, Dr. McKusick restructured it when he took it over in 1957. He organized pediatricians, neurologists, ophthalmologists, and others into a group informed by the burgeoning new field of genetics. Under that umbrella, they conducted groundbreaking research and were enabled to communicate more effectively with each other and with patients. For many years, McKusick also presided at annual dwarfism symposia at Hopkins where physicians, patients, and their families met informally and attended informative workshops; McKusick led the genetics workshop for laypersons, communicating an available, kindly presence.

His relationships with his colleagues were equally beneficent. In 1997, Francis Collins, director of the National Human Genome Research Institute, related his feelings about McKusick's winning the Lasker prize to him: "I think in many ways we all sort of feel in some part as though we are your kids and so we're honored and delighted and thrilled."[73]

McKusick arrived at Hopkins as a medical student in 1943 and remained for his whole medical career. In earlier years, he studied heart sounds and murmurs and published "a fat book" called *Cardiovascular Sound in Heart and Disease*. His first genetics volume, *Heritable Disorders of Connective Tissue*, was first published in 1956.[74] The phrase, "heritable disorders of connective tissue," first coined by McKusick, became the accepted term used to describe the association of such superficially disparate conditions as Marfan syndrome and certain dwarfing disorders. His observation of heart patients had led him to study the genetics of Marfan syndrome, while his work with Old Order Amish patients in nearby rural Pennsylvania had led him to explicate their common dwarfing conditions. In 1999, Johns Hopkins united nine existing medical centers to form a new institute called the McKusick-Nathans Institute of Genetic Medicine, thereby honoring two pioneering physicians who "transform[ed] a fledgling scientific specialty into the driving force of medicine."[75]

Without the framework provided by McKusick's most famous work, *Mendelian Inheritance in Man,* procedures such as amniocentesis, DNA fingerprinting, and gene therapies could never have been conceptualized.[76] His ability to convince the March of Dimes Foundation in 1970 to finance the creation of a map of human genes jumpstarted the process; the U.S. government began to involve itself in 1985, and eventually an international coordinating body was created. In 1988, the Human Genome Organization (HUGO) was established to oversee gene-mapping research. Its 220 founding members asked McKusick to be its first president.[77]

Many had met through the annual genetics seminar initiated in 1958 that still operates every July in Bar Harbor, Maine. Called "The Short Course in Medical and Experimental Mammalian Genetics," McKusick founded it to compensate for what he regarded as "the woeful state of genetics education in medical schools."[78] In 1960 it became a joint venture of the Jackson Laboratory and Johns Hopkins University, supported by the March of Dimes. For the next forty years, an ever-increasing number of scientists made a summer pilgrimage to that small waterfront town in Acadia National Park, sharing the latest information and establishing personal contacts with colleagues who would go on to initiate significant genetics research projects.

McKusick credits a lengthy teenage hospitalization for first attracting him to medicine; Collins jokes that perhaps the fact that McKusick is a twin inspired his curiosity about genetics. Whatever its origins, his career burgeoned under the influence of an inquiring mind, concern for patients, and remarkable stamina. His satisfying family life as the father of three, and especially his marriage to Dr. Anne McKusick, who shares many of his interests, no doubt helped provide the stable structure for his commitment to research and service. Now retired, she was a highly respected clinician in the area of connective tissue disorders and arthritis at Johns Hopkins. Although his schedule has abated, there is no question of McKusick's retiring. He sees few patients, but continues to write, lecture, and consult, even when ostensibly on vacation. Some years ago he told his assistant that the day he retires is the day that he will die.[79]

The Greenberg Center for Skeletal Dysplasias at Johns Hopkins was created in 1982 as an offshoot of the Moore Clinic; it has been significant for the research and treatment done there, but also in training American and foreign physicians. Among those trained at the centers are Drs. David Danks and John Rogers of Australia, Malcolm Ferguson Smith and Martin Nelson of Great Britain, Peter Harper of Wales, Michael Wright of Scotland, and Gabriela Reppetto of Chile. From their Hopkins experience, they gained not only a specific body of knowledge but also a model for integrating research with humanistic treatment that enhanced the care of persons with dwarfism in their home countries.

The Greenberg Center

No medical chronicle is complete that fails to mention the financial problems that always plague ambitious enterprises. For many years, the treatment of dwarf patients at the Moore Clinic at Johns Hopkins was subsidized by research funds provided by the National Institutes of Health (NIH). Routine treatment and even expensive surgeries for patients without adequate health insurance could often be justified as part of vital research studies. In time, however, NIH began to withdraw its support, causing budgetary constraints.

Even before 1980, shortfalls had been met through contributions solicited by Kay Smith, McKusick's assistant, principally from persons who had benefited from surgeries at the Moore Clinic. These funds helped needy patients, paid doctors' travel expenses to LPA conferences, etc. Eventually this fund was officially established as the Kathryn K. Smith Foundation. Smith sent letters asking for contributions once a year, usually in the spring.

The largest contribution, however, had a different origin. One morning, Alan Greenberg, CEO of the brokerage house Bear Stearns, read an article in the *New York Times* about an achondroplastic child treated at the Moore Clinic. Touched by her story, Greenberg sent $150, asking that it be spent on something that might make the girl happy. As was her custom, Smith wrote to Greenberg, thanking him and telling him more about the patient. He wrote back and said, "If this child ever needs anything, just let me know." They kept in touch, and whenever someone at the clinic had an unmet need, she called him, and he would send a gift (somewhere between $500 and $1,700 was the common range). The gifts became ever more welcome as funds grew sparser.

One day, as Smith was taking a bath, the telephone rang. It was Greenberg, who volunteered, "Kay, I want to do something for the little people." She asked, "What do you want me to do?" He answered resolutely: "Establish a foundation—I'll give you $250,000!"

The next day Smith was on the train to New York, formalizing an agreement. Greenberg visited the clinic at her request and McKusick's, and then he and his family attended an LPA conference. In a *New Yorker* article he joked, "You give Kay Smith $150 and you end up giving $3 million." Mr. Greenberg's funds helped to support patient care and a training program for physicians, as well as to assist several LPs with college and medical school fees.

Despite this heartwarming tale, the Greenberg Center faced an uphill battle as it struggled to maintain its financial health and restore its earlier congenial ambience. After geneticist Dr. Julie Hoover-Fong was appointed as clinic director in 2004, however, her talent and infectious enthusiasm gave the center a lift. Dee Miller, the caring senior clinic coordinator, evaluates patients' needs and schedules appointments with specialists for the approximately 900 patients currently on the clinic rolls.

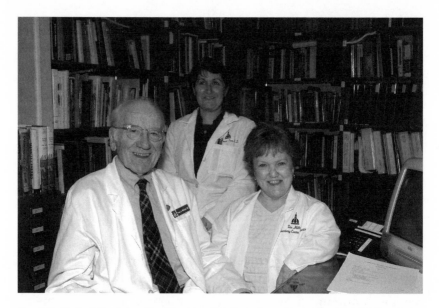

Fig. 1.5. Staff of the Johns Hopkins Hospital Greenberg Center for Skeletal Dysplasias (left to right): Dr. Victor A. McKusick, director; Dr. Julie Hoover-Fong, clinical director; Dee Miller, senior program coordinator. Photograph courtesy of the Greenberg Center.

Dr. Clair A. Francomano

Versatile clinical and molecular geneticist Clair A. Francomano has successfully joined her scientific and humanistic concerns, making significant contributions to basic genetic research, as well as exploring quality-of-life and ethical issues. Her achievements led to her election as president of the International Society for Skeletal Dysplasia, a post she served in from 2001 to 2003.

After receiving her M.D. from Johns Hopkins and completing fellowships, she went on to join the Johns Hopkins School of Medicine faculty in the departments of Medicine and Pediatrics in 1984. From 1994 to 2001, she served as chief of the Molecular Genetics Branch and clinical director of the National Human Genome Research Institute. She later joined the Human Genetics and Integrative Medicine Section of the NIH/National Institute on Aging, where she is presently a senior investigator and chief of the Human

Genetics and Integrative Medicine Section in the Laboratory of Genetics.

When I interviewed Francomano in 2000, I was aware that she had played a central role in the 1994 discovery of the gene for achondroplasia.[80] Although scientist John Wasmuth at the University of California at Irvine ultimately located it and has been credited, many articles mentioned the significant role of Francomano and her colleagues at Johns Hopkins. I hoped that she could translate for nonscientists just what it meant to "discover a gene."

It turned out that when Francomano was only a junior in high school she had received a scholarship to a genetics laboratory at Victor McKusick's annual summer institute in genetics in Bar Harbor. She again encountered McKusick as a medical student at Hopkins. In her first year, she investigated dwarfism in the Amish community and spent three summers doing research. At the 1979 LPA national conference in Lancaster, Pennsylvania, she met Joan and Bill Hare (members of the group). "Then I was hooked, emotionally and intellectually hooked," Francomano remarked. "It became my life's work."

Her involvement grew throughout her residency and a later fellowship, and her research interests expanded. Some of her myriad articles deal with overarching concerns of genetics; others confront the genetic conundrums of individual conditions and implications for treatment.[81] Major advances occurred in the early 1990s, when Francomano and her interdisciplinary team, supported in part by the Greenberg Endowment, searched for the genes for achondroplasia and pseudoachondroplasia and did genetic mapping to locate nail-patella syndrome, a more uncommon disorder. They also studied neurological and respiratory problems in children, establishing guidelines for treatment.

During her tenure as chief of the Medical Genetics Branch at the NIH, the program grew from three persons to sixty-three. Projects spanned the full range of heritable disorders of connective tissue. In her summary for the National Human Genome Research Institute, Francomano noted that identifying genes represents only the beginning, and that it would take much time and energy to elaborate the relationship between phenotype (how the condition looks when expressed in an individual) and genotype (its appearance in the gene).[82] It is not sufficient to note the impact of the condition's most influential gene: in considering the mutated gene of achondroplasia, for example, it is necessary to assess the interaction of a variety of genes that contribute to differences in each individual's appearances and health profile.

How does one "discover" a gene? In the past, the journey was long and arduous. The whole genome had to be inspected slowly and carefully for the "moving target," the mutated gene. The process has been compared with searching a village, locating a single house, then a room, and finally the obscure area of that room where the gene may be hidden. In the case of achondroplasia, Francomano explained that there are 400 markers that allow an investigator to scan the genome. Her group, and a French group, had scanned and excluded more than 335.

At the same time, Wasmuth, searching for the Huntington disease gene, noticed from their reports that the gene Francomano suspected was responsible for achondroplasia was in the same area as the likely location of the Huntington gene. When he tested 16 achondroplastic individuals, he found that 15 had the identical notation at the far end of chromosome four, confirming Francomano and colleagues' surmises.[83] Looking for one gene, Wasmuth had been rewarded by stumbling on another; his perspicacity allowed him to verify his find. They determined that more than 97 percent of persons with the condition had a mutation in the transmembrane domain of the FGFR3 gene on chromosome four; mutations of that gene also affect other conditions, including hypochondroplasia.[84]

This event became a paradigm for the speeded-up time scheme that would revolutionize the field. Francomano noted that it had taken ten years to find the Huntington gene and six months for the final identification of the achondroplasia gene. Her investigations were part of a greater drama of discovery whose climactic moment occurred in June 2002 when Dr. John Craig Venter of the Celera Corporation, the private foundation that mapped the genome, and Dr.

Francis Collins, who directed the National Human Genome Research Institute, a public consortium, crowned their competitive efforts by announcing jointly that scientists had come close to sequencing the entire human genome. A *New York Times* special science issue, in an article entitled "Now the Hard Part: Putting the Genome to Work," highlighted the daunting problems that would have to be confronted before mechanisms for gene replacement could be implemented.[85]

Dr. Francomano explained that treating deficiencies with circulating proteins, such as those involved in growth hormone replacement, was less difficult than understanding and manipulating the mechanisms of bound proteins. Circulating proteins, such as those made in liver and bone marrow, can more easily be replaced or supplemented. In cartilage and bone, particular sites are difficult to target. One must express protein and then solve the problem of getting the promoter (the part of the gene that regulates expression) to function at the same time or place in order to alter the mutated gene. Because FGFR3 is expressed in growth plate cartilage, it would not be simple to alter it.

Francomano noted other questions scientists were asking: Should the procedure be attempted before implantation, in the embryo, or by injecting cartilage after birth? Should we do something just because we can—or must we discuss the implications beforehand? Like Wasmuth, she had struggled with issues stemming from the discovery. Neither of them believed that the general population should be tested for achondroplasia, lest that identification lead those ignorant about dwarfism to abort. Now that so many more genes have been identified, ethical questions have become more urgent.

Johns Hopkins became the first medical center to offer in utero testing for achondroplasia. Francomano developed the evaluation program, using chorion villus sampling and counseling. Because Hopkins had long experience serving a dwarf population, its patients were less afraid than the general public about having a dwarf baby. Dwarf or mixed couples were typically not concerned about whether their children would be of short or average stature; the principal benefit of investigation with two achondroplastic partners is to learn if a fetus was "double-dominant" (with a mutant gene from each that would mean early death).

Because prenatal testing for dwarfism was a new procedure when Dr. Francomano initiated the program, potential attitudes toward performing it were unknown. Her concern led her to assess attitudes of LPA members.[86] Individuals with achondroplasia and family members generally viewed the procedure as suitable for identifying lethal double-dominant genes but far less acceptable to terminate a pregnancy based on a diagnosis of either achondroplasia or average stature. Spurred by such issues, Francomano agreed to lead medical ethics sessions at the Medical Genetics Short Course.

The major enterprise Francomano had headed, the Skeletal Genome Anatomy Project (SGAP), was designed to improve understanding of the pathology of relatively rare skeletal disorders and to illuminate the processes that affect skeletal growth and aging. She finds the National Institute on Aging, to which she moved in 2002, satisfying because of its expertise in designing and implementing longitudinal studies. She has an umbrella protocol to study clinical and molecular aspects of the skeletal dysplasias while still looking for genes and mutations in several different connective tissue disorders.[87]

She also studies the causes of morbidity and mortality in different forms of connective tissue disorders, including dwarfism. Although she continues to study mice that carry the thanatophoric dysplasia type II mutation to offer insight into what FGFR3 overactivation does to the brain, in March 2004 she got the go-ahead to study the increased mortality rates in mid-adult life in achondroplasia.[88] She is eager to obtain information about older adults, which has heretofore been sparse.

Dr. David L. Rimoin

Dr. Rimoin holds the Stephen Spielberg Chair of Pediatrics at Cedars-Sinai Medical Center in Los Angeles and is director of the Medical Genetics-Birth Defects Center and its International Registry for Skeletal Dysplasia. Sought after for his expertise in many areas of research, he was the founding president of the American College of Medical Genetics (ACMG) and of the American Society of Human Genetics, and a founder of the International Skeletal Dysplasia Society. He is past president of American Society of Human Genetics, the ACMG Foundation, and the Western Society for Pediatrics Research, as well as a long-term member of the LPA Medical Advisory Board. He has been honored by election to many distinguished groups.

The achievement for which Dr. Rimoin will probably be best remembered is his work as principal coeditor of *Emery and Rimoin's Principles and Practice of Medical Genetics.* The fourth edition, which was called a landmark book by the *New England Journal of Medicine,* was published in 2002. It had been twenty years since it was first published, and this updated three-volume classic was hailed as the only comprehensive work in the field, a resource that no medical geneticist could practice without. It details the past five years of remarkable scientific progress and contains chapters that help shape the practitioner's approach to clinical treatment.

Rimoin is one of the most talented of the many geneticists and other physicians who trained at Johns Hopkins and thrived in Dr. McKusick's orbit. During our telephone interview in 2000, I spoke with him about that period of his career. He said that he counted himself very fortunate to have trained under and worked with McKusick, and commented particularly on McKusick's ability to allow students to run free with their ideas and go off on their own particular tangents.

In this atmosphere at Hopkins, Dr. Rimoin was able to make a major contribution to the understanding of isolated growth hormone deficiency. His early studies included one in which he identified normal pathology of cartilage in achondroplasia and defined the abnormalities present in many of the other dysplasias. His investigation of disturbances in growth hormone metabolism led to his publication in 1971 of *Genetic Disorders of the Endocrine Glands,* a work that would become a classic in its field.[89] Rimoin came to recognize that there was also a paucity of information about the skeletal dysplasias in the medical literature, and he began to nurture what would become a lifelong interest in that area.

His fascination with genetics had been apparent from an early age. At 17 he participated in the honors genetics program at McGill University. After his medical training at Johns Hopkins, he secured his first faculty position at Washington University where he ran the genetics clinic. He moved on to Harbor General in Los Angeles in 1970 and to Cedars-Sinai in 1986. He helped to develop the $2.2 million Skeletal Dysplasia Center at Harbor-UCLA and the International Skeletal Dysplasia Registry. The skeletal dysplasia unit sees more than 200 dwarf patients a year.

A scion of the McKusick tradition's triune commitment to research, clinical work, and teaching, Rimoin has been a major force in shaping the field of genetics; he is particularly notable for his involvement with the renditions of the International Nomenclature for Constitutional Disorders of Bone, now updated every other year. I asked him what countries maintained research and treatment centers for skeletal dysplasia; he mentioned France, Germany, Switzerland, Belgium, Great Britain, South Africa, Argentina, Brazil, Uruguay, Israel, and Australia. Rimoin is often called on to consult on difficult cases at various hospitals. Shriners Hospital for Children, Honolulu, for example, has had him review their dysplasia cases at an annual genetics clinic. As a result of its success, he has conducted a telemedicine clinic that allows him to examine more than twelve patients a day.[90]

The consultation process is enhanced by Cedars-Sinai's International Skeletal Dysplasia Registry, a referral center for research into diagnosis, management, and etiology of skeletal dysplasias. Physicians are invited to submit clinical summaries, X-rays, ultrasound tapes, tissue specimens, DNA, etc., to be evaluated for definitive diagnosis and for future use in collaborative research and publication.[91] Currently, the registry accumulates 600 cases a year from around the world and has collected more than 9,300 cases.

More optimistic and less circumspect about the future of gene therapy than many patients and physicians I had spoken with, Dr. Rimoin was engaged by the prospect of "fooling Mother Nature and getting around it." He recognized the difficulties of developing treatments and once commented, "You need a smart bomb to get the DNA to the right place, and a smart detonator to set it off at the right time, and for the most part those mechanisms are not yet available."[92] Although no absolute time frame can be promised, he nevertheless envisions significant progress in the next decade, including investigators working on turning off the receptor for achondroplasia, exploring problems related to bone growth, and looking for drug treatments.

Rimoin indicated that he trusts persons' ability to make up their own minds about whether and how to use recent scientific discoveries and surgical methods. Whether these choices relate to childbirth or limb lengthening, he feels individuals might legitimately make different choices. If, for example, a dwarf couple was told which of their fertilized eggs would result in a dwarf child and which an unaffected offspring, they had a right to decide how to proceed. Whatever internal struggle might be involved, it was theirs to resolve.

He felt similarly about the limb-lengthening controversy. He believes that each young person (in general, between the ages of 12 and 20) should be given the facts and the opportunity to consider the decision. Initially opposed to the procedure, after meeting contented patients at the 1988 achondroplasia conference in Rome, and later observing the Villerubias method in Spain, which reduced lordosis and increased spinal volume, he and his colleagues decided the method was worth trying. All too often, he feels, whether genetic questions or specific treatments are involved, the most vocal and sometimes the most negative voices may command the most attention. Couples have been talked out of treating their pituitary dwarf children with growth hormone, for example, he noted, even though that treatment can improve general well-being along with height. Rimoin encourages pundits to relax and let the people involved make up their minds about what is best for them.

Rimoin is involved in many respected colleagues' research activities, and he has spoken up about the political and economic aspects of genetics. He recommends convincing managed care that preclinical diagnosis is cost effective; establishing a genetics-biotechnology company with profit sharing like the one Cedars-Sinai had established; and organizing a course in medical economics for house staff, as he himself had done, with participation of the hospital legal team and others.[93]

He is not afraid to challenge prevailing opinion, endeavoring to study each matter carefully, then to see that research and treatment are performed properly. His critical intelligence, boundless energy, and forceful personality have combined to make him a recognized leader in his field; in 2000 he was appointed cochair of an influential national health policy committee and has served as one of only twenty-five persons on another committee designed to influence clinical research funding and regulatory issues over the next decade.[94]

Dr. Cheryl S. Reid

Geneticist Cheryl Reid is well known to members of LPA, especially for her lucid presentations of the etiology and treatment of breathing problems, both at annual conferences and in the pages of *LPA Today*. Dr. Reid is a stimulating presence at regional meetings in the New Jersey area and at conferences as far away as Canada. Formerly head of the Genetics Division at Cooper Hospital/University Medical Center in Camden, New Jersey, for 11 years, she now has a private practice in Moorestown, consulting on a variety of conditions for persons with dwarfism and children with developmental disabilities and other genetic disorders. She continues to serve on the consulting staff of five southern New Jersey hospitals and is an adjunct professor in genetic counseling at Arcadia College (formerly Beaver College) in Glenside, Pennsylvania.

Dr. Reid has an especially rich background in the history of medical anomalies and its relationship to medicine and art. As a child, she had been interested in both science and art; at one point she had considered becoming a medical artist. She had always responded to symmetry and asymmetry in art and nature. When exposed to persons with malformations, she had felt a mixture of emotions, but first and foremost had wondered "why it was like that." In addition, she had had a friend with no thumbs. This was one of the catalysts that led her to think about how people with physical differences were able to adapt. Her involvement with the question persisted throughout her college years, while her study of music and theater contributed to an appreciation of difference.

After deciding on a medical career, she trained in pediatrics at Montefiore Hospital in New York City, where she was introduced to its large treatment program for persons with craniofacial defects. These patients presented surgical challenges and significant problems of sleep apnea. After the distressing deaths of two patients, she resolved to pursue her special interest in apnea, figuring out how to prevent death and help patients live better lives.

At the time there was no specific course of study in birth defects, so, recommended by mentors at the March of Dimes, she was offered a genetics fellowship at Johns Hopkins. Stimulated by the atmosphere, she began to examine the questions engendered by her previous work with patients with craniofacial defects.[95] She wondered particularly why babies seemed to have more problems with respiratory disorders than older children. In 1982–83 she initiated a research project investigating who was most at risk and why.

She and her colleagues investigated three factors that seemed most salient: (1) small chest cage; (2) problems with breathing during sleep due to constricted nasal passages; and (3) abnormal breathing patterns due to chronic compression of the upper spinal cord.[96] In 1987 they published their findings, definitively demonstrating the value of neurological and respiratory evaluations of children with achondroplasia.[97] She also took part in developing standard curves for chest circumference in achondroplasia, making evident the relationship of chest circumference to respiratory problems.[98] She has continued to speak at regional and national LPA conferences, helping families recognize symptoms that signal the need for treatment. Building on the research of Reid and others, surgeons such as Dr. Benjamin Carson at Johns Hopkins have designed innovative operations for babies at risk for foramen magnum compression. The mortality rate for achondroplasts under the age of five has been reduced to just 1 percent.[99]

Reid's experience with apnea research is a good example of how progress occurs in such a field. In the early 1980s there had been considerable difference of opinion among dwarfism specialists at centers in Baltimore, Houston, Madison, and Los Angeles about the nature, incidence, and seriousness of apnea. As a result of multicenter research, consensus was achieved and findings disseminated. Individual physicians became confident about the meaning of symptoms and able to recommend appropriate care.

Among the benefits of the centers' research was improved judgment about hydrocephalus. It is now less likely that shunts will be inserted when not absolutely necessary. Judgment about when to recommend decompression at the back of the neck is also much more accurate, and the skills needed to perform the surgery more widely available. In the last two decades, Dr. Reid has seen a significant increase in the knowledge and ability of Medical Advisory Board physicians. Studies continue to be published in the United States and abroad refining and evaluating treatments (including tonsillectomies, adenoidectomies, and spinal surgery for breathing disorders).[100]

Dr. Reid, like several other Medical Advisory Board members, spoke of feeling grateful for what people in LPA have taught her and being pleased to be a part of such an important enterprise. Her broad knowledge, her analytic mind, and her superior communication skills have proved invaluable in patient treatment and education.

Dr. Steven E. Kopits

CLINICS
Michael Bachstein

When I am four a crippled hospital
Peels me out of my parents' arms
To make me better. I wring my mother's neck

For safety, knowing this is not
What they said would happen, that they
Are as unnerved as I am to see their mangled only son stripped
    from their love
Into the cracking-plaster bowels
Of this place, into a row of endless cages
Where children no stronger than their parents'
Worst fears lie writhing, waiting for the legs

Their doctors have promised. I have made it
Perfectly clear ever since breakfast
That I want to stop there again on the long
Way back, at that same roadside place
Where I slurped up my hungry hot oats this morning
And they said we'd be sure to, but now
They just stand there growing smaller as some
White-headed woman with her glasses on a chain
Around her neck takes me down the long green
Hallway frowning, and they are still waving goodbye
As we turn the ugly corner and disappear, and what
If I never get my legs and they forget me?[101]

Dr. Kopits, the renowned orthopedic surgeon, whose death caused much grief in the dwarfism community in June 2002, is recognized as having known more than anyone else about the orthopedic problems of dwarfs. He was also exquisitely tuned in to children's emotional nuances. Kopits felt boundless responsibility to the thousands of patients he treated and committed his life to their well-being.

Although Kopits performed surgery on adults, children represented 90 percent of his practice. The poem above captures some of the feelings Kopits's young patients experienced. Extraordinarily empathic, Kopits strove to make each child comfortable physically and emotionally, through respectfully delivered information or playful joking, as circumstances dictated. He paid precise attention to every diagnostic detail as he planned and performed complex surgery that often meant the difference between mobility and permanent dys-

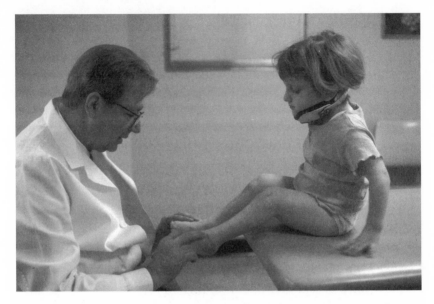

Fig. 1.6. Dr. Steven E. Kopits with a young patient. Photograph courtesy of Roger Miller, Roger Miller Photo, Ltd.

function. Similarly, during evaluations, approaching surgery, and during convalescence, he created a caring climate for his patients.

At the International Center for Skeletal Dysplasia at St. Joseph's Hospital, his professional home from 1978 to 2002, the specially designed seating units were lower and less deep to accommodate the bodies of dwarfs; there were also seats for average-statured relatives. Door handles and bathroom fixtures were similarly adapted. The environment declared, "This world is designed especially for you!"

Staff members were similarly welcoming, but it was Dr. Kopits's warm greeting that completed the sense that one had come to the right place, and all would go well. Personal accounts often mention his first words: "What a *beautiful* baby!" This signature remark was no less genuine for perhaps being a considered stratagem. This baby was as precious and wonderful to him as he hoped it was to the parents. Often the family had traveled a great distance and previously encountered impersonal or pitying physicians.

Born in Hungary in 1936, Kopits was the son and grandson of orthopedic surgeons. The family, trying to escape Europe toward the end of World War II, were captured by the SS, and then fled through Austria, France, and Spain. Unable to gain entrance to the United States, they went to Argentina. Kopits went to medical school there and later completed a surgical internship at Union Memorial Hospital in 1964 and an orthopedic residency at Johns Hopkins from 1965 to 1968.[102] His surgical experience began much earlier, however, when, like child apprentices of earlier eras, he stood by his father's side while he performed operations. Kopits explained:

"I was raised to respond to disability. My father was one of the pioneers in treating people who had osteogenesis imperfecta—the 'pretzel people.' We had the crippled people of Barcelona and Buenos Aires eating at our table all the time. They were the people you would see pushing themselves along the streets on platforms. Some had brilliant minds, brilliant, and were reduced to begging. They were my father's friends. When he retired, after practicing medicine for 60 years in eight countries in five languages, he said that the most important lesson he had learned was to love his patients."[103]

His experience echoed his father's, in confirming for him that one could be a truly good doctor only by being involved. Innumerable patient testimonials attested to the fact that this love was returned. Nine-year-old Joshua Phillips wrote:

"We went to see Dr. Kopits for a pre-surgery checkup. This involves measuring each and every bend in my body. . . . Dr Kopits is a funny man. He makes my doctor appointments fun by joking with me and playing along with all my jokes. Whenever Dr. Kopits comes on the children's floor at the hospital, everyone is glad to see him. We start saying, "Dr Kopits on the floor" and laughing at how funny he walks toward us. He is always ready to laugh and hug every child around."[104]

"I can't imagine what my life would be without him," wrote a teenage patient, Meredith Segal, detailing her participation in school government, Drama Club—and even the softball team. "I would probably be confined to a wheelchair, unable to walk, stand, or take part in the everyday activities that most people take for granted. I am not saying that being a little person is easy (I have my rough days),

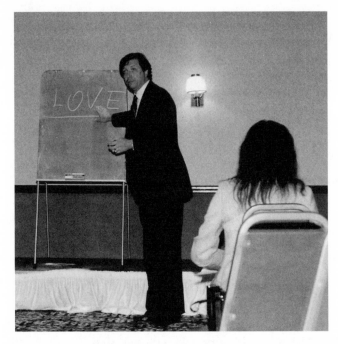

Fig. 1.7. Dr. Steven E. Kopits at First International Conference of Little People, in Washington, D.C., 1982. Photograph courtesy of Julie Rotta.

but Dr. Kopits has given me something that could easily have been out of my reach—the chance to be somebody. . . . I know that no matter how long I have to wait my turn to see him, he is always generous with his time as he is with each patient. He is always there to help me and to comfort me. Dr. Kopits is a credit to his field and is doing exactly what he was meant to do. . . . I am hoping and praying that other doctors will follow in his footsteps."[105]

It was not uncommon for Dr. Kopits to be described in superlatives, as "truly a saint," as Clinton Brown III of New York, a diastrophic dwarf, termed him. Brown's parents despaired of finding a solution until they found Kopits when Clinton was 22 months old. In the next four months, Dr. Kopits performed ten surgeries on his lower limbs: "He gave hope to a couple of scared parents and showed them that there was a bright light at the end of a presently dark and gloomy tunnel."[106] Brown believes that had he not met Dr. Kopits, he probably would have died before his eleventh birthday. As he grew older, he became increasingly aware of the ten- and twelve-hour surgeries Kopits performed, his research stints in his office till midnight—and the hundreds of children "given the gift of a better life because one man cares."

Brown remarked, "I remember one time this past summer, as I was lying in bed after surgery and crying because of the pain, Dr. Kopits walked into my room. The minute I heard his voice and saw him, a feeling of serenity came over me. I don't know how he did it, but for the while he was with me, the hurt seemed to vanish."[107]

Dr. Kopits had spent ten years at Johns Hopkins, from 1968 to 1978, becoming increasingly engaged by the orthopedic problems of dwarfs. He had performed hundreds of surgeries, inventing procedures when need arose. He found that by the time surgery was performed, irreversible deformity and even paralysis had occurred. Concluding that technical innovation was not sufficient, Kopits developed a program of "planned management" to anticipate problems and intervene at the optimal moment.

To illustrate the problem, he described his experience with 19-year-old Kathy Penland, whose rare condition, Strudwick dysplasia, had led to limb weakness that mystified physicians in North Carolina. When Penland came to him, she was "getting paralyzed from the neck down. Her hips were a shambles. Her knees, spine, ankles . . . each one added to the problems of the others."[108] He immediately braced the vertebrae so that they could be properly aligned, fused her neck and then did her hips, which he described as "almost at the point of no return."

As concerned as he felt about Kathy and the 52 other patients in his practice with Strudwick dysplasia, he was appalled when someone who could have benefited went untreated: "I have one patient whose parents refused the surgery. The child sits like a pretzel. Her spine is so deformed she bends over double. Her neck is dislocated. She is panting for air. I have known her since she was 2. Do you know how that hurts me?[109]

Dr. Kopits's immense empathy at least as much as his visionary approach caused him to leave Johns Hopkins in 1978 to establish the In-

ternational Center for Skeletal Dysplasia at St. Joseph's Hospital in
Towson, Maryland. Many could not understand why anyone would
leave an institution with the reputation and resources of Johns Hopkins to become a solitary practitioner at an obscure hospital. Certainly there were unfortunate consequences—working an impossible
schedule, he lost close contacts with colleagues—but the move also
had benefits. Kopits had become determined to devote his surgical
practice exclusively to little people; this restricted scope was not an
option at Hopkins. Furthermore, a packed schedule of complex
surgery requiring endless hours of operating-room time would always represent an economic deficit for a hospital. This was particularly true of a population consisting of often-uninsured patients with
severe disabilities. Kopits hoped that the charitable character of a
Catholic institution would facilitate his serving this special population properly. To a considerable degree, it did.

Just one example: when he first met Juliana De Souza in Brazil, her
arms, legs, feet, and hands had already begun to grow twisted; she
could only scoot along the floor on her backside or pull herself along
on a toddler's tricycle.[110] It took 84 hours of surgery to allow her, at
19, to stand upright and walk. Her older sister Katia, also a diastrophic
dwarf, had been even more seriously impaired when Dr Kopits met
her—her spine so damaged that she was losing the ability to breathe.
He referred her to a surgeon in Minneapolis, and her life was saved.
Juliana's surgery was made possible by Dr. Kopits's waiving his fee and
convincing the hospital to accept her as a charity case—absorbing
costs of $350,000.

In addition to creating his specially adapted office space, Dr. Kopits was able to set up the Pierre House where out-of-town families
could stay for a nominal fee or arrange for a foundation to pay for a
longer-term guest suite. As his reputation grew, patients flocked to
him. His roster of active patients peaked at more than 1,500, with persons arriving from 41 of the 50 United States and 26 foreign countries:[111] no one else in the world had devoted himself to dwarfism
conditions alone or had Kopits's pure skill and knowledge.

His insightful 1976 article "Orthopedic Complications of Dwarfism" suggests how his experience informed his decision making. In it he discussed achondroplasia, pseudoachondroplasia, metaphyseal chondroplasia, diastrophic dwarfism, Morquio syndrome, and spondyloepiphyseal dysplasia congenita. Although he learned considerably more in the quarter of a century that followed, seeds of later understanding were apparent. For example, he noted that in Morquio syndrome, cervical myelopathy, when present, resulted in a progressive lack of endurance to physical exertion at about 4 to 6 years of age. In the past, difficulties the child experienced on uneven terrain or managing distances were often mistakenly attributed to the increasingly prominent knock-knee deformity; thus surgeons performed lower limb osteotomies, after which some patients never regained independent ambulation due to myelopathy.

Kopits recommended alignment osteotomies at 8 to 10 years, saying that these surgeries had the best permanent results (skeletal growth does not progress much beyond then). But he focused on the necessity for spinal surgery, noting that severe problems resulted if cervical myelopathy was not addressed as soon as it appeared—with cord compression often causing progressive weakness of the upper limbs and trunk, chronic respiratory failure, and early death. He also discussed the question of doing bone fusions to correct ligamentous laxity of wrists and ankles, suggesting the procedure was difficult due to unavailability of cancellous bone. Often, instead of fusion surgery, he used plastic splints. I cite this illustration to illuminate his thinking, focus on timing, and consideration of alternatives. He studied outcomes and modified procedures as evidence accumulated. He also invented surgical instruments, such as the steel "halo" for Morquio patients, now in use by others and named after him.

Anyone familiar with diastrophic dwarfism is aware of frustrations with repeated, not fully successful, surgeries for clubfoot. In 2000, Vita Gagne, originator of the comprehensive Diastrophic Web Page on LPA Online praised his multifaced analysis of diastrophic dysplasia (DD) and the surgical techniques he developed in treating hundreds of DD patients. She was grateful that her son, a diastrophic dwarf, had been lucky enough to be one of Dr. Kopits's patients:

We all talk about how Dr. K. treated the whole person, not just the parts that needed his healing talents, but the first two years of Stefan's life were what proved it for us. Stefan was a very active baby and Dr. K. did his darndest to allow him to be so. During his surgery year, Stefan only had to be kept down for 6 weeks in the beginning and 6 weeks at the end—in between Dr. K. fixed up Stefan's casts so that he could stand and walk. At first he didn't intend that Stefan should do this, but once he saw that unless Stefan was chained to my side at all times, he was going to stand and walk, Dr. K. adapted his own ideas to suit Stefan's personal needs.[112]

Kopits had long accumulated detailed longitudinal information about his patients; the dwarfism community had awaited the results ever since his first correspondence to patients in 1980. At that time he had written a letter appealing for funds to complete a preliminary stage of research. He described advances he had made in the treatment of bowleg deformity and presented the conundrum of the variations in spinal cord compression that cause back problems among persons with achondroplasia.

By 1980 he had operated on 90 patients for bowleg deformity with six combinations of procedures, searching for the perfect method to prevent recurrence. In only 10 percent had the deformity reappeared, and he scheduled regular visits to check on growth. The objective had been the correction of postural alignment and improvement of gait. Analyzing the intricacies of problems relating to the spine proved much more difficult. He designed a prospective study to clarify how the curve of the back in achondroplasia relates to the degree of compression of spinal cord and nerves. He had already performed 650 examinations by then, generating 286,000 pieces of data, in the hope that he could discover why patients were more or less symptomatic— how the back's curvature and other factors influenced later back and leg problems.[113]

The world waited and wondered why no publications appeared. The project was held up by the absence of the prodigious funding required for such a large-scale enterprise, as well as the scarcity of time

Kopits was able to purloin from patient care. Nevertheless, for the next two decades he accumulated and analyzed data. By the time of his death in 2002, almost 500 cases of bowleg correction had been accumulated, demonstrating to his satisfaction that aligning the system resulted in less pressure on knees and backs. Ten thousand X-rays were digitalized, and a great deal of other information collected in an effort to suggest optimal timing and effectiveness for various procedures.[114]

With the help of Dr. Bruce Barton, a biostatistician, and David Jonah, a medical illustrator, Kopits undertook a series of scientific papers presenting the results of his bowleg deformity research. In addition, videotapes he made during his last ten or twelve years of surgery were gradually being edited and annotated for other physicians. The professionals involved in taping and editing accepted low or no fees.

Dr. Kopits had hoped to have finished and published his research by 2000. However, in January 1999, he broke a shoulder; the seizure that caused his fall had been caused by a brain tumor. He underwent brain surgery and radiation and a shoulder replacement. Kopits's illness realized the worst fears that patients had expressed for decades. They had seen the toll that very long work days had taken on his health—the bright, ebullient young man had aged greatly by his sixties, and his face and body betrayed his exhaustion. He had not been able to find a capable, like-minded physician to share his practice and had assumed the workload of at least two persons.

During the period of convalescence that preceded his death, Dr. Kopits was able to focus a bit more on research. When his cancer recurred in the summer of 2001, he knew he could no longer responsibly continue doing surgery: he made suitable referrals to patients and supervised two data-analysis teams. He began to narrate his surgical videotapes to make them available to medical schools and patients. Since Dr. Kopits's death in 2002, Dr. Barton and Mr. Jonah have been working steadily on a series of scientific papers presenting the investigations of bowleg deformity; videotapes and articles about Morquio syndrome and diastrophic dwarfism are being edited and should become available during the next year or two.

In the meantime, even at major centers in the United States, there is a dearth of surgical experience with rare conditions. It will take some time for the journal articles to find their way through review to publication. Even afterward, one mother wonders, in a hurried managed care climate, how many surgeons will be committed enough to continue the search for innovative, effective techniques?

At Dr. Kopits's funeral at the Cathedral of Mary our Queen in Baltimore, there was an honor guard of LPs, most of them Kopits's former patients. His brother George mentioned his selflessness in a moving eulogy: "He routinely overcommitted himself, and then, with unmatched tenacity he delivered—always with a smile or a joke." George Kopits spoke of Steven's devotion to family—his elderly parents, four children, and seven grandchildren—as well as to the Hungarian community and his parish. Like others, however, George concluded that Steven Kopits's greatest passion had been the care and healing of little people. A few patients had become physicians themselves—among them Dr. Jennifer Arnold, a pediatric resident at Children's Hospital in Pittsburgh, and Judith Badner, M.D., Ph.D., a geneticist and psychiatrist specializing in psychiatric genetics at the University of Chicago. Another former patient, gastroenterologist Dr. Kenneth Lee, remembers how honored he felt when Dr. Kopits allowed him to assist at one of his surgeries.

Dr. Michael C. Ain

When Dr. Ain was featured on *20/20* and on the ABC documentary "Hopkins 24/7" in 2000, he was already something of a celebrity. He had been profiled in the *Baltimore Sun* and *Johns Hopkins Magazine*, and the documentary *Dwarfs: Not a Fairy Tale*, in which he was featured, was in preparation. The media had sought him out for his success in defying the odds: an achondroplastic dwarf, he had succeeded in becoming an orthopedic surgeon at prestigious Johns Hopkins.

The preceding accounts emphasize the obstacles Ain had to surmount to attain his present position. After attending Phillips Academy, he went on to Brown University, where his interest in medicine crystallized. He credits his experiences as the patient of some compassionate physicians with stirring his desire to become an excellent doctor. An energetic person who had played varsity baseball and done wrestling and weightlifting at college, he felt drained when, despite good credentials, he was rejected by all of the 30 medical schools he applied to: "I was scared. I was angry. It was the only time I hit the wall. . . . It was the only time I felt trapped."[115]

Perhaps the fact that Ain majored in math, not science, may be seen as contributing. However, because interviewers raised questions about his strength, his ability to reach his patients' bedside, and the probable difficulty of his gaining respect, he strongly suspected bias. Determined to improve his standing, he returned to Brown and earned two A's with distinction in science courses; he did physiological research that was later published. This time he applied to twenty schools. He was rejected by all but one—Albany Medical College.

Dr. B. Barry Greenhouse, then an associate professor of anesthesiology, was taken with Ain, whom he termed a good student and a compassionate, decent young man who would be a credit to the medical profession. Despite success at Albany, Ain again faced obstacles seeking a residency. He had a strong interest in pediatric neurosurgery and was confident that, as an experienced woodworker, he had the manual skills required. He was turned down for the neurosurgical programs he desired most and even for surgery residencies at low-status institutions. The same remarks about his stamina and likely difficulty gaining respect were expressed—this time overtly. Once again, however, Albany Medical College accepted him for a five-year residency in pediatric orthopedics, where he excelled.

Dr. Paul Sponseller, chair of pediatric orthopedics at Johns Hopkins, wanted to strengthen the department's skeletal dysplasia program and was looking for someone well trained in children's orthopedics, and chose Ain for a fellowship. Hopkins had enjoyed a reputation for preeminence in the treatment of dwarfing conditions for four decades. Although with the establishment of the Greenberg Center it had renewed its commitment, its orthopedic component had suffered from the departure of Dr. Kopits. By the 1990s, there was an urgent need for a surgeon willing and able to focus on the complex orthopedic problems of dwarfs, especially children.[116]

Ain was recognized as a skilled pediatric orthopedist who could also offer a perspective gained through life experience. At first he resisted: "It's the last thing in the world I wanted to do because it's like looking in the mirror every day." But Dr. Allen Carl, his mentor at Albany, had told him about a newspaper article he had read about the father of a daughter with achondroplasia. The father had felt reassured about his daughter's future after meeting a physician with the same condition at a party. Dr. Ain realized that *he* had been that physician! "So at that point, without sounding corny, I thought, there are a lot of good hand and joint surgeons. If I could have an effect, help people, or be able to sympathize and understand certain issues, maybe that's why God wanted me to become an orthopedic surgeon."[117]

I spoke with Dr. Ain by phone in 2000 before his long day of surgery.[118] Media attention had often focused on his struggles in seeking to become a physician; later interviewers were more apt to inquire about his dual role as dwarf and physician to dwarfs, as well as the specific details surrounding his work as an orthopedist. Ain indicated to me that his sense of being part of the dwarfism community had developed relatively recently. He had gone to just one LPA meeting as a child, but since he has been at Hopkins he has begun to attend conferences, serving at its workshops and medical clinics; he is now a member of the Medical Advisory Board. Another development has brought him personally closer to the group: one of Ain's daughters, Alexa, has achondroplasia. Her younger sister Kayla is average-statured as is his wife Valerie, a nurse.

Dr. Ain had between 700 and 1,000 patients on the rolls: 20 percent of them were dwarfs, of whom approximately 70 percent were children. Although the largest number had achondroplasia, he had recently performed surgeries on persons with a wide range of diagnoses. He has learned that although surgeries for persons with skeletal dysplasias have much in common with those performed on average-statured individuals, they also have unique features that necessitate creating new guidelines and strategies. He has noted, for example, that adults with achondroplasia who need extensive decompression surgery often do not need fusion during the procedure, but average-statured individuals do. Also, many short-statured patients have premature arthritis and require joint replacements; in those instances special custom implants must be designed, with the help of Dr. Frank Frassica, a professor of orthopedics who specializes in musculoskeletal oncology and trauma, and a company that designs the prosthetics and instruments required.[119]

Ain has coauthored an article about reoperation for spinal restenosis in achondroplasia, based on eight Hopkins cases.[120] He mentioned that until recently surgeons had been hesitant to reoperate, fearful that the surgery might not help or do more harm than good. However, in recent years, understanding of spinal conditions has grown and treatment has altered. In the past, surgery was performed on only one or two spinal levels; today, knowledgeable surgeons increase efficacy by operating on more levels than those obviously offending. Among Ain's recent articles are one on hip arthroplasty in skeletal dysplasias and another on spinal fusion for kyphosis in achondroplasia.

During our phone conversation, while discussing the problem of spinal stenosis in achondroplasia, Ain noted the three major questions addressed when a patient presents with distressing symptoms: Should we operate? If so, which levels shall we decompress? Shall we include a fusion? Radiological evidence does not provide all the answers, and clinical evidence, while most crucial, is often difficult to evaluate. Although this situation also prevails among average-statured individuals, it is particularly important for dwarfs to seek physicians experienced with skeletal dysplasias when contemplating surgery.

I was surprised to hear that Ain was the only surgeon in the Department of Orthopedics who operated on pediatric patients with skeletal dysplasias. He indicated that much of what he had learned was self-taught, but that he had been fortunate enough to have neurosurgeons Daniel Rigamonti and Benjamin Carson and chief pediatric orthopedic surgeon Paul Sponseller as colleagues. Carson is the famed neurosurgeon featured on "Hopkins 24/7" removing much of one hemisphere from the brain of a 4-year-old with debilitating seizures. Carson has devised a delicate foramen magnum surgery that relieves spinal compression, thereby reducing the rate of SIDS in achondroplastic infants. He thins the bone down "to the thickness of a cornflake": this procedure has been enormously helpful. Carson has written two compelling autobiographical works that reflect his humanitarian vision.[121]

Although Ain and Kopits never discussed the matter, I knew they differed on the implication of bowleggedness. Half of all achondroplasts have significant bowing. Dr. Ain believes many of them do not need any treatment.[122] Melissa Hendricks, author of the *Johns Hopkins Magazine* article "Aiming High," quotes him as mentioning that a supposed link between bowing and arthritis is based on research involving average-statured patients; he thinks because achondroplasts have shorter limbs, they may not be subject to the same degree of risk. Dr. Kopits, on the other hand, believed the surgery had great potential for reducing pressure on joints and improving gait.

No doubt their differing views were influenced by both professional and personal experience. When he was eighteen, Ain had an osteotomy to straighten his bowlegs: his limbs had to be broken and reset, and he remained in a body cast for several months, experiencing considerable pain. Although his surgery had been prompted by a wrestling accident, prophylactic surgery for bowleggedness, especially at a younger age, is common. (Surgery done at the age of four typically takes under an hour, necessitating only a few days with complete bed rest and a couple of weeks of recuperation. Most of Dr. Kopits's surgeries were of this nature and performed on very young children.)

Dr. Ain and biomedical engineer Edmund Chao are currently studying the problem by creating a computer model of bowleggedness; Ain is also researching persons with achondroplasia who are 40 years old and older to assess correlations between degrees of arthritis and bowleggedness. It is to be hoped that the results of his research and Dr. Kopits's will bring surgeons closer to consensus.

Other controversies, such as limb lengthening, involve attitudinal as well as purely medical factors. Although Ain is not totally averse to the procedure, he himself does the surgery only for individuals who have one leg shorter than the other. He is concerned about the complications associated with limb lengthening and opposed to parents making the decision for preadolescents. Also, he has commented, "Most of the people I've seen who had it are stiffer—they don't run faster or jump any higher, they're just taller."[123]

Research is one exciting part of Dr. Ain's professional life, but while accumulating its long-term results, he is sustained by the daily satisfaction of transforming so many persons' lives. He has commented, "The kids are fantastic to work with. You do wonderful things and you help a lot of people doing it. I wouldn't trade my job with anybody." I nevertheless wondered how he could manage all-day surgeries; I knew how difficult it is for most persons with achondroplasia to stand for long periods without pain or numbness. Ain answered matter-of-factly: "*Most* surgeons are very tired at the end of a long workday— I am too. It comes with the territory."

Dr. Judith G. Hall

When Dr. Judith G. Hall was named to the prestigious Order of Canada in 1999, the *Canadian Pediatric Society News* declared that there was scarcely room for another honor or accomplishment.[124] Currently professor of pediatrics at the University of British Columbia Children's Hospital (having stepped down as head several years ago), Hall has been named one of the thousand best doctors in North America by *American Health* magazine, received the British Columbia Science Council's Gold Medal, and been inducted into the Johns Hopkins Society of Scholars and the British Columbia Science World Hall of Fame. She is also the winner of the New Frontiers in Research Award for her work on inherited conditions in children. A former president of the American Society of Human Genetics, she helped found the American Board of Medical Genetics. Born in Boston, she spent nine years at the University of Washington, and then served as professor of pediatrics and medical genetics at the University of British Columbia, as well as physician-in-chief at the Children's and Women's Health Centre of BC.

Hall is familiar to LPA members through her popular informal presentations at the "ladies' tea" that is a regular feature of the annual conference, and a variety of communications that she has prepared for members over the years: a study of gynecological problems of women, a paper about anesthesia for dwarfing conditions, another on nutrition, and an item about the handy practical device called "the bottom wiper" that persons with short arms can use for bathroom hygiene. This last innovation demonstrates that no problem is too pedestrian to merit Dr. Hall's attention.

However, she is equally at home discussing complex aspects of her two specialties, pediatrics and genetics. During our telephone interview, she spoke of her interest in the "natural history" of conditions, explaining that she approached given disorders not as fixed entities, but rather as they developed and changed over time. She illustrated with an example drawn from arthrogryposis, a group of conditions in which multiple joint contractures are present at birth, in the classic case affecting hands, wrists, elbows, shoulders, hips, feet, and knees.[125] (She had become expert in this group of disorders at a time when few physicians studied it.) She explained that if you don't move your joints, organs don't develop: when lungs don't develop, for example, one can't swallow—and so it is very important to get a baby to move. Similarly, if you stretch a cell, it changes its properties. One must be aware of all these interactions and the potential paths for development over time if one is to treat a condition properly and provide timely physical therapy.

Another example: when fetuses are small and the placenta does not supply enough blood flow, the fetus puts out receptors to pull in sugar and sodium. A process that is useful during the fetal period may promote a dangerous situation later—leading to hypertension and heart disease. Therefore, the clinician must be alert to the potential problems of each stage. Dr. Hall recommended an important article about dwarfing conditions that specified the problems for which a child needed to be monitored.[126] She lamented that research grants were rarely given for natural history studies, because she believes they would influence appropriate treatment, as well as the functions of the genes themselves.

Once, asked about her greatest achievement, Dr. Hall replied, "Translating advances in genetics in order to provide better care and more options for families."[127] Her commitment to informing patients and families on health issues and assisting with practical matters are reflected in her teaching and in chairing conferences such as *Child Health Care in the Twentieth Century.* Hall has written several hundred articles, contributed fifty chapters to larger works, and edited or coedited several books. One of these is *Human Malformations and Related Anomalies,* a major reference work about birth defects that discusses diagnosis, pathogenesis, history, and approaches to treatment and prevention.[128] She has also coedited three other important works: *Arthrogryposis,*[129] *Handbook of Physical Measurements,*[130] and *Organelle Diseases.*[131]

These works represent a synthesis of an enormous amount of research and clinical practice over three decades. Scanning her bibliography and noticing articles about topics such as children of incest and counseling for adoptees, one may well wonder how one individual can have written about such a wide range of subjects. Hall maintains that all these topics had simply crossed her path at different times. If one has difficulty summing her up, it is probably best to adopt her own definition: "a clinical geneticist primarily interested in congenital anomalies, genetics of short stature and connective tissue abnormalities, with a particular interest in the natural history and clinical heterogeneity of these disorders."[132] Hall was among the first to focus on these areas, crucial to assessment and treatment; later works, such as *The Management of Genetic Syndromes* (2000) edited by Suzanne Cassidy and Judith Allanson, reveal a similar approach, highlighting more than twenty genetic syndromes, including a number of dwarfing conditions. [133]

Her pleasure in scientific inquiry is evident in her articles: in one, "Mendel Might Get Dizzy,"[134] she asserts that a mutation is not what it used to be and describes changes in thinking about heritability that occurred in the past several years. She has helped unravel some genetic mysteries in twinning (monozygotic twins are not truly identical) and heritability because she has recognized that an insight about one disorder is apt to ripen as a result of painstaking familiarity with many others.[135] It came as a surprise to many investigators to discover that one can get a recessive disorder from only one parent if that parent has contributed two chromosomes with the disorder to the genetic mix. Dr. Hall translates: "Everyone thought, 'Well, the dad wasn't the dad but he *was* the dad, and what happened was that this child got both chromosome 7s from Mom.'"[136]

Although Hall recognizes the hazards implicit in deciphering the genome, she is more apt to dwell on potential benefits. Once genetic screening has permitted us to identify most diseases and tracers have been designed to track cell functioning, we should be able to grow organs from our own cells and correct problems we are now just beginning to understand. She is less sanguine about retrovirus gene therapy, which she describes as "overrated." She emphasizes that there are good reasons it has proved difficult to design and accomplish. "My own bias is, if you can learn to turn genes back on or off, it is better to do that than to repair." She explained that in the case of hemoglobin, for example, if one could turn back on a fetal gene that had functioned until shortly before birth, when an adult gene took over, it might be possible to relieve a condition such as sickle-cell anemia.

Ultimately, the "downstream issues" are the ones that interest her most. It makes little sense to her to try to correct a single gene before understanding the full spectrum of what is involved as its expression plays itself out over time. She is convinced, for example, that a skeletal gene such as the one for achondroplasia, because it is present also in the brain, doesn't affect only the skeleton—it may have implications for issues such as obesity and temperament. One must understand how a gene works in relation to everything else before tampering with it. Functional genomics or proteomics take complexity into account.

When Dr. McKusick seconded Hall's nomination for the British

Columbia Science and Technology Award, he noted that the contribution "likely to have the most far-reaching implications is her work on folic acid supplements." In a strongly worded article summarizing evidence that folic acid taken before conception or early in pregnancy could prevent a variety of birth defects, Dr. Hall had recommended changes in individual women's behavior and public policy.[137]

In an interview for the *Canadian Medical Association Journal* in 1999, she identified two important personal influences: she credited her mother's "infectious curiosity and hard work" as providing a model, and Bruce Cattanach's study of uniparental disomy in mice as transforming her thinking about nontraditional types of inheritance.[138]

When Hall worked at the University of Washington, salaries had often depended on grants, and tenure positions were unavailable. At 40, concerned about her three children's future, she heard that the University of British Columbia was looking for a clinical geneticist. She considers it the best move she ever made. It afforded her ample opportunity to use her clinical and research skills, and she also benefited from being a part of the Canadian health care system, which she praised enthusiastically.

Back in Washington, families whose children had genetic anomalies were often forced to pay out of pocket. Families found themselves forced into bankruptcy. Canada provides health care to everyone, using funds equal to only 9 percent of the GNP, whereas the United States, using 14 percent, leaves a substantial portion of the population with inadequate or no coverage. During her twenty years in Canada, Hall had also been impressed with the quality of care—one might have to wait for treatment, but not unduly.

Hall's concern for patients is omnipresent, but especially so when she discusses the controversial issues of prenatal diagnosis and abortion, as well as when she mentions the special relationship between women physicians and their female patients. She feels it is vital to have women physicians available to discuss sensitive gynecological and sexual issues. She had been pleased to conduct research on women's health problems and to speak with young and older women about a variety of medical and other concerns. She concluded our interview by mentioning how she valued the persons she had met through LPA: "I think that part of human nature is to have to struggle, and that real people learn from their struggle. Ordinary people may struggle over pimples and hair—or depression. So many people with short stature are real with their struggles. Of course, I don't want people to suffer: I really feel torn. But some of the finest people I know have been persons with skeletal dysplasias—their lives enhanced by their struggles."

Dr. Charles I. Scott

Dr. Scott, long-term chair of the LPA Medical Advisory Board, is known especially for his well-regarded CIBA pamphlet on dwarfism and an influential article in the March of Dimes Birth Defects Series, entitled "Medical and Social Adaptation in Dwarfing Conditions."[139] He also helped to edit *Dwarfism: the Family and Professional Guide,* an invaluable work published originally by the Short Stature Foundation and later made available through LPA.[140]

I met Dr. Scott at his office at the duPont Institute for Children in Wilmington, Delaware, which was festooned with Christmas cards and photographs of families and children he had treated. He was easily drawn into reminiscences about his thirty-year stint as chair of the Medical Advisory Board. Created around 1969, it had developed gradually and informally. The group discusses current issues, reviews research proposals of members, exchanges information, participates in clinics, and responds to requests from physicians and patients worldwide.

In 1968, when Dr. Scott was a teaching fellow at Johns Hopkins, Ellie Jones, an LP from Gloucester, New Jersey, contacted Dr. McKusick. In those days, individuals with short stature were commonly assigned only three labels: achondroplasia, Morquio, and midget. At that time, there were up to twenty-three fellows working in some capacity with Dr. McKusick at Hopkins, including pediatricians, surgeons, anthropologists, dentists, and a variety of others. Working closely together, many became friends, and some took field trips to LPA regional meetings and other events. Dr. Scott accompanied Kay Smith and Dee Miller, the LP who is now coordinator of the Greenberg Center, on weekend drives to Atlanta; Pittsburgh; Flint, Michigan; and elsewhere.

Eminent radiologist Dr. Len Langer helped create what would become an enduring relationship between LPA families and physicians, working from "the shadow world of X-rays," to help refine diagnoses and make them more accurate. During that era, when the March of Dimes was contributing heavily to investigations of what was then referred to as "birth defects," many meetings were held at Hopkins, with participants from Europe and all over the world. After the fellows dispersed to jobs across the country they would consult each other: "Have you ever seen anyone like this," one physician would say? "Oh yes, I've seen two," the other might respond. Before DNA swabs, such consultation was invaluable; even now, enduring relationships have made it much easier to reach accurate conclusions.

Other physicians currently prominent in the field trained with the original group, as Dr. Rich Pauli did with Dr. Hall when she was in Seattle. However, most of these remarkable colleagues, whom Dr. Scott referred to as "the dinosaurs," are no longer serving in their former leadership positions, though Drs. Francomano and Reid are still active members of the LPA Medical Advisory Board (fig. 1.8). Although some younger persons are joining the Medical Advisory Board (Dr. Gary Bellus, an accomplished laboratory investigator and clinician in Denver; Dr. Pauli, at the University of Wisconsin; and Dr. Ain at Johns Hopkins), there is no new generation like the group trained at Hopkins in the golden era. Federal and private monies for clinical training have largely dried up, and fellows such as Dr. Michael Wright, a dwarfism specialist and skilled, personable geneticist who returned to England after his training, do not have the same collegial cohort to rely on.

At the same time, the need for attention to dwarfism has grown enormously. Dr. Scott receives countless e-mails from perplexed

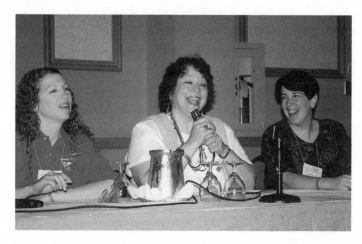

Fig. 1.8. Drs. Cheryl Reid, Judith Hall, and Clair Francomano at the 1994 Little People of America National Conference in San Antonio, Texas. Photograph courtesy of Julie Rotta.

physicians and parents, and he fields inquiries from as far as Slovenia, Maui, and Bosnia. With Dr. Kopits's office closed, Dr. Scott and his colleague Dr. Will Mackenzie, a renowned orthopedist and neck and spine surgeon at duPont Hospital for Children, have had to deal with an increasing case load (fig. 1.9).

Scott is semiretired, however, and is concerned about who will eventually replace him. He sees patients two days a week and is quick to help physicians at other institutions with a diagnosis or to suggest books to colleagues or patients. He is particularly enthusiastic about Jill Krementz's series, which includes *How It Feels to Live with a Physical Disability,* and recommends a few genetics works that he regards as indispensable. Among his own contributions, he cites the developmental scales for achondroplasia, available in *Dwarfism: The Family and Professional Guide.* He feels strongly that the duPont system of scheduling each child to see a geneticist every six months for the first six years assures proper support and medical care. Scott regularly advises a child not gain more than three pounds a year before puberty, helping to guarantee a lifetime of fewer orthopedic problems.

A few days after my visit to Dr. Scott, the local LPA chapter tried, as it had intermittently before, to establish a center in the New York area. Barbara Brullo (now Spiegel), then president of the Mets chapter, and I met with Dr. Jessica Davis, geneticist at Presbyterian New York Hospital who had close connections with the original Hopkins group, and later with Dr. Cathleen Raggio, a pediatric orthopedist with special expertise in osteogenesis imperfecta, at the Hospital for Special Surgery (HSS) (these two institutions have a close working relationship). We raised the possibility of establishing a dwarfism center that followed the Hopkins model.

They agreed to assess the knowledge base and interest of other staff, and several doctors "signed on." Maria Telesca of the Long Island chapter had contacted Alan Greenberg, the benefactor of the

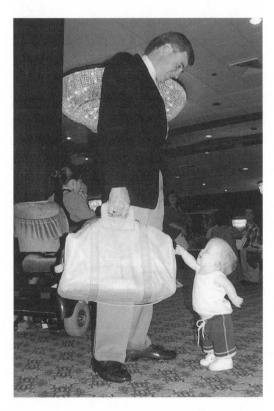

Fig. 1.9. Dr. William Mackenzie, orthopedic surgeon, Alfred I. duPont Hospital for Children, Wilmington, Delaware, at the 1995 Little People of America Conference in Chicago. Photograph courtesy of Julie Rotta.

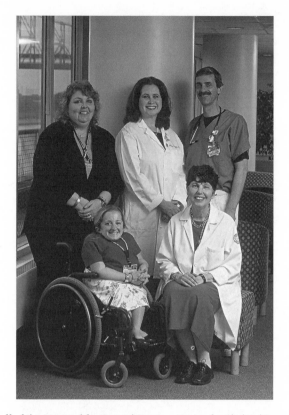

Fig. 1.10. Staff of the Hospital for Special Surgery Center for Skeletal Dysplasias (left to right): Lorraine Montuori, C.S.W., social worker; Cathleen Raggio, M.D., orthopedic surgeon and codirector; Richard Slote, R.N., nurse coordinator; Tara Shea, M.S., clinical coordinator / genetic counselor; Jessica Davis, M.D., clinical geneticist and codirector. Photograph courtesy of Hospital for Special Surgery

Hopkins Greenberg Center, about her distress that no adequate facility existed in the New York area for her own treatment. Greenberg and his wife, Kathryn, volunteered to help fund the proposed HSS clinic for the next several years.

On 13 February 2003, several members of the New York and New Jersey chapters of LPA met with the enthusiastic Davis and Raggio—now the codirectors—to discuss the path of the new Center for Skeletal Dysplasias. The two were committed to the holistic approach practiced by the original Hopkins group. The center opened in May 2003 and has begun to serve an increasing number of pediatric and adult patients.

There are other physicians who deserve lengthy consideration, among them Drs. Richard Pauli, William Horton, Leonard Langer, and other eminent European physicians. Experts in other areas of short-stature research and treatment, such as endocrinologist Robert M. Blizzard, a renowned figure in the history of growth hormone, have been unfairly ignored. I trust nevertheless that the spirit of these and others who have guided the extraordinary transformation of dwarfism research and treatment has been captured.

Joan O. Weiss

Some years ago, the parent of an infant dwarf daughter told me she was enormously impressed with the medical care and the atmosphere at the Moore Clinic at Johns Hopkins: "Everybody is a social worker there—even the doctors!" Still, the physicians understood that a doctor's ability to tackle social and emotional issues was limited. Therefore, every initial evaluation, and most subsequent appointments, included a visit to the social worker.

For many years that person was Joan Weiss. She came to know families intimately, sometimes seeing them through crises engendered by surgeries. The normal wear and tear of marriage and family life is intensified by having to cope with a disability. Patients and their families formed vital relationships with Weiss, and not being treated as anonymous, not being directed to yet another new face to whom they must reveal confidential matters, increased their openness.

Weiss's individual counseling role was crucial, but she also initiated several projects helpful to a broad patient population. In 1979 she co-authored with Dr. John Rogers, an Australian physician at the clinic, a booklet for new parents called *My Child Is a Dwarf*. At that time there was scant nontechnical literature available, and the Human Growth Foundation was the only other source of useful printed matter. The brochure answered frequently asked questions and helped families to approach the experience of raising their child more positively. Recently, LPA has revised the brochure, retitling it *A Whole New View*.

In 1971 Weiss, along with Kay Smith, Dr. McKusick's assistant, organized the Short Stature Symposia held annually at Johns Hopkins from 1971 to 1984. They were inspired by Weiss's belief that there was a tremendous need to address psychosocial concerns. Although the symposia featured workshops on medical concerns, they also offered workshops for new parents and siblings, and others about sexuality, vocational concerns, and preparations for college. A number of them provided opportunities to discuss personal issues. At lunch or coffee hour, individuals and families connected and sometimes established enduring friendships. Most attendees were from the Northeast, but many came from the mid-Atlantic region, and a few from the South. Although LPA had held national conventions since the late 1950s, it had not always had the extensive program of workshops it currently does—the Hopkins symposium model provided the impetus.

In addition, Weiss conceived the PACT (Parenting and Communications Training) program offered at Johns Hopkins in 1982 for parents of children with dwarfism. The weekend sessions focused on sensitivity training and strategies for outreach to new parents. PACT parents, by contacting hospitals, physicians, and social agencies, hoped to refer newcomers to an experienced family who could provide vital information and support. In the New York City area, for example, attendees contacted geneticists and obstetricians at fifty hospitals, stimulating years of referrals. Although the program was offered only twice, many of its graduates continued to play important roles in the dwarfism community.

Weiss began her social work career at family agencies, focusing on adoption placements and individual and couple counseling. However, she has devoted most of her work life to the psychosocial aspects of medical genetics. Her years at Johns Hopkins and her experience with various genetic disorders helped convince her of the need for a true partnership between consumers of genetic services and health care providers. In 1986, convinced support and advocacy groups could benefit from joining into a strong disability community, she helped found the Alliance of Genetic Support Groups, now called the Genetic Alliance.

She codirected the Human Genome Education Model Project and is on the steering committee of the GenEthics Consortium of the Greater Washington Area and on the boards of several national and regional genetic support groups. After helping to establish many such organizations, she coauthored *Starting and Sustaining Genetic Support Groups.*[141] Weiss is also author or coauthor of many articles in the field of genetics. One that touches on some of the dilemmas created by recent scientific advances is "Genetic Discrimination: Perspectives of Consumers" published in *Science* in 1996.[142]

At annual LPA conferences she counsels individuals and leads workshops dealing with personal and emotional matters. (She has led similar workshops for the Restricted Growth Association in Great Britain.) In more than a quarter of a century since she first worked at Johns Hopkins, and fifteen years on the LPA Medical Advisory Board, she has come to know hundreds of members. She remains energized by these enduring human relationships, reminders of why the organizational work she spearheaded matters.

Dr. Selna Kaplan

Dr. Kaplan is a pediatric endocrinologist who played a vital role in introducing human growth hormone as a treatment for hypopituitary dwarfism. She has also held important positions in various professional organizations. These contributions will be detailed later, but to capture the quality of Dr. Kaplan's clinical approach and to offer readers a dramatic example of the contrast between inept and skillful medical management, I begin by describing the vital difference to my own life and my daughter's that her presence made.

It was Dr. Kaplan who confirmed Anna's diagnosis of achondroplasia a few weeks after her birth, after examining the X-rays and photographs that she had asked me to send. Without her guidance, I would no doubt have had to tread a far more tortuous course. Both before and after hearing from her, I had a number of distressing experiences with doctors. The neonatologist at the major New York City hospital where she was born misdiagnosed her, stating she had a "fifty-fifty chance of having a condition that would lead to retardation and early death." Only after taking X-rays and reviewing them did he correct his diagnosis and, moments before we left the hospital, call us into his office and inform us that she had achondroplasia. He gave us a sketchy, inaccurate account of what that unfamiliar term meant.

His discomfort was apparent. He never used the word *dwarf* and, after consulting a medical book in our presence, informed us that she would be "under five feet" (the average height of females with achondroplasia is actually about four feet, with little variability). He asked me if I had any short women with large heads in the family and subsequently sent a forwarding letter to other physicians in which he noted "my peculiar habitus." When, a few months later, I wrote to him suggesting what I wished he had done and telling him about my route to Johns Hopkins, he failed to reply, despite my having requested a response.

Two separate pediatric endocrinologists to whom I was referred within the first two months were not at all helpful. One, a woman, observed, "It doesn't have to matter that much—women can wear heels." While I was making these appointments locally, I also contacted Dr. Kaplan in California. I had known her all my life—our mothers were cousins and close friends. I knew Selna was an expert in the field of dwarfism, a clinician and a faculty member at the University of California at San Francisco School of Medicine.

She responded with a special delivery letter that confirmed the diagnosis and introduced me to the Human Growth Foundation and to LPA, saying members "have an active social life and happy times together. They teach children the self-confidence to live with their problems. It is important since these children are of normal intelligence and display all the normal activities and capabilities of normal children. . . . I know that it may be difficult for you not to feel depressed about this 'happening to you.' Perhaps you don't. Either way, you must remember whatever her problem is, your daughter needs your love, affection, attention and guidance as does any child. She will be less bothered by her shortness than you will."

None of the several doctors I had encountered had mentioned these groups. Their referrals had provided neither helpful information nor emotional wisdom and tended to minimize any difficulty or communicate discomfort and pity. Selna's advice set us on a felicitous path. Hers was my first sensible, encouraging encounter with the medical profession. She also sent brochures and invited me to ask for more information. I followed her suggestion and attended a Human Growth Foundation chapter meeting, where I was encouraged to make an appointment at Johns Hopkins. Later I joined LPA.

Dr. Kaplan's career was inextricably intertwined with the development of growth hormone therapy. She had completed her internship at Bellevue and residency at Kings County and gone on to Columbia in 1958. There she began research with Dr. Melvin Grumbach in the field of pediatric endocrinology. Growth hormone had recently been isolated and methods of making it both pure and potent had been developed. In 1955 and 1956, growth hormone–deficient children began to be treated with hormone obtained from human pituitaries. One of Dr. Kaplan's first assignments was to organize a system to allow her research group to set up a group of pathologists who would provide the glands. This canvassing allowed the Columbia clinic to treat between five and ten patients a year.

Dr. Maurice Radin in Boston and Dr. T. H. Li in Berkeley were also conducting significant research. Competition for glands was intense, and other researchers would sometimes outbid the Columbia group. There were also no accurate tests yet to identify which patients had isolated growth hormone deficiency. Once a National Pituitary Agency was established, researchers were required to submit proposals to NIH in order to be assigned growth hormone. Kaplan was chair of the Columbia committee that selected projects and approved grant proposals.

There were occasional families who did not appear for the regular blood tests required to obtain treatment, but most did, eager to watch their children grow to normal heights. The system was in many respects artificial and cumbersome, but it did provide free treatment to many who needed it. The most frightening, devastating period of Dr. Kaplan's life, she reflected, occurred in 1985 when it was discovered

that some batches of human growth hormone had been contaminated. Some patients began to develop a devastating illness called
Creutzfeldt-Jakob disease (CJD), a rare, infectious autoimmune disorder causing debilitation and death. A person killed in an auto accident whose pituitary had been harvested, it was belatedly discovered,
might not have manifested symptoms but could have still passed the
disease on to the patients.

For years, Dr. Kaplan had been telling patients that HGH was the
safest drug we have, so, receiving the news at a meeting, she was
shocked. "This meant we had to go home, distribute the names of patients and start calling them. It was the worst time of my life. Parents
asked, 'Does my child have it?' and there was no way we could answer
with certainty because the effect of the virus was a slow one—it might
take ten years to develop."

Dr. Kaplan was president of the International European and
United States Pediatric Society when a joint symposium was organized to make decisions about using human pituitaries. The United
Kingdom, the Scandinavian countries, and the United States discontinued use, but some countries believed the issue was limited to rare
batches and that they did not have the problem. France kept using a
contaminated product for two years longer, resulting in twenty or
more patients dying very quickly. One patient in California and one
or two patients in New York died.

The crisis led NIH in 1985 to the prompt approval of synthetic
growth hormone, which had been tested during the previous four
years. Those patients with compelling needs were treated immediately; others had to wait six months, but finally safe and plentiful
growth hormone became widely available. The only difficulty was establishing guidelines and convincing insurance companies to pay for
treatment.

Once quantities of growth hormone became commercially available, there was an explosion of research aimed at finding out to what
extent it could improve the height of children who were not growth
hormone deficient—children with constitutional short stature, Turner syndrome, and bone dysplasias. Seventy to eighty percent of short-

statured children showed immediate improvement. However, only a small percentage of those with initial improvement ended up with a greater final height than might have been projected without treatment. One possible strategy, Kaplan ventured, might be to treat children earlier and stop treatment before puberty, thereby maintaining the increase, rather than have them go through puberty quickly and cease growing.

Studying the relationship between growth and puberty has been helpful in treating persons with Turner syndrome. By postponing treatment with sex steroids, previously given to girls with Turner syndrome at 12 or 13 years of age to induce secondary sex characteristics, until 14 or 15, these girls have grown two to four more inches. Despite the disappointing results with bone dysplasias, the literature is still replete with studies from many countries making claims for the efficacy of HGH in this group. Kaplan points out that only carefully designed studies that include projections of *final* probable heights, rather than early improvement, are trustworthy.

She also spoke of a variety of problems associated with deciding who ought to receive growth hormone. Since it has become more widely available, many families with constitutional short stature or even families of children who are projected to be of average stature now apply for treatment; they often represent the greatest number of applicants. Dr. Kaplan, without moralizing about her viewpoint, makes it clear that she does not feel that everyone who is short should be treated.

Dr. Kaplan herself is no more than five feet tall. That fact may contribute to her ability to confidently assure parents that height is not the be-all and end-all for success. Nevertheless, she is sympathetic with those crushed that they will be of average or less than average height. Although the family of a youth with these feelings might be advised to seek psychological help, in most instances, families who have already presented themselves at a clinic seeking growth improvement are not apt to view the suggestion favorably.

Girls, in Kaplan's experience, are less apt to be sensitive about their height, especially compared with boys in school settings that emphasize competitive sports. She has seen instances of positive personality change and confidence come from boys' increased stature. Nevertheless, she is acutely conscious of the ethical concerns involved in manipulating a natural process. Only a very small percentage of children are permanently handicapped by being short, she believes: If they have received support, they end up reasonably well off. Recent research concurs.[143]

Among other delicate problems that clinicians face is deciding how to define growth hormone deficiency, thereby enabling a patient to be eligible for treatment and insurance. Treatment for Turner syndrome may cost as much as $30,000—$45,000 a year; young short-statured patients may pay as little as $10,000 a year. Cost is dose dependent, approximately $225–$250 per 5 milligrams. Although insurance companies must pay for growth hormone deficiency in childhood and adulthood and for Turner syndrome, because these treatments are regarded as medically necessary, they balk at paying for what may be constitutional short stature. It has not been simple for physicians to designate growth hormone deficiency. A decision was made to set a value at a higher level than originally, to qualify marginal candidates—those with "insufficient growth hormone." It becomes tempting to repeat tests so as to select the lowest value and secure a patient's eligibility.

Knotty questions such as these represent a minor though troublesome aspect of a rewarding career like Dr. Kaplan's. Mostly, she focuses on research and treatment aimed at improving the lives of patients. As I discussed with her the pleasures of her profession, she spoke of the satisfaction she had experienced working with patients over many years' time. In some instances, she has gone on to treat the children and grandchildren of some of her original patients with growth hormone deficiency. She has kept in touch with many former patients, enjoying being part of the fabric of their lives—in some instances attending their weddings. In addition, she has enjoyed the intellectual stimulation of research and writing, both individually and in association with colleagues, about a variety of endocrine conditions. She has received awards from the Endocrine Society and been past president of Lawson Wilkins Pediatric Endocrine Society.

Back in the early 1950s, Kaplan had difficulty getting into graduate school, let alone medical school, despite excellent undergraduate performance and recommendations. Female, Jewish, a graduate of Brooklyn College rather than an elite school, and quite short, she had to overcome many obstacles before gaining admission to a doctoral program and then medical school at Washington University in St. Louis.

After her research at Columbia, Kaplan relocated to UCSF with Dr. T. H. Li, her close colleague and friend. Now in her 70s, she is officially retired, but treats some patients; previously, she published articles on hypopituitarism, hypogonadism, and other matters involving hormones and metabolism. She coauthored the article "The Growth Hormone Cascade," which describes the long-term results of growth hormone treatment and contains a comprehensive bibliography.[144] A good overview also appeared in John Monson's *Challenges in Growth Hormone Therapy*, but for the most recent information about growth hormone developments, the best resource is the Web site of the Lawson Wilkins Pediatric Endocrine Society.[145]

LIMB LENGTHENING

After the birth of a dwarf child, one of the first questions often asked is, "Can anything be done?" usually meaning, "Isn't there any way to make her grow taller?" Growth hormone was appropriate only for persons with endocrine disorders; there was no remedy for bone disorders. But suddenly, in the late 1980s, television and magazines were awash with reports of a miraculous solution. *Donahue, 20/20, Time,* and the *Washington Post* described the procedure and featured dwarf children who would now attain nearly normal height.

Media attention flagged, then revived, as procedures were refined. In 1998, *Oprah* featured limb lengthening in her series on modern medical miracles. Children and young adults could be enabled to grow 9 to 12 inches, achieving a final height between 5 and 5½ feet instead of between 4 and 4½.

The first articles tended to have heart-wrenching titles such as "Enduring Agony, A Boy's Made Taller."[146] It describes the odyssey of Mary Tarabocchia, who had desperately searched for a remedy for her son's dwarfism. She had taken him to doctors for hormone injections at two and to Lourdes for the baths, with no benefit. She had visited any number of physicians who had encouraged her to accept him as he was, but she feared that the world would not do so. After U.S. doctors rebuffed her, considering the procedure too risky, she raised funds from friends and neighbors and took 9-year-old Anthony to Italy for limb-lengthening treatment. She slept on a cot by his bed as the doctors turned the screws each day on the painful system of wires and braces. Listening to the screams of other children, while massaging her son's legs, she doubted her decision, but was reassured when, asked if he was happy, he responded, "Yes, because now I am bigger and kids don't make fun of me."

Another article, "In New Jersey: A Boy Grows Towering Tall," described 14-year-old Reza Garakani.[147] His parents, a psychiatrist and a psychologist, were recent immigrants from Iran. Although his father cautioned he might have to endure several years of pain, Reza elected to proceed. The article depicts him as animated by his response to the pity and ridicule he had experienced and by his guilt at the pain his condition had caused his family. He is described as surviving on painkillers and a great deal of mind control and courage. Later accounts are apt to be less emotionally fraught, in part, because of improved pain management and also fewer young children among the patients.

Although there is now also an "internal nail" method, that procedure is not suitable for the very short limbs of most dwarfs.[148] The most common method uses a fixator (a metal framework that runs the length of the section being stretched) that is pinned onto the bone.[149] Under general anesthesia, a cut is made through the bone shaft, and within several days new bone starts to form at the fracture site. Instead of allowing the fracture to heal, the cut ends are pulled apart, about a millimeter a day. The fixator holds the bone steady and straight. This process continues for several months until the bone reaches its desired length: physical therapy is offered when the bone can bear weight. Patients report varying degrees of pain, worst if infections develop; uncomfortable muscle reactions (cramps and twitching) are common, and physical therapy is often arduous. Some centers report the pain has now lessened; Dr. Rimoin reports that the Villerubias technique used at Cedars-Sinai involves little pain.

Limb-lengthening procedures are now offered as late as young adulthood. Originally, only leg lengthening was done; now, in recognition of the fact that longer arms are required for symmetry and function, both legs and arms are done, legs first. The surgeries can cost between $80,000 and $130,000. Although similar surgery has long been used for congenital problems, or limbs shattered in accidents, and these still represent the largest part of the practice of specialized centers, only in recent decades have orthopedists begun to adapt these techniques for lengthening the limbs of dwarfs.[150]

Limb lengthening was attempted by Codovilla as early as 1905, and external fixators were initiated by Dr. Joseph Bittner in 1929.[151] In the 1930s and 1940s, circular fixators were described in German and Russian publications; the Wagner method was used in the 1970s. All proved impractical because of complications.[152]

Beginning in 1951, a new method was devised by Professor Gavril Abramovich Ilizarov in Siberia. Starting with a small laboratory, he experimented first with animals and later with humans, developing an innovative distraction (bone-stretching) technique. After years of obscurity, his contribution was honored with the Lenin Prize for Medicine in 1978. By 1982 he was in charge of an institute with 1,200 beds, 12 operating rooms, and research laboratories. More than a million patients have been treated using his methods.

In 1983 Ilizarov directed the first course explicating his methods in Lecco, Italy, before 300 specialists. Orthopedic surgeons made pilgrimages to Ilizarov's center, as well as to centers in Italy and Spain. De Bastiani and his colleagues in Verona proposed variations using a technique known as monolateral fixation.[153] Orthopedic surgeons Victor Frankel of New York and Dror Paley of Toronto were among the physicians trained in Kurgen, Italy, and Spain; they organized conferences in New York and Washington in 1987 and 1988. Paley later moved to Baltimore and established the Maryland Center for Limb Lengthening and Reconstruction; now called the International Center for Limb Lengthening and Reconstruction (ICLLR), it has expanded into a modern facility at Sinai Hospital, Baltimore.

One of the most notable voices raising questions about limb lengthening was Dr. Steven Kopits, who felt that it did not merit use as a "cure" for dwarfism.[154] He indicated that the procedure had a higher rate of complications than any other orthopedic surgery, including neurological damage, foot-drop deformity, and stiff ankles. He questioned its effect on muscles and nerves and increased loading across a joint. In one notable case he observed a teenager who had surgery in Italy and was taller, but who now walked spastically.[155] Kopits also felt that because dwarfs often required other essential surgery, the risks of limb lengthening, which he considered cosmetic, did not make sense; he was wary of "the never-ending quest for normalcy." When the First International Conference on Achondroplasia was held in Rome in 1986, Dr. Judith Hall commented that more research was required to investigate safety and long-term results of this potentially remarkable procedure and that a new highly trained cooperative team was necessary for positive results.[156]

Today, Ilizarov centers have proliferated in many countries, and the procedure, with variations, has become common in the United States. Dr. Mark Dahl at the Minneapolis Limb Length Center and Dr. C. Robert Rozbruch at New York's Hospital for Special Surgery are among the physicians who have the most expertise with limb lengthening. Drs. Paley and Herzenberg at the ICLLR have continued to refine their techniques; their center treats more patients than any other. Cedars-Sinai in Los Angeles, although treating only a small number of patients, is recognized for its effective use of the Villerubias method.

Because opting for limb-lengthening procedures suggests a person is attempting to trade one identity for another, the choice is filled with existential resonance. Although someone who has the surgery may no longer experience himself as a dwarf, not all dwarfism's marks disappear. It also is retained in the genes and may need to be reconfronted in the next generation. And yet, the fantasy beckons. A disabled person can join the "normals." A very short person can physically extend her reach and meet the world on equal terms.

From the first, the dwarfism community was circumspect. In 1988 the Board of Directors of LPA issued a lengthy statement to the press, citing medical complications, pain, and uncertainty about long-term effects on joints and lower back as among the risks that made the procedure questionable. It noted that dwarf children, raised in a supportive environment, do well and achieve success in adult roles and asserted that happiness, success, and quality of life are related to self-esteem and accomplishments, not height.[157] So that surgery would not be used inappropriately to correct what was in fact a social problem, the board also suggested that parents not make the decision while their children were too young to give informed consent. Despite all these reservations, the organization stated its desire to see the procedure become safer and more effective for those who did choose it.

By 2000, centers abounded worldwide, with most surgeries performed on persons with achondroplasia or hypochondroplasia, because those with rare diagnoses often have orthopedic problems that make them unlikely candidates. The 1990s studies generally reported lower complication rates, but disturbing observations persisted. One account of surgery performed on twenty-six patients with short stature reported transient pain in 70 percent, infection in 45 percent, drop foot in 35 percent, and stiffness of the ankle in 30 percent and the knee in 15 percent.[158] Others noted complications such as incorrect alignment of lengthened bones or weakness of foot flexion.

A thoughtful study comparing several methods concluded that surgeries should be done only at established centers.[159] Such centers make efforts to correct persistent problems, as when the ICLLR noted that a device monitoring nerve function during limb lengthening significantly reduced nerve-stretch injury, a serious complication.[160] In 1999, Herzenberg and Paley, discussing procedures performed on twenty patients with skeletal dysplasia between 1987 and 1994, reported that very few patients had permanent sequelae and that even these declared themselves very satisfied with their results.[161] By now between thirty and forty patients have successfully completed various stages of treatment, generally with good outcomes.[162]

They have offered their reasons for considering their method superior to the Villerubias technique and have prepared detailed materials of their differing strategies for juveniles versus adolescents.[163] An Israeli study discovered significant sex differences and recommended that males begin surgery at 8 years old and females at 15 to achieve maximal skeletal growth.[164]

Even established centers do not escape problems. In 2001, Aldegheri and Dall'Oca in Verona reported that among 140 patients with short stature whose average gain in length was 18.2 ±3.9 cm, 43.8 percent had complications and 3.8 percent had sequelae. The authors discuss the difficulty of achieving the benefits of the surgery, the strong commitment required by families, and the severity of those permanent sequelae.[165] The hazards are even worse when single practitioners or clinics with just a few patients attempt the surgery. Many persons in the dwarfism community have encountered at least one or two individuals who have undergone the procedure and been left with unequal limbs, nerve damage, or dysfunction. Even the ICLLR experienced one heartbreaking case of paraplegia; they attempted to reverse the situation and could not, although they have learned from it.[166]

At the same time, there have been affecting accounts of satisfaction with the procedure. Gillian Mueller has often discussed her experience at the Maryland Center (now the ICLLR).[167] Although it had its difficulties, for the most part she found the pain minimal, experienced only one complication, and is pleased to be more than five feet tall and able to be physically active, without the daily problems of short stature. Of the more than 2,500 people that her surgeon, Dr. Paley, and his partner, Dr. Herzenberg, have operated on (most with conditions other than dwarfism), she is convinced that almost all were better off than when they began. At the same time, she believes that whether to have the surgery is a personal decision and that different choices should be respected.

Until recently, most members of LPA, although they too spoke of respecting choice, have been apt to be more critical. Although only a small number of adolescent LPs elect the procedure, and only one child of a dwarf adult is known to have had it, some attitudes were softened by the decision of Dr. Rimoin to initiate a limb-lengthening program at Cedars-Sinai. Initially strongly opposed to such surgery, he attended a conference in Europe and was impressed with the physical results and positive patient response. After studying Villerubias's work in Barcelona, he concluded that the Villerubias method was the most benign. It was less painful, and, by cutting some tendons and rotating the femurs, Villerubias had proved able to reduce spinal curvature (lumbar lordosis) while lengthening the upper legs.[168] This tends to reduce stenosis, thereby preventing the problems of back and spine that so many dwarfs begin experience by their third or fourth decade.

Dr. Rimoin accepts only patients 12 years of age and older and includes psychological counseling in his program, which Dr. Paley has ceased to include, except in cases of constitutional short stature. Although recognizing that limb lengthening is not appropriate for everyone, Rimoin wants to see that it is accomplished well for those who elect it. When I asked him about the complication rates, he surprised me by responding, "One hundred percent!" He explained that although some difficulties occurred in all cases, for the most part, the problems were not permanent. But neither Rimoin nor the Cedars-Sinai surgeons took any complication lightly. I asked Rimoin whether the reduction of lordosis and stenosis could possibly be done without the lengthening. It seems that it cannot; along with cutting tendons and rotating femurs, success of limb lengthening depends on concomitant stretching of limb, muscle, and tissue.

Dr. Rimoin does not seek to expand the Cedars-Sinai program, which is extremely demanding and labor intensive for staff members and families. But he is quick to note that not a single person has indicated that they would not do this again if presented with the choice. It is not the fact that they can now reach things that turns out to be the most salient benefit, but as one patient commented, "I can now look people in the eye when I talk to them." The surgery, called "cosmetic" by its detractors, may offer the advantage of not having to overcome inherent social distance.

The few studies of emotional implications are hard to evaluate. An Italian group comments that adolescents and young adults with achondroplasia suffered greatly from feelings of inferiority and negative social experiences and enjoyed much more favorable self-perception after the surgery.[169] Even the investigators seem a bit perplexed by the results, noting, "the very positive finding seemed incongruous with the reality that all subjects still had disproportional body configurations, prominent scars on their legs, and in one case poor ambulation following limb lengthening."

Here the social reality of attitudes about dwarfism may be significant. It seems that in some countries (Italy is a notable example) not meeting prevailing standards for beauty is experienced as disastrous (even among physicians), and even imperfect physical amelioration can bring psychological relief. In the United States, on the other hand, particularly for dwarfs who have experienced positive identity through LPA, cultural norms can seem less oppressive.

At the same time, in Denmark, a benevolent, open-minded society in which the government pays for limb lengthening, several members of the Restricted Growth Soceity of Denmark have elected to have limb lengthening and remained active in the group. Simon Eriksen, for example, a young college student, is the organization's Web master.

By 2002 a new dialogue could be discerned on the LPA Dwarfism List. One person compared the ELL (extensive limb lengthening) procedure with the cochlear implant surgery now available to the deaf and hard of hearing; the choice of limb lengthening was no more a betrayal than being able to hear as the result of a cochlear implant. Though still expressing satisfaction with their dwarf identities, a few others wondered aloud why, if surgery or lenses for blindness were acceptable, ELL should not be. One individual who had undergone the surgery complained about LPA's previous lack of helpfulness in offering her information and wondered if she would now be discriminated against at conferences. An older member noted that if the treatment had been available in the sixties and early seventies, he "would have done it in a heartbeat."

In December 2002, LPA revised somewhat its official position on ELL, stating it would help patients and families make informed decisions and "provide warm and open membership access" for those who undergo ELL, while still resisting its marketing purely for cosmetic purposes. Still, both LPA and the Medical Advisory Board remain cautious about its desirability. Ambivalence is reflected in the fact that Dr. Herzenberg of the ICLLR was scheduled to meet with the Medical Advisory Board at the 2003 LPA conference, and then "disinvited." Clearly, it remains difficult for LPs and their physicians to appear to encourage a relationship with surgeons who are engaged in altering the configuration of bodies that that persons with dwarfism have struggled to affirm.

Although there have been no formal studies of psychological or quality-of-life outcomes, there have been anecdotal reports, positive and negative. In April 2004, I spoke with Mary Tarabocchia and her 27-year-old son, Anthony, who at age 9, during a 13-month stay in Italy, had limb-lengthening surgery with Drs. E. Ascani and G. C. Giglio.[170] One of the first Americans to have the procedure, he was subsequently treated by surgeon Victor Frankel at the Hospital for Joint Diseases in New York, completing it at age 13.

Mrs. Tarabocchia, a warm, communicative woman, recalled how she had agonized over the decision about whether to have the surgery; relatives had visited from Italy and had encouraged her to do so, and a discussion with the Italian physicians had suggested that results would be best if done early. All the while, Anthony was speaking frequently about "wanting to be like the other kids." She was concerned that as an adult he might reproach her if she did not take advantage of a possible treatment. As she recalled the experience, she mentioned the enormous care that had been necessary—how she fastidiously tended the pin areas to avoid infections, and how, during the Italian period, it had been difficult to watch his pain.

Both Mary and Anthony are nonetheless glad about the decision. He attended Mercy College and Pace University and is currently a financial analyst. Anthony is now 5'3", has long-standing friendships, and says he feels quite comfortable with himself. He is able to engage in some sports, including tennis, although he does tire after walking half a dozen blocks. Like Gillian Mueller, who formerly worked at the ICLRR and now is on the staff of Hillary Clinton, he seems to have no regrets.

I have met a few others who are less pleased, who had incomplete surgery, resulting in uneven limbs, nerve sequelae, depression, or all of these. It seems to me that both the quality of the surgical care and the previous mental health of the individuals were significant factors. Sometimes individuals who elect the surgery in late adolescence or early adulthood may have unrealistic expectations, believing that height gain will "fix" other troubled areas of their lives. Overall, however, it seems that the majority of patients queried by their physicians express satisfaction with the surgery and its outcomes.

Despite great improvements in procedures and changes in attitudes, however, some of the questions raised earlier remain. The demands of the surgery and the expense, as well as uncertainty about the long-term effects on joints, limbs, spine, and quality of life, are apt to result in its not being used widely. It is very unfortunate that centers have not reported investigations of long-term physiological and psychological outcomes. Dr. Herzenberg and his colleagues at the ICLLR have begun to publish accounts of their work, but Herzenberg points out that it is difficult to report conclusively about long-term outcomes because the first limb-lengthening surgeries were completed less than 15 years ago. Even at European centers, where many surgeries were completed more than two decades ago, adequate reports are lacking. Focused on performing and analyzing the procedures, most surgeons did not set up prospective studies. Psychological, quality-of-life, and identity issues seem to have been particularly neglected.

One of the few centers evidencing concern about these issues has been the Cedars-Sinai group. Dr. Rimoin reports that all patients have declared that they are delighted they had the surgery and would definitely do it again; he feels that the careful selection process, which considered prospective patients on the basis of their psyche and family situation, contributed to the positive results. The Cedars-Sinai group hopes to publish a psychological follow-up survey by 2005.[171]

To illuminate the discussion, which now often seems to proceed in the same speculative fashion that it did a decade or more ago, a multicenter database and collaborative studies are needed. Follow-ups to evaluate long-term physiological outcomes and interviews to assess patient quality of life and explore any remaining concerns would seem a desirable element in any limb-lengthening center's program. Also, it is possible that just as individuals and families in dwarfism groups have benefited from the support of others, ongoing groups might be formed to ensure that persons who elect the surgery do not have to "go it alone." Even without formal groups, informal contacts among prospective, current, and former patients who desire it might be facilitated.

OTHER SURGICAL DEVELOPMENTS

The notoriety achieved by the limb-lengthening procedure has obscured the importance of other surgical advances made or significantly refined in the field of dwarfism:

1. improved lumbar surgery for spinal stenosis, preventing paralysis and/or pain, and improving mobility.
2. innovative spinal surgery in the foramen magnum and upper cervical spine areas, remedying limb weakness and failure to thrive and preventing paralysis and sudden infant death.
3. improved osteotomies for bowleggedness, and hip and knee surgeries.
4. diagnosis of hydrocephalus and surgical implant of drainage shunt when necessary, aiding brain function and preventing failure to thrive.
5. new treatments for obstructive apnea, including monitoring oxygen levels and, as necessary, removing adenoids, using a CPAP or BiPAP device, supplying oxygen, or a tracheotomy.

Surgical advances such as these and promising developments in the use of enzyme and gene therapy may alter the medical landscape dramatically during the next several decades.

THE EFFECT OF MEDICAL PROBLEMS
ON THE LIVES OF DWARFS

One would need an anthology of anecdotes written by patients, families, and physicians to properly convey the emotional consequences of medical problems. There are even some conditions that require a baby to have one or more surgeries during the first year. It is difficult to sustain the joy of the birth of a child, or maintain one's energies, while grappling with medical emergencies. In addition, persistent effort and ingenuity are required to struggle with insurance companies or convince the bureaucracy to finance a baby nurse while parents work.

Now that some hazards of various early childhood conditions are better understood, breathing problems are monitored more carefully, and a small but significant percentage of young children undergo adenoidectomies, tonsillectomies, tracheotomies, or surgery of the cervical spine. Some have shunts installed in an attempt to ward off ear infections and potential partial deafness. Some young children have osteotomies to correct or inhibit bowing. Even parents of the many children who encounter few or no problems are often anxiously watchful.

The tensions that begin for some families in childhood become an inevitable part of life for many adults. Children and adults with a variety of bone dysplasias often must undergo a series of surgeries. Those with osteogenesis imperfecta deal at all ages with unpredictable fractures, pain, and mobility problems. Children with hypopituitary deficiency require almost daily injections; by adolescence they are given the task of injecting themselves and often wrestle with decisions about how long they are willing to persist with this uncomfortable procedure to achieve optimal height. Girls with Turner syndrome face a similar situation and, in addition, must come to terms with questions relating to their inability to bear children. Other more rare conditions involve a wide variety of complications.

New troublesome symptoms may appear over the years. Persons with achondroplasia, for example, frequently have a certain amount of transitory discomfort or numbness, and they and their doctors must decide whether and when to perform surgery, a daunting dilemma.

Deteriorating joints and aching muscles are characteristic of many conditions, and in addition to helpful measures such as glucosamine or anti-inflammatory drugs, physical therapy, therapeutic massage, or acupuncture, various surgeries, including joint replacements, are sometimes required. Although some persons ride the waves of an inexorable next surgery well, rearranging their lives and viewing the interruptions as just a "nuisance," few can manage a succession of bodily assaults without some feelings of depression or indignation Whether the body's disobedience and pain are temporary or chronic, they become an inextricable part of a little person's identity.

A sense of humor helps. Mary Carten, a former LPA president and coeditor of the Diastrophic Web site, begins an article: "I'm currently recovering from my latest hip replacement of the original replacement! Yup, that's what I said, replacing the replacement, or bringing in the second team!" She finds herself instructing her "two young, friendly smiling (rehab) therapists: Oh, did I mention that I was their *first dwarf encounter?* Once the staff stopped coming in to take turns to look at me, we were finally able to get past 'show and tell.' I was subjected to the usual visits by curious staff members (those required and those not required). I even had a visit from the local 'shrink'!"

Returning to work, she was grateful for the marvelous surprises that her ADA-conscious colleagues at Banc One had arranged, such as lowered furniture and a lowered ATM machine. Unfortunately, less pleasant surprises followed, including a knee problem, and later a life-threatening situation, compounded by inept emergency-room treatment by physicians unfamiliar with her condition.

Such calamities can get people down, but they can also invigorate and teach perseverance and empathy. Many onlookers are amazed by the resilience of children, in particular, wondering why repeated surgeries, bouts of pain, mobility restrictions, and other health limitations rarely prove to be crushing blows. Vita Gagne, co-webmaster of the Diastrophic Dynamics site, believes that perhaps because these young people must take ten steps to others' three, the techniques developed to meet physical challenges carry over into other areas, raising their frustration threshold.

INSTITUTIONAL PROBLEMS OF THE MEDICAL SYSTEM THAT AFFECT MEDICAL INSTITUTIONS AND DWARFS' ACCESS TO CARE

This chapter has spotlighted many capable and compassionate physicians. However, complaints of incompetent, uncaring physicians abound—those who are inattentive when the patient is attempting to explain a situation, or who are unable to admit their limitations. Probably the greatest medical problem faced by persons with dwarfism is access to expert medical care. Sometimes the individual lives far from a treatment center, and therefore doctors' visits become major expeditions that are unmanageable for many families. At least as formidable are the financial obstacles. The costs of complex surgeries are exorbitant, and if the patient is not covered by good insurance, surgery may be unavailable.

Some insurance plans still leave the patient with a substantial co-payment. Major teaching or charity institutions may be able to write off some of the medical care, but not all. Many patients simply do without needed treatment; others raise funds from family, friends, and churches, or they get some assistance from LPA. Many get by with inadequate care from less experienced practitioners; botched surgery, unfortunately, is not rare. Some expert surgeons frequently forgo or reduce their fees, but the cost of operating rooms and hospital beds cannot always be written off.

One significant exception in the United States is the Shriners system of twenty-two hospitals offering free care to children younger than 18 years who require orthopedic treatment, including surgery. Its annual budget for the year 2000 is $540 million.[172] Only in a few European countries, notably in Scandinavia and Germany, is surgery generally available without cost to all who require it. Despite its much vaunted medical system, Canada is often not able to offer expert prophylactic, nonemergency medical surgery, and long waits are all too common.

My discussions with Medical Advisory Board members alerted me to another institutional dilemma.[173] By consulting with patients at annual LPA conferences, physicians risk problems: licensure is granted by individual states, not the federal government. Legally, visiting doctors have no status at medical facilities in the local community where the conference takes place. Occasionally, a patient has become ill and needed to be taken to an emergency room, and LPA physicians have been shown disrespect or turned away because they were not locally licensed. When a patient seen at a conference applies for disability insurance or coverage for surgery and requests a letter from a consulting Medical Advisory Board member, that letter may be dismissed because it is written by a physician from another state who has seen the patient only once, even if he or she is one of the most renowned authorities in the specialty.

The advent of e-mail has created further problems. Many patients, especially those living in remote locations, contact specialists and send them X-rays. Although they are more expert than doctors in a small Kentucky town or a village in Transylvania, these specialists' opinions are not covered by their malpractice insurance. Should something go wrong, the LPA consultant could be subject to a lawsuit. Also, a tactful letter to a local physician explaining that the specialist has examined the patient at a conference or spoken by phone and viewed her MRIs may engender her home physician's ire.

Some form of national licensure is essential, as are agreements with managed care companies to expedite claims on a national basis. Better formal and informal lines of communication must be facilitated between experts and local doctors. Finally, as the volume of potential consultations at conferences, and by e-mail and telephone, increases exponentially, ways must be found to compensate specialists for unpaid services now expected of them.

Some solutions will require political action. Recently, LPA, along with the Genetic Alliance, the National Organization for Rare Diseases, and the National Partnership for Women and Families, has been part of the patients' rights dialogue on Capitol Hill. Legislation has been passed permitting referral to specialists outside a managed care network, as long as that managed care plan does not include an appropriate specialist. However, networks often resist referring dwarf patients to other centers, arguing that their own specialists are sufficiently qualified, although they have treated few or no dwarf patients. With an adequate appeals process in place, dwarf patients could appeal or sue to gain access to necessary expertise.

LPA has crafted an official policy paper entitled "Treating the Complications of Dwarfism in a Managed Care Environment" to educate physicians, health care administrators, and policymakers about how LPA defines quality care for individuals with dwarfism. It recommends that physicians have experience and practice as part of a multidisciplinary treatment center. Cara Egan, LPA National Health Policy Advisor, keeps up with developments in Congress that affect patients' rights; she engages the dwarf community when an advocacy campaign becomes necessary.

THE IMPACT OF GENETIC AND OTHER
SCIENTIFIC DEVELOPMENTS ON ACTUAL
TREATMENT IN THE FUTURE

When Dr. Francis Collins and Celera, a private company led by Dr. Craig Venter, announced on 26 June 2000 that the scientific institutes they headed had finally decoded how complex strands of DNA are arranged to program the biological destiny of human beings, this accomplishment was deemed at least as monumental as space exploration.

However, scientists and nonscientists soon realized that most practical uses of the information lay far in the future. The subtle interactions of genes and the attendant biochemical and molecular processes needed to be interpreted before the function of any gene could be modified. The next challenge, delivering a "genetic repair kit," would not be simple.[174] Any treatment would have to penetrate a large, specific number of cells long enough to finish its work, while not arousing the cells' natural tendency to reject loose bits of genetic material. An effective delivery system had to be devised that would bypass the body's immune system, protecting the beneficial gene and doing no harm.

One innovative direction was highlighted at a conference of the Coalition of Heritable Disorders of Connective Tissue in Washington, D.C., in November 2000. A group of scientists representing a wide range of disorders concluded that identifying a gene or studying a cell was not all that really mattered. To understand the pathogenesis of any disease throughout its lifetime or throughout the life of the person, one had to understand the communication that takes place in the matrix, the connective tissue between the cells.

The matrix plays a role in strengthening and binding the cells. It also enables the proteins within to communicate to others inside and outside the cells, while connective tissue and cells complete the process of differentiating functions, becoming spine, eyes, muscles, and so on.[175] Investigating the matrix should help clarify why some mutations result in severe diseases and others in milder diseases and what causes phenotype variability, areas not well understood.

Bodin and Hershey, the journalists maligned earlier for a variety of errors, were not good prognosticators when they remarked: "When scientists have learned all the secrets of our mysterious glands it is not improbable that midgets, and their strange cousins, the giants, will go the way of the dodo, the dinosaur, and the pterodactyl, themselves the victims of faulty glands, into oblivion."[176]

Given the inevitable appearance of new mutations, one need not feel apprehensive about the disappearance of dwarfs from the planet. Even if it tried, no obstetrics department could field a program that would identify and alter the vast cascade of genetic differences, given the frequency and complexity with which they present themselves. Although conditions such as hypopituitarism or mucopolysaccharidosis represent more likely and closer targets than chondrodystrophies, it is certainly reasonable to conceive of influencing some aspects of bone (e.g., bone strength, troublesome in most skeletal dysplasias). Jacqueline Hecht, Ph.D., who led the research team that discovered the genetic link to pseudoachondroplasia, has noted that the cartilage oligomeric matrix protein (COMP) gene is vital for normal bone development and function.[177] She discovered that in pseudoachondroplasia the normal COMP gene changes or mutates, causing the condition. If this mutation could be blocked, associated growth problems and joint replacements could be avoided.

In 1998 a collaboration agreement was signed between ProChon Biotech, Ltd., an Israeli company, and SUGEN, Inc., an American biopharmaceutical company, to develop small-molecule drugs.[178] Research is currently in progress at the Weizmann Institute in Israel and elsewhere that attempts to block the mutant FGFR3 signals that cause conditions such as achondroplasia. Nevertheless, although an increasing number of articles have reported developments, geneticists such as Dr. William Horton are well aware that "a cure" is not yet at hand. He cautions that therapies on the horizon that promote normal bone growth by targeting the overactivity of the mutant FGFR3 receptor are theoretical at this point and must be tested rigorously before being approved as safe and effective.

He summarizes the three approaches being investigated: (1) reduction of the tyrosine kinase activity of the FGFR3 by using chemical inhibitors; (2) a variation that uses an antibody generated in the lab that targets the receptor from outside the cell and prevents it from being activated (in achondroplasia, the excessive signals slow bone growth); (3) the Yosada approach, which proposes to interfere with the propagation of growth-inhibitory signals "downstream" of FGFR3 by using a naturally occurring substance called C-type natriuretic hormone. All have the problem of targeting the therapeutic agent to the bone without adversely affecting other tissues that need FGFR3 to regulate important functions.[179]

Just the possibility that interventions could lead to affected persons becoming significantly different has raised unsettling questions about how each individual feels about retaining or altering his or her identity. The goal of fixing the most troublesome aspects, but still retaining the desirable ones, remains elusive.

EUGENIC CONCERNS

Far more unsettling than imminent genetic intervention are the potential consequences of in utero diagnoses. A futuristic piece called "The Genetic Report Card" in the *New York Times* anticipates a time when, with one thumbnail-sized chip, embryos could be scanned for a wide collection of genetic conditions.[180] The rudiments of that screening already exist in a procedure called preimplantation genetic diagnosis that enables parents to screen and select embryos. Tests are now very expensive ($12,000 to $15,000 with in vitro fertilization); available for only several dozen conditions, they are used mostly by parents who already have an affected child.

Even now, genetic testing is available for more than 300 diseases or conditions in more than 200 laboratories in the United States.[181] Diagnoses are made on the basis of amniocentesis, ultrasound, and placental chorion analysis. The Department of Health and Human Services has established a Secretary's Advisory Committee on Genetic Testing that has recommended federal legislation and public education and input be used to exercise more effective oversight of genetic testing. Although the most extensive processes are performed only at a few labs, some tests identifying dwarfing conditions are widely available.

The primary technique used for short stature has been ultrasound, although with this method prenatal misdiagnosis has already proved to be a neglected but significant problem.[182] Dr. Rimoin responded to an article about a misprognosis on a 22-week fetus that resulted in termination of pregnancy, with the comment, "You cannot make a diagnosis of hypochondroplasia at 22 weeks!"[183] He believes that misdiagnosis is uncommon and only takes place in inexperienced hands.

There are ways to reduce errors, but even accurate information presents an ethical dilemma, and turmoil may accompany patient-doctor interaction. What happens when prospective average-statured parents are told that their child is going to be a dwarf? For parents who have no experience with dwarfism, the decision to abort may be a foregone conclusion; others may do more soul searching. A good genetic counselor can be invaluable.

The stance of the physician is vital. At the 2000 LPA conference genetics workshop, physicians acknowledged that attitudes of doctors delivering the news to prospective parents could be significant. If a doctor was familiar with the disability in question, for example, the parents might be more inclined to go forward with the pregnancy. If he or she was unfamiliar, or clearly viewed the potential birth as tragic, the parents would be more likely to abort.

An article entitled "Doctors: Don't Want No Short People 'Round Here" discusses a poll conducted after the controversial abortion of a 32-week-old dwarf fetus in Australia. This survey of obstetricians found that support for making abortion available for fetuses diagnosed with dwarfism was 100 percent at 13 weeks.[184] It fell to 14 percent at 24 weeks, but remarkably, 70 percent of geneticists and obstetricians who specialize in obstetrical ultrasound thought abortion should be available at 24 weeks if dwarfism was diagnosed.

The original news report seemed to suggest that the doctors *supported* having abortions. However, a correction by Julian Savulescu, the ethicist who performed the survey, said that the physicians believed only that abortions should be made available, not necessarily facilitated.[185] A deeper inquiry would be required to glean what subtle and overt messages had been communicated. True neutrality is rare. Dr. Clair Francomano has spoken out against routine screening for achondroplasia, feeling passionately that it makes abortion a more usual procedure when it is detected.[186]

As far as I know, there have been few direct efforts to influence the attitudes of clinical specialists, but there have been attempts to personalize the decision-making process for prospective parents. Some institutions have procedures for introducing couples whose fetuses have been diagnosed with dwarfism to parents of dwarf children or to adults with that diagnosis.

Wendy Ricker and Betsy Trombino, mothers of thriving adult LPs, and professionals in the areas of mental health and disability, are uneasy about this procedure. Ms. Trombino articulated the wrenching dilemma that she and others had faced in speaking with parents who were confronting a decision. The encounter tends to be profoundly emotionally draining for all concerned. It also poses an ethical problem. One's tendency as a dwarf or the parent of a dwarf is to present a positive picture. However, the diagnosis may consign individuals with numerous complications to an arduous life course. The task of presenting a balanced view when emotionally involved is daunting. Even though the family makes the final decision, one cannot escape feelings of responsibility. Parent volunteers have sometimes withdrawn later, despite their conviction that children with dwarfism have the right to be born.

Tom Shakespeare, short-statured disability scholar and bioethicist, holds that termination till now has been treated as acceptable because the perspective of parents has prevailed rather than that of persons with disabilities. He has been opposed by social scientists such as John Gillott who argue that it is worth noticing that parents of disabled children usually choose not to repeat the experience, as they must bear the financial and emotional strain. Gillott maintains that those with the responsibility must be listened to, and comments, "Shakespeare's argument amounts to a demand that disabled activists be allowed to hold parents, and society, to ransom."[187] Although distinguishing himself from old-style eugenicists, Gillott notes that society has no hesitation in condemning a drunk driver who causes a disability; therefore, it should not praise a woman who knowingly gives birth to a disabled child. Eliminating diseases and deficiencies improves the lot of humankind, a wholly reasonable stance, he believes.

Partisans on both sides have less trouble agreeing in certain clear-cut situations, such as the determination that a fetus is "double dominant," carrying lethal genes from two achondroplastic parents, and therefore destined for early death. This situation occurs in approximately 25 percent of births where both parents have achondroplasia. The new technology permits early detection, sparing the parents a lengthy pregnancy with a devastating outcome, if they so choose. A study of 189 persons with achondroplasia and 136 of their relatives indicated that the groups were remarkably similar in their interest in testing for double dominance and their unwillingness to consider termination based on a diagnosis either of achondroplasia or average stature.[188]

More problematic is the situation in which persons affected by a condition are given the chance to avoid passing on that gene. Simon Mawer presents a compelling scene in the novel *Mendel's Dwarf*, in which the protagonist has the choice of which embryo to select from among eight that have been created through in vitro fertilization.[189] Some prospective parents with genetic conditions are now being given the option of having a child through in vitro fertilization, and choosing the embryo without the mutant gene. I know persons with a genetic condition who have been offered and rejected this option, accepting the possibility that the child would inherit their condition. All such persons are forced to grapple with how they feel about their own lives and to contemplate a similar future for their offspring. Dr. Rimoin did not know of any dwarfs who had been offered the choice but indicated there was no technical impediment to prevent it being an option.

What other questions may arise is uncertain, but some profound ethical issues are already upon us. So far, routine testing is done for only a very few disorders, most notably Down syndrome. The rate of abortions for Down syndrome in Great Britain is approximately 95 percent, Dr. Gregory Wolbring reveals. A biochemist, molecular biologist, and disability activist who teaches at the University of Calgary, Wolbring has assembled some of the most interesting material currently available on issues relating to the interface of genetic technology, disability, and ethics.[190] His own disability, his limbs foreshortened because of thalidomide, greatly limits his mobility, but it also means he has been able to martial his scientific knowledge in the interest of a cause he cares about passionately.

Excellent, wide-ranging analyses of ethical issues have been raised by genetic advances.[191] A cogent position paper from one advocacy group, the Campaign against Human Genetic Engineering (CAHGE), asserts that preimplantation genetic diagnosis represents a serious threat, and strict regulation guidelines must be developed.[192] The central thesis of this and other disability rights groups is that society's effort to prevent the birth of children with genetic impairments is driven by misinformation about disabled people's lives. Many adults without disabilities hold the view that disabilities are tragic and believe that it would have been better had the affected persons not been born. Even persons with severe disabilities, on the other hand, most often do not experience their lives as tragic and are pleased to be alive. CAHGE, like many disability groups with similar positions, presents its program as an effort to forestall what it calls "consumer eugenics" and encourage careful decision making by individuals and government groups.[193]

John Wasmuth, who discovered the gene for achondroplasia, declared that he thought prenatal screening for the gene should not be offered to average-statured parents. He feared that procedures might begin to be widely used to eliminate any person deemed inferior or unfit. Having denounced the eugenics movement of Nazi Germany (which had many adherents in the United States), many wondered whether we should stand by while it was revived under the auspices of the medical establishment.

As a result, LPA revitalized its education campaign for the medical community and general public, emphasizing that giving birth to a dwarf child should be a cause to rejoice:

We are teachers, artists, lawyers, doctors, accountants, welders, plumbers, engineers and actors. We represent every nationality, ethnic group, religion and sexual orientation. Many of us have secondary disabilities as well. We are single and married, with families with spouses, parents and children who are average sized and dwarfed, biological and adopted. . . . We have been educating society and the medical community about the truths of life with short stature and working to dispel commonly held myths. With the discovery of various genes and mutations causing dwarfism, our educational and advocacy efforts have become ever more important in the face of a rapidly changing genetic frontier.[194]

Thus LPA fired its first salvos against the threat of being treated as undeserving of life. Participants at a genetic ethics workshop at the 2000 LPA conference expressed their concern about abortion of fetuses with skeletal dysplasias and other genetic conditions, as well as selection of embryos via in vitro fertilization. Genetic privacy and the potential for gene therapy were also discussed. Ruth Ricker, former LPA president and disability activist, has addressed similar knotty questions.[195]

Tom Shakespeare's RGA Genetics Survey Report is a provocative study of attitudes toward restricted growth; it includes his statistical analysis as well as respondents' personal comments, contrasting attitudes of 74 short- and average-statured members of the British restricted growth community. Approximately 40 percent of parents, friends, and relatives believed that genetic discoveries would have positive effects for the dwarf community, whereas only 20.6 percent of short-statured persons were that optimistic. A telling 34 percent of short-statured individuals and 50 percent of average-statured persons were uncertain about whether potential outcomes were apt to be positive or negative. Although only 7.9 percent of average-statured respondents would consider aborting a fetus with restricted growth, 25.8 percent of short-statured respondents would.[196]

There is good reason for the membership to be concerned about the response of physicians, the press, and the general public to news about genetic disorders. Misinformation and reminders of negative attitudes toward dwarfing conditions are still common. A 1992 *New York Times* article described persons with Turner syndrome in a discouraging fashion as only "looking like a girl," and possibly being mentally retarded.[197] (In fact, most women with Turner syndrome have promising prospects.) Although a Letter to the Editor countered

the misinformation, one wonders which description readers will remember.

Perceptive critics recognize that eugenic thinking does not affect
only the small percentage that are never born, although their loss
could be monumental; it may also cast a shadow over dwarf survivors,
who may be viewed with greater misgivings once it becomes common
practice to eliminate others like them. Simi Linton, author of *Claim-
ing Disability: Knowledge and Identity,* has used the term "preventa-
bles" in expressing her concern about the negative impact this group
of individuals would experience.[198]

Len Sawisch, the influential member of LPA who helped establish
the Dwarf Athletic Association, is a psychologist, writer, and some-
time stand-up comedian. As a child he at first responded enthusiastically to the March of Dimes commercial, "Help wipe out birth defects in your lifetime." However, he later found it a very frightening
concept: "On the one hand we are spending thousands and thousands
of dollars every year as a society to incorporate individuals who are
considered to be handicappers, people like me who are to be mainstreamed into society. On the other hand, we're spending thousands
and thousands of dollars every year to avoid people like me being
born."[199]

Sawisch communicates the irony that he is expected to participate
fully in society at the same time that he is encouraged not to be here
at all. He affirms that the greatest changes that need to be made are in
attitudes, those of society and of disabled individuals themselves.

It has become increasingly evident that no medical decisions are
purely medical and that an authoritarian model can no longer serve.
The intimate relationships that develop during the course of a lifetime lead many physicians who have dwarf patients to adopt a holistic approach; they do not treat spines and ears and limbs, but short-
statured individuals, and their empathy energizes them toward new
discoveries and improved quality of care.

In much of Africa, Asia, and South America, and even in rural and
urban areas in the United States, there remain persons overlooked by

the medical revolution. There is a dearth of trained specialists with sufficient expertise to treat dwarfing conditions. One wonders whether the current generation of physicians, beginning their medical careers with substantial debts from educational loans, will be as likely to seek out challenging but less lucrative hospital positions. Medical Advisory Board chair Dr. Richard Pauli commented, "Unfortunately, the most critical and most difficult to come by is a physician who will really commit to becoming expert and taking responsibility for a clinic of this sort. Our health care system currently tends not to support that kind of commitment, which is, unfortunately, not terribly remunerative."[200]

The future course of persons with dwarfism will depend on themselves and their physicians, but also on many others who must join them in political advocacy if competent treatment is to become widely available.

2 ～
PSYCHOSOCIAL ASPECTS

It is not unusual for dwarfs to express dismay about strangers' mistaking their physical differences for lower intelligence or personality defects. Their protest is epitomized in the eloquent statement made by Julie Rotta that appears on the cover of Joan Ablon's groundbreaking work, *Little People in America* (1984): "We are a contradiction in packaging, for encased in our small bodies are not small minds, not small needs and desires, not small goals and pleasures, and not small appetites for a full and enriching life."[1]

Many dwarfs would claim that the only factors distinguishing them from others are physical appearance and limitations in reach and mobility. Do outsiders presume differences that do not exist, or are there in fact significant differences that individuals with dwarfism simply deny? Do they differ from the average statured in personality and life satisfaction? The following verses by Czech poet Rainer Maria Rilke (1875–1926) capture the often-unspoken assumptions that many outsiders have made about how dwarfs view themselves. The poem is from a series called "Voices," which includes "songs" intoned by such unfortunates as a beggar, a widow, a blind man, and a leper.[2]

THE SONG THE DWARF SINGS

My soul is perhaps level and good;
but my heart, my crooked blood,
all that gives me pain
that I can't bear upright.

My soul has no garden, has no bed,
it just hangs on my sharp skeleton
with a terrified beating of wings.

My hands too—nothing will come of them.
How stunted they are: Look,
tenaciously they jump about, clammy and hard,
like little toads after a rain.
And the rest of me is
worn out and old and despondent.
Why does God hesitate
to toss it all onto the dungheap?

Is he perhaps angry with me for my countenance
with its sullen mouth?
Yet it was so often ready, deep down,
To become entirely light and clear;
but nothing ever came as close
as the enormous dogs.
And the dogs—they don't have it to give.

This wrenching poem expressing the dwarf's self-deprecation also conveys his poignant awareness that underneath he has a good soul. Some readers may be mystified by Rilke's reference to dogs. Innumerable Renaissance paintings depict dwarfs and dogs together; for this speaker, the animals' companionship is an inadequate balm for loneliness.[3] The stereotype of solitary, unhappy dwarfs is a recurrent image in the arts, and it reflects what many in the general public, even today, perceive as the likely self-image of dwarfs.

In the past several decades, however, researchers have endeavored to explore the psyches of dwarfs in a very different manner, trying to set aside stereotypes and cast light on whether persons with dwarfism indeed depart from the norm in various respects. Most studies, like this review, focus primarily on persons affected by skeletal dysplasia, growth hormone deficiency, and Turner syndrome, in large measure because these groups are accessible to researchers through dwarfism organizations.

One 2003 government publication offers a helpful overview and bibliography, citing literature related to both physiological and psychological aspects of dwarfism in children.[4] Several other works also offer essential background and new evidence about the psychosocial world of adults. Medical anthropologist Joan Ablon, in *Little People in America,* reports the results of in-depth interviews with twenty-four members of Little People of America (LPA). In quoting them at length, she identifies the major issues that dwarfs contend with. In her sequel, *Living with Difference,* she focuses on the varying reactions of parents to discovering that their child is a dwarf and provides useful summaries of earlier research.[5] Her insights derive from a more personal, in-depth analysis than most studies.

Stabler and Underwood's *Slow Grows the Child* (1986) contains fourteen influential articles drawn from a 1984 symposium on psychosocial aspects of growth delay. It explores the cognitive and psychological correlates of a number of dwarfing conditions. *Growth, Stature, and Psychosocial Well-Being,* edited by Eiholzer, Haverkamp, and Voss (1999), revisits some of these issues; in addition, it offers research findings about whether short stature in and of itself represents a handicap or disadvantage, either for healthy persons or for those with chronic disorders. Martel and Biller's *Stature and Stigma* (1987), although more limited in scope, offers an interesting, mostly negative, picture of the impact of short stature on the lives of young male college students. Originally a doctoral dissertation, it contains valuable references.[6]

Among the myriad of journal articles, just a few recent studies, unlike most early investigations, have surveyed large numbers of subjects and have been careful in their use of methodology. Of special interest are the following: Stabler and his associates' reports on growth hormone–deficient children (1994, 1996, 1998); Stace and Danks's in-depth study of a population of children and adults with chondrodystrophies in Victoria, Australia (1981); and Hunter's 1998 investigation of psychosocial aspects of individuals with chondrodystrophies from Australia, Great Britain, the United States, and Canada. All these works contain excellent reviews of the literature. Two admirable studies of single skeletal dysplasias are Ablon's of personality in osteogenesis imperfecta (2003) and Gollust, Thompson, Gooding, and Biesecker's of quality of life in achondroplasia (2003).[7]

INTELLIGENCE

Many studies of intelligence in persons with dwarfism have appeared during the past several decades. Perhaps one reason why dwarfs as a group were formerly assumed to have intellectual deficits is that there are indeed a number of subcategories in which there is significant cognitive impairment, among them cretinism (IDD), Down syndrome, several mucopolysaccharidosis and mucolipidosis syndromes, and Russell-Silver syndrome in which approximately half of those affected have some cognitive impairment.[8] In individuals with intrauterine growth restriction, 8–10 percent do not catch up postnatally, and intellectual development is also affected.[9] Psychosocial dwarfism, also called deprivation dwarfism, failure to thrive, or Kaspar Hauser syndrome, is often marked by severe retardation or variability in intelligence influenced by environmental factors. Space limitations prevent doing these categories justice here; fortunately, much information is available both on PubMed and organization Web sites.

Numerous studies of other categories have found that persons with dwarfism are of average intelligence, although there are provocative differences within and between groups that become apparent when one looks more closely at these disorders. A pattern of scholastic underachievement that researchers grapple with but find difficult to understand is often present and extends across categories.[10]

Most early investigations used a relatively small number of subjects, and few used control groups. One of the best early studies is Drash, Greenberg, and Money's 1968 study that compared four syndromes of dwarfism.[11] It included thirty-six patients with hypopituitary dwarfism, thirty-eight with Turner syndrome, seven with achondroplasia, and fourteen with deprivation dwarfism. The first three groups had average intelligence, and intelligence in the last group was significantly impaired. In both the Turner and achondroplasia groups given the Wechsler Intelligence Test, children scored higher on verbal than performance categories.

Before too long, however, investigators realized that the psychosocial group was too different from the others to merit comparison, and basic information about the other groups' characteristics made superficial comparisons between groups unnecessary.

Intelligence and Skeletal Dysplasia

In the 1960s and 1970s, researchers were still uncertain about whether the intelligence of dwarfs departed from the norm, and if so, how. Rogers, Perry, and Rosenberg, in a frequently cited 1979 study done at Johns Hopkins, reviewed the IQ data on sixty-eight preschool and school-aged children.[12] The mean IQ of nineteen school-aged children with achondroplasia was 96; the mean IQ of twenty-two children with a dozen other skeletal dysplasia diagnoses was 104. Although both means are in the "normal" range, investigators wrestled with the discrepancy. They suggested that studying unaffected siblings of achondroplastic children might offer further clues. Although concluding that children with skeletal dysplasias do not differ from the norm in intelligence, they advocated appropriate counseling so that each individual might be viewed according to individual strengths and limitations, not short stature alone. This last bit of advice remains eminently sensible.

The study's finding of average intelligence scores has repeatedly been confirmed. In a 1996 article, Low, Knudsen, and Sherrill found that intellectual development is typically normal in individuals with achondroplasia, cartilage-hair hypoplasia, diastrophic dysplasia, and SED tarda and congenita.[13] Intelligence had also been termed normal in acromesomelic dwarfism (Langer et al., 1977).[14]

Because, by the 1980s, it had seemed well established that intelligence in most dwarfing conditions was within the normal range, researchers seemed to lose interest. However, in the 1990s, noting contradictions in the earlier work, and subtleties overlooked, some investigators began to use new assessment approaches. The unraveling of the genome and the existence of new technology offered promising innovative methods.

Low et al. had commented that in some cases of achondroplasia, notably among male children, parental anecdotal evidence seemed to indicate an increased number of learning disabilities. Unfortunately, they did not discuss this observation further. They also reported that only in hypochondroplasia, for reasons unknown, did there seem to be a 10 percent rate of mental retardation. I might have accepted this conclusion, had I not come across a careful study of twenty-seven cases of hypochondroplasia in the Skeletal Dysplasia Registry, which found that mental disability had *not* proved a factor in a single case. The British researchers Wynne-Davies and Patton consequently concluded that earlier respected studies had at the very least overestimated its occurrence.[15]

To see if greater clarity could be attained, Dr. Gary Bellus and his colleagues conducted a preliminary study of 300 patients with suspected diagnoses of hypochondroplasia.[16] They performed diagnostic testing to determine whether subjects carried the FGFR3 mutation (N540K) associated with hypochondroplasia. About half did and half did not. Patients and families were asked to fill out a questionnaire about whether there was any history of learning disabilities, developmental delay, or neurological problems. About half the patients in each group reported problems, most commonly with speech delays and unspecified developmental delay. This is a much higher occurrence than one would expect from randomly selected children and young adults. Some had no deficits, however.

The researchers were cautious about overinterpreting results because they had relied only on subjective data (no actual developmental evaluations had been performed), so they suggested that formal studies be undertaken to include both genetic testing and cognitive and developmental evaluation. In the meantime, they recommended careful monitoring and early intervention as needed.

Similar questions have arisen regarding achondroplasia. Investigators have begun to assess brain function in order to cast light on the relationship between brain abnormalities, medical symptoms, and intellectual functioning. They hypothesize causes for the reduced mean IQ in achondroplasia that Rogers had noted and the academic difficulties affecting *some* achondroplastic children that families have observed.

In a 1993 study, German investigators G. Brinkmann et al. compared thirty children with achondroplasia to three control groups: their next-born siblings, thirty children with other forms of dwarfism, and thirty children of normal height.[17] They found that achondroplastic children had more frequent histories of delayed motor development, retarded speech development, and lower verbal scores. They concluded that the lower scores are probably related to conductive hearing loss caused by middle ear infections that affect speech and reading ability and by hypotonia that affects muscle coordination. The researchers do not entirely rule out hypoxic or high-pressure-related cerebral dysfunction, although they believe that would probably affect overall intellectual functioning, not simply verbal functioning.

Although this study is one of the very best, and a rare controlled study, it focuses on *group* scores; it does not report differences in past medical history of low-scoring and high-scoring individuals. Surprisingly, although personality tests were given, their results are not reported, at least here.

A promising approach has been used in two small prospective studies of intellectual development in achondroplasia. In 1991, Hecht, Thompson, and University of Texas colleagues evaluated thirteen achondroplastic infants with psychometric testing to determine mental and motor performance.[18] The most important positive finding is that severe respiratory dysfunction seemed to play a significant role in lowering intellectual potential. Because at the time of this investigation many researchers had just begun to understand the early neurological and respiratory problems associated with achondroplasia, this study helped to confirm the importance of their work and the crucial role of early medical, and sometimes surgical, intervention.

In a 1991 follow-up study, Thompson, Hecht, and new collaborators report on the neuroanatomical and cognitive status of sixteen children with achondroplasia, seven of whom had been included in the earlier investigation.[19] Investigators found that, although cognitive abilities at school age were average, mild deficits were seen in visuospatial tasks, similar to a hydrocephalic comparison group, as well as some gross motor coordination deficits. They conclude that despite generally adequate cognitive skills among these early-school-aged children, children with achondroplasia should be evaluated individually, because they are at risk for cognitive, academic, and motor deficits. The results of this longitudinal study should provide further information about the relationship of the variables to scholastic achievement.

A considerable range in intellectual ability exists among individuals with achondroplasia. Although some difference is accounted for by inherited family traits, it may become increasingly possible to avert losses in function. Recent awareness that both hearing problems and apnea are present in a significant number of children with achondroplasia, for example, suggests that in at least some instances these deficits may have an impact on learning and proper assessment is essential.

I contacted Dr. Nora Thompson for insight into the subtleties of learning disabilities in achondroplasia. She indicated that the Texas group had not encountered the lower group verbal scores that had been reported by Brinkmann et al. In the Texas sample there were as many children with higher verbal than performance IQ scores as the reverse. However, the researchers did not perform an analysis comparing children with and without learning problems. Dr. Thompson cited a number of individual cases, some with fine motor coordination problems that had reduced Performance scores, and others with various unique features. She concluded that it was difficult to postulate a "typical profile of skills and deficits in achondroplasia," but that parents should be advised that risks for language and learning problems are elevated.

Many persons with achondroplasia have not encountered language difficulties; in fact, they have demonstrated superior verbal skills in scholastic and professional endeavors. However, even some accomplished individuals have had significant academic struggles. Parents and specialists suggest that there is at least a subgroup of seemingly bright achondroplastic children ("street smart," personable, and whizzes at computer tasks) who have problems with written materials and avoid reading. Apart from standardized IQ tests, careful evaluations are needed to illuminate the specific processing problems that interfere with learning.

Of course, the greatest challenge is to provide medical and educational assistance where needed. Many parents and affected individuals have expressed their distress about learning problems to teachers, psychiatrists, psychologists, or counselors to no avail. Because measured IQs were at least average, individuals' problems were minimized. One psychiatrist, for example, after testing a poorly achieving adolescent, declared that she did not have "a classic learning disability." In his report, he described her large head and short stature in pejorative terms and attributed her performance problems, with no specific evidence, to her being distracted by concern about her stature. In fact, she was functioning happily in her family, in LPA, and at an after-school job. School had been her only nemesis. The evaluation had held out hope and dashed it.

Underachieving children, often mislabeled "just lazy" by counselors, are apt to be demoralized and in need of assessment and advice. For the minority of achondroplastic dwarfs with inadequate language skills and reading comprehension, comprehensive longitudinal studies of cognitive functioning are needed, and more thoughtful individual assessments must be done in the meantime. Families whose children have mysterious learning problems must address the "conspiracy of denial," contributed to by the fact that dwarf youngsters would rather not acknowledge a second stigma, and professionals tend to jump to psychosocial interpretations.

Intelligence and Growth Hormone Deficiency

Some of the same issues arise among those with growth hormone deficiency (called *hypopituitary dwarfs* in older literature). Many studies assess the relationships between IQ and achievement, personality, and behavior. A majority report average intelligence in the group, with differing ranges of variability, often accompanied by scholastic underachievement. Among the factors held responsible in early studies are poor work habits, tendency to tire easily, short attention span, school phobia, and need for approval.[20] Some recent research mentions unspecified learning disabilities and attention-deficit disorders (Sartorio et al., 1996).[21]

Overall, intelligence in growth hormone–deficient (GHD) children tends to be average or close to average. However, achievement does not always keep pace, and sometimes personality factors appear to contribute to impaired performance. In one of the better studies, Siegel and Hopwood (1986) report their findings, then attempt to explain differences between fifty-five GHD children and earlier studies.[22] They find that their subjects evidence greater variability in verbal and performance scores than previous groups and also evidence difficulty with visual-motor integration, suggesting neurological immaturity.

Siegel and Hopwood explored two conflicting conclusions from previous studies. Some researchers had suggested that GHD children failed to live up to their intellectual potential because of poor self-concept and psychomaturational lag; a smaller number had found lower achievement to be the result simply of generally lower IQs. But when Siegel and Hopwood distinguished subgroups, they identified other explanations for achievement problems. Some children, they concluded, had done poorly either because of low ability or cognitive deficits; a smaller number might have done better if not for poor self-esteem. This study suggests that most children with hypopituitary conditions do feel good about themselves and are functioning at a level consistent with ability, but in questionable cases, comprehensive psychological assessment is in order.

Siegel and Hopwood's study confirms that investigators need to identify subcategories and mark individual differences in cognitive structure, growth hormone deficiency measurement, personality variables, parenting, and social milieu. If the group is not large enough to provide a proper statistical analysis of variables, at least in-depth interview analysis might supplement the data and suggest appropriate clinical measures and remediation for individuals.

The much-anticipated results of a National Cooperative Growth study by respected researchers Brian Stabler and his colleagues of children being treated for growth hormone deficiency were reported in several articles between 1994 and 1998.[23] The largest, most comprehensive study of this diagnostic category, it administered tests of intelligence, academic achievement, social skills, and behavioral variables to 166 children referred for growth hormone treatment. That group was assessed and found to contain 86 with growth hormone deficiency and 80 others with normal or near-normal GH levels, who were classified as having short stature of unknown origins (idiopathic short stature [ISS]).

The investigators again reported that mean IQs in this group were at least average, but achievement scores were significantly lower. They were more likely than an average-statured comparison group to have been retained at least a grade or receive special education services in reading, spelling, or arithmetic. One-third of the group evidenced a learning disability, and achievement did not improve with growth hormone therapy. This was true of both growth hormone-deficient and idiopathic short stature samples.

The researchers are unable to explain the reasons for achievement problems in these children from well-functioning families of medium to high socioeconomic status. They conclude that perhaps the test battery was inadequate for assessing the skills component. Psychosocial factors are not implicated, because, in general, the underachieving group is distinct from those with personality and behavior problems. The various other studies that note the gap between intelligence and achievement in GHD rarely cite specific cognitive problems. Abbott et al. (1982) are among a very few researchers who have reported a consistent finding of disturbance in visual-motor integration.[24]

Stabler and his associates question, finally, whether short stature itself predisposes the GDH and ISS groups to learning problems, or whether these parents are simply more likely to seek help. Whatever the explanation, these studies offer cause for concern about unidentified learning disabilities in this population and suggest that growth hormone treatment alone cannot improve achievement. Possible confounding biochemical factors such as low blood sugar, differences in height, or the nature of the treatment itself are not assessed. Unfortunately, an opportunity was also lost in not directing more attention to assessing specific cognitive sources of the learning disabilities.

It is not likely that another study on this scale will be undertaken soon. One wonders whether it might be possible to reexamine the data and tease out other differences between individuals in this study who were more successful or less successful academically, obtaining independent learning disability evaluations for a small sample of subjects.

In 1984, Holmes, Thompson, and Hayford had reported that 23 percent of the short-statured children with growth hormone deficiency, constitutional delay, and Turner syndrome that they had studied were experiencing underachievement, behavior problems, and grade retention, despite average intelligence.[25] It is troubling that two decades later the mystery of underachievement seems not much closer to resolution.

Intelligence and Turner Syndrome

Turner syndrome, a chromosomal short-stature condition in females that is marked by estrogen deficiency, pubertal delay, and infertility, presents a characteristic intelligence pattern. On the Wechsler Intelligence Scales, girls and women with Turner syndrome tend to be average in verbal scores, but below average in performance because of poor functioning on subtests relating to perceptual and spatial organization.[26] Steinhausen and Smith's comprehensive review suggests that data from females with Turner syndrome confirm previous findings that spatial perception is sex linked and biologically determined.

A compelling feature is their disclosure that, as late as 1959, it was believed that all patients with this condition were mentally retarded or below average in intelligence. The authors suggest that girls with Turner syndrome were overrepresented in institutions for individuals with mental retardation because of physical appearance. In addition to short stature, girls with Turner syndrome sometimes have a webbed neck, low posterior hairline, prominent ears, and a small mandible. Most are not "slow." Later studies have indicated that any measured deficit in full-scale IQs is attributable to low performance (visuospatial) scores not verbal scores.

Training can make a difference and should be provided at an early age. Typically, schools have been quicker to provide assistance with reading skills than with visuospatial deficits, which more likely to affect girls. Many women with Turner syndrome are extremely successful in their fields, which include law and a variety of high-profile, demanding occupations. Because verbal skills are most essential to academic pursuits, the visuospatial learning problems have not generally compromised scholastic success.

Intelligence and Constitutional Short Stature

The few studies limited specifically to constitutional short stature in children tend to find them not statistically different from children of average stature in intellectual functioning, academic achievement, or visual-motor performance.[27]

The Relationship between Height and Intelligence in the General Population

There is a small positive correlation between height and intelligence in the general population, as demonstrated in such studies as the British National Health Examination Survey (1985) of 7,119 children and 6,768 adolescents ($r = 0.18$ on the Wechsler Intelligence Scale for Children [WISC], $r = 0.19$ on the Wide Range Achievement Test;

$r = 13$).[28] However, when the same subjects are tested years later, and height increases in some, intelligence does not increase accordingly. This finding is a caution to those who might mistakenly conceive of growth hormone therapy as a way to increase intelligence in those with constitutional short stature.

Wilson and his colleagues ask why there should be any correlation at all between height and intelligence. They mention various intrauterine and postpartum medical factors, as well as social factors such as parental expectations of children corresponding to size rather than age. This last hypothesis is hard to substantiate, because studies do not do an analysis of variance to assess the contribution of medical and psychological factors to intelligence. Even in major studies, potential contributing factors such as birth order, kidney disease, and socioeconomic status to height-intelligence correlation are rarely assessed. In a rare study of living conditions in Sweden in 1991, Peck and Lundberg found that the prevalence of short stature was significantly related to a number of adverse conditions in childhood: economic hardship, large family, and family disunity.[29] Although their study does not include intelligence, and correlation does not prove causality, it reminds us that the same factors that have an impact on height may have an impact on intellect as well.

Intelligence and Psychosocial Dwarfism

Just how important environmental factors are in determining intelligence is apparent in the plethora of studies of psychosocial failure to thrive (PFTT). According to Burgin, approximately one-third of abused children are stunted in growth by at least two standard deviations.[30] There is considerable evidence that when they are removed from their homes and placed in a hospital setting, they make substantial gains in both height and intelligence. To what degree these benefits of "rescue" are maintained back at home depends in large measure on whether successful intervention has led to improved family dynamics. Although neuroendocrinological disturbance is involved in some cases (subnormal values of growth hormone are sometimes found in children with PFTT), treatment with growth hormone offers only very short-term improvement. As Burgin notes, differences in GH values seem not to be the cause but the result of the illness and can therefore be used as one marker of progress.

It is difficult to choose among the thousand or more studies of aspects of psychosocial dwarfism. Its impact on intelligence was first identified by Powell and his colleagues in 1967.[31] Money and associates, also at Johns Hopkins, found that the mean IQ of a group with this condition was 66 in abuse and 90 after rescue; the greatest change occurred in a girl whose IQ was measured as 36 at the age of 3 years, 11 months, and 120 at the age of 13 years, 11 months.[32] Later investigators confirmed the evidence for the condition; some, such as Green, Campbell, and David (1984),[33] found no consistent relationship between endocrine levels and retardation and catch-up growth on removal from an inimical environment.

Other later researchers, such as Skuse and Gilmour, have suggested that there is a subcategory called hyperphagic short stature, a stress-related condition with changes in GH levels, which they are trying to distinguish from other groups of psychosocial dwarfism.[34] Their hyperphagic group has an IQ of 76; the nonhyperphagic, an IQ of 93. Strangely, although their article is entitled "Psychosocial Short Stature: Follow-up to Adolescence and Adulthood," it focuses exclusively on childhood and adolescence. One of the great mysteries is what has become of the persons described with these conditions in later years. If intelligence is so dramatically affected in a condition such as PFTT, there is little doubt that similar effects must be present to a lesser degree in the conditions previously mentioned, as well as in others. However, the contributions of familial and socioeconomic factors defy precise measurement when their role is not as dramatic, and other factors are at work.

It must be remembered that the field of intelligence testing has a checkered history; even some of the best-known names in the field have been charged with error or locked in disagreement. Binet, the father of intelligence testing, emphasized that such tests were a practical device, not intended to bolster any theory of intellect or define an innate or permanent state.[35] Their appropriate use, he believed, was not for ranking children with normal intelligence, but rather for identifying those whose difficulties could be helped with training. Later approaches became increasingly politicized, and psychologists such as Howard Gardner and Robert J. Steinberg offered new approaches to viewing varied aspects of intelligence.[36] Far more important than single numbers supposedly reflecting generalized intelligence—a "g" factor—are the learning style or disability and the assessment of physiological and psychosocial factors affecting performance.

Individual intelligence tests such as the WISC and the Wechsler Adult Intelligence Scale (WAIS) are rarely used in studies anymore; however, they and more specific measures for diagnosing learning difficulties are invaluable in clinical practice and should be used in association with medical and neurological instruments to lead to informed counseling, treatment, and tutoring as needed.

PERSONALITY

Although intelligence may offer challenges in assessment and interpretation, it is relatively straightforward compared with areas such as personality, psychological adjustment, and quality of life. These factors are rarely adequately elucidated by the usual assessment tools, questionnaires, and rating scales—whereas in-depth interviews offering a more complete picture have not often been used. Methodology is improving, however. Haverkamp and Noeker (1998) at the University of Bonn are endeavoring to perfect questionnaires for parents of short-statured children which contain more sensitive scales for evaluating this population. Gollust et al. (2003) used Likert scales in connection with their survey and standardized indices of self-esteem and quality of life.[37]

Early investigators, charting completely unfamiliar terrain, sometimes compared more than one diagnostic category. The 1968 study by Drash et al. investigated personality differences in ninety-five dwarfs with four differing diagnoses.[38] They reported that children with hypopituitary dwarfism tended to lag in psychomaturational development, with such defense mechanisms as withdrawal, inhibition, and dissociation. However, these tendencies seemed to be moderated if the family had treated the child according to age rather than size.

The researchers found some psychomaturational lag in persons with Turner syndrome, but deemed them reasonably well adjusted, despite some tendency to be overly compliant, and lacking in verve, spontaneity, and activity level. Their somewhat stolid temperaments, investigators concluded, are a help to the young women as they face the realities of infertility and differences in appearance. The few individuals with achondroplasia were described as displaying a "hearty, cheerful, and optimistic personality," with least maturational lag. Those with deprivation dwarfism were described as evidencing bizarre behavior, including eating disorders and regurgitation, retarded speech, aggression, and very poor school performance.

Most early studies did not find dwarf children and adults (other than those with psychosocial dwarfism) to be significantly impaired psychologically. Brust et al. (1976), in their study of eleven dwarfs with achondroplasia and five with hypopituitarism, in general, found the group to have secure identities as "little people," pleasant interpersonal styles, and satisfactory life adjustment.[39] They found that male dwarfs evidenced more emotional distress than females, although a later study reported that females experienced more problems.[40]

Subsequently, investigators usually considered the diagnostic categories independently of each other. Several large, more sophisticated studies did comment on variability and sometimes benefited from interviews. Ablon's *Little People in America* offers cogent reviews of the pre-1984 literature and identifies major issues.[41] Only a few valuable studies have appeared in recent years.

Personality and Growth Hormone Deficiency

Since the advent of synthetic growth hormone treatment in the 1980s, many children with GHD start treatment shortly after birth, growing to average height or taller. It is therefore difficult to compare early or later studies, and later studies do not always indicate at what stage of treatment subject may be.

At least one early study implicated family constellations as the source of poor emotional adjustment. Noting children's use of denial as a defense mechanism, and their tendency to manifest gender identity problems in adolescence, Kusalic and Fortin (1975) reported that a high percentage of family members evidenced covertly rejecting attitudes.[42] However, this finding is not frequent.

Although many children and adults with GHD have been found to function well, many investigations have reported characteristic personality problems (immaturity, inhibition, anxiety, poor learning skills, and poor self-concept), and it has been suggested that because their facial appearance makes them look younger, hypopituitary dwarfs are sometimes treated accordingly. Parents sometimes complain of "babyish" behavior; investigators identify treating children according to size rather than age as the greatest parenting hazard.

The earliest studies were the most negative. In a study of seventeen pituitary dwarfs, Money and Pollitt (1966) deemed that only seven were adequately adjusted, stressing immaturity and lack of aggressiveness.[43] Although a few researchers such as Steinhausen and Stahnke (1977) and Drotar et al. (1981) found that these children compared well in general adjustment to a matched control group, most identified a number of emotional and behavioral problems.[44] Drotar emphasized poor response to frustration.

In a 1980 study, Stabler et al. concluded that social judgments were less adequate in the hypopituitary group, although improved under competitive conditions.[45] The authors posited that the children's limitations in sports, and greater exposure to teasing, might produce anxiety and withdrawal and a fear of confrontation. Allied problems were found to persist into adulthood, with Stabler et al. publishing two studies of GHD adults (1992 and1996) that indicated that they were more reactive to stress and had greater social phobias and poorer psychological adjustment.

More and more, biological roots of observed psychopathology were sought. Stabler and associates' 1998 study had found that GH treatment had had no effect on intelligence and achievement; however, it seemed to have a marked effect on behavioral measures. After three years of growth hormone treatment, GHD children showed significant improvement on subscales such as somatic complaint, anxiety/depression, attention problems, social problems, thought problems, and aggressive behavior. (Social competence, however, did not change.)

Because the GHD group showed improvement that children with idiopathic short stature did not, the investigators concluded that the changes were likely to be biochemically mediated. They suggested that pituitary-limbic pathways might also be involved, affecting attentional behavior. They cited previous evidence that blunted GH secretion is associated with traits of shyness, anxiety, and inhibition. Uncertain whether psychotherapeutic effects of the growth hormone treatment will endure, they echo the recommendation of Eminson et al., that GH therapy be combined with cognitive-behavioral counseling, the combination perhaps more effective than either treatment alone. By 2001, Stabler had become increasingly impressed by the complexity of quality-of-life issues occurring throughout the life span and recommended a variety of medical and psychosocial strategies.[46]

Researchers in many countries have found that psychosocial problems in GHD children often persist into adulthood (Dean et al., 1986; Sartori et al., 1986; Stabler et al., 1992, 1996; Nicholas et al., 1997).[47] These investigators are troubled by the fact that hypopituitary adults have a low marriage rate, high unemployment rate, and significant psychosocial problems. The Stabler group tends to believe that GHD and stature alone cannot account for everything; they speculate that perhaps catecholamines or cortisol may be at least partially responsible for the psychosocial problems of patients with multiple hormone deficiencies. In addition, patients with adult-onset GHD experience similar psychological and quality-of-life problems. Although investigators speak of the need for multidisciplinary intervention, only rarely are attempts reported (Glatzer et al., 1987)[48]; neither do sociological aspects receive much attention.

Even the most interesting studies can be difficult to evaluate. For example, one study that compared isolated and multiple pituitary deficiencies found differences in reactions to stress between groups, but these categories are usually not identified separately.[49] Factors such as final heights of patients, age of treatment onset and its length, and similar variables are rarely noted in psychosocial behavior studies. Family status may be reported, and a personality instrument used, but personality data usually are limited. Interviews are rarely included, and because precise biochemical and other characteristics are not compared, it is difficult to know what has enabled the individuals with the most satisfying quality of life to achieve it.

Nevertheless, the quality of the studies has improved, and their tone has tended to be more positive. One encouraging article reviewed studies that reported that GH replacement therapy had proved useful in improving quality of life for at least some adult patients (McGauley et al., 1996).[50] A Magic Foundation brochure prepared for persons with a diagnosis of GHD either in childhood or adulthood offers guidance:

> Feeling tired, listless, easily fatigued, and having a lack of motivation are often reported by patients. Some individuals also report feeling anxious, irritable, losing interest in sex, and pervasive sense of gloom and pessimism about their lives. Because of these effects, persons with GHD may tend to avoid contact with others, show signs of stress in their marriage, and experience a gradual increase in their productivity at work. Quality of life begins to decline and the affected individual often suffers in silence. This brochure is provided to help you understand these feelings and what actions you can take to improve your life.[51]

Among recommended remedies are further GH replacement therapy, medication to control anxiety or depression, participation in a support group, and psychological counseling.

I called the Magic Foundation to inquire whether the group saw studies as accurately describing members with GHD. Gail Duca, GHD division consultant, recognized that the studies reflect real problems, but she knows many individuals who have fashioned satisfying lives for themselves. One young man came immediately to her mind: recently married at 24, he had benefited a short while ago from a cycle of growth hormone treatments that had given him renewed vigor. Duca felt that because GH replacement therapy was now provided at a much earlier age, it was apt to transform the previous profile of low energy and psychosocial problems. Although treatment of GHD adults had been helpful, she said, the current generation of children would demonstrate dramatically that affected persons could attain a better quality of life.

Duca credited the Magic Foundation for offering information and support that led to her own 6-year-old son's positive development. Information exchanged among parents, she felt, had led to discoveries unnoticed in formal studies. Parents' identification of problems, such as high occurrence of asthma, attention-deficit/hyperactivity disorder (ADHD), and speech delay among GHD children, might lead to earlier and more effective treatment. These parents' experiences suggest some possible sources of reported underachievement.

Duca indicated that adults who received GH replacement therapy in childhood were not as well represented in Magic Foundation leadership positions as were parents of affected children. I speculated that whether they had "heighted out" of dwarfism because of successful treatment or been discouraged by minimal height increases, this group may have found the memory of that period difficult and preferred to detach. (It remains to be seen whether the generation now coming of age will respond differently.) Persons with skeletal dysplasia, who have less choice, are more apt to seek others like themselves and willingly serve as role models. Physicians acquainted with GHD adults who have remained very short indicate that many have rewarding lives, although some do not. What variables have made the greatest difference (biochemical, familial, temperamental, or societal) are unclear.

Personality and Turner Syndrome

McCauley et al. (1986, 1987) conducted some of the best-designed and most carefully executed studies of social functioning in children and adolescents with Turner syndrome.[52] They posit that social interaction is impaired by difficulties with spatial relations, attention, and short-term memory, especially with visualization and interpreting facial affect. Studies cite problems with lack of assertiveness and peer relationships, recommending early intervention and training. Although children with Turner syndrome have lower self-esteem, they do not exhibit clinical depression.

Downey et al. (1986, 1989) found that adult women with Turner syndrome did not evidence more serious mental illness than average, but enjoyed less-than-optimal mental health in daily functioning.[53] Problems were more likely to be manifest as anhedonia and withdrawal than in acting out, as with alcohol and drug abuse. Women with Turner syndrome were more apt to be sexually inexperienced, dating and marrying later when they did achieve these milestones. There was a tendency to minimize discontent.

Other patients reported more serious psychiatric problems and impaired self-esteem, overtly expressing dissatisfaction (McCauley, Sybert, and Ehrhardt, 1986).[54] Another, larger study found low self-esteem, conservative sexual attitudes, and less sexual activity (Pavlidis, McCauley, and Sybert, 1995). However, individuals with a better health status reported a better self-concept and greater sexual satisfaction.[55] Other studies have also emphasized variability and indicate the need to identify risk and protective factors (Ross, Zinn, and McCauley, 2000). They suggest that neurocognitive deficits may prove somewhat reversible with estrogen treatment.[56]

During the past decade, articles about the psychosocial aspects of French, Italian, and Swedish women with Turner syndrome have also appeared (Toublanc et al., 1997[57]; Calo et al., 1993[58]; Sylven et al., 1993[59]). Although results vary, with the French women attaining a higher level of education and the Italian women attaining almost full employment, between 80 and 90 percent of the women in these two groups were unmarried; most still lived at home and were not sexually active. The Swedish study, conducted by an OB-GYN department, focused on the feelings of grief hospital patients expressed about their infertility. Several American and European studies have emphasized the importance of professionals and support groups in addressing psychosocial issues.[60]

One overview suggests that women with Turner syndrome have had difficulty achieving their full potential and, lacking self-confidence and parental support, have often chosen civil service careers, assuming they would not marry (Dorholt et al., 1999).[61] However, the more positive the body image, the better their psychological well-being and life satisfaction. It may be, as some physicians have suggested, that those persons who have more complications related to Turner syndrome (cardiac problems, hearing loss, or learning deficit) are at greater risk.

The mature women who play leadership roles in the Turner Syndrome Society have forceful personalities, have developed strong friendships with each other, and serve as role models for the younger ones. Many, such as attorney Gertrude (Trudy) McCarthy, with whom I spoke in May 2001, have achieved rewarding, productive lives. McCarthy believed that the most satisfied individuals often do not come to the attention of researchers. She reports that questions such as "Can I have a relationship?" and "Can I have children?" have been more vexing than short stature for women with Turner syndrome. Sometimes, individuals have not been well enough socialized; however, she believes that estrogen and growth hormone treatment have eased sexual identity concerns, low self-esteem, and relationship questions that vex women with Turner syndrome. It will take ten or fifteen years, she believes, to fully see positive results. Another research issue being addressed is accumulating morbidity and mortality statistics, which is of particular concern to older members.

McCarthy mentioned three factors that she believes play a vital role in individuals' lives—the quality of familial relationships, interactions with pediatric endocrinologists, and participation in the Turner Syndrome Society. Shirley Poirier's essay on the Turner Syndrome Society's Web site offers an interesting personal account.[62]

Personality and Skeletal Dysplasias

Persons with skeletal dysplasias, especially achondroplasia, have tended to be described as reasonably well adjusted. The aforementioned Drash, Greenberg, and Money study describes achondroplastic children as extroverted: "The proverbial cheerfulness of the achondroplastic dwarf was evident in the majority of the nine children in the present group. . . . They were unexpectedly accepting of their situation, optimistic and generally happy with life. Despite the rather grotesque appearance with which some were afflicted, they did not appear 'crushed' by their predicament."[63]

What a difference thirty years has made in researchers' attitudes, methodology, and conclusions! Words such as *grotesque* and *afflicted* would not be found today, nor would impressionistic allusions to "proverbial cheerfulness." Nevertheless, these individuals are still described as "constantly active, sociable, jovial and cheerful sometimes to the point of euphoria."[64] Perhaps the greater physical vigor and energy level, in contrast to other groups of dwarfs being studied, influenced early investigators. Later studies and self-reports of persons with achondroplasia do not confirm this observation.

In the Brust, Ford, and Rimoin (1976) study mentioned earlier, eleven achondroplastic adult dwarfs and five hypopituitary dwarfs were interviewed. The majority of subjects professed themselves to be happy or content, though noting that they were occasionally depressed or irritable. Only one subject described himself as generally depressed. Nevertheless, both clinical judgment and self-report dispelled Money's notion that persons with achondroplasia are constitutionally cheerful: "Some are, some aren't, and some act that way," was the general consensus.[65]

In this group, eight of sixteen were married, and most were employed, attended school, or were homemakers. Any problems emanated from outside experiences, such as employment discrimination. Independent psychological testing confirmed the relative absence of psychological problems and the presence of secure identity. Interestingly, the mean IQ was 120, 105 for the hypopituitary group, and 125 for the achondroplasia group.

In Ablon's study, despite previous problems, subjects enjoyed considerable life satisfaction.[66] Their group profile was skewed toward higher intelligence, and half were either professionals or skilled workers. All but five were currently married, and all but three owned their own homes. As LPA members, they had accepted their difference and found group support. Demographics varied: none were from wealthy backgrounds; eight were from comfortable economic backgrounds; the rest were working class. Their geographic origins varied from farm to town to big city; none felt overprotected. Approximately half had at least some college, with women having more education than the men. The men seemed to have felt the need to prove themselves economically at an earlier age. In addition to a strong work ethic, every dwarf Ablon has met, male and female, has highlighted marriage, which she considers "a legitimization and normalization rite for a population disenfranchised from many of the taken-for-granted, normal social rituals of our society."[67]

Briefer accounts of psychosocial milestones that dwarfs and their families must traverse successfully can be found in several articles written in the 1960s and 1970s, addressed to the dwarfism community, professionals, or the general public.[68] Although they note the need to develop strategies for dealing with ignorant or abusive strangers, they communicate that a dwarf child who has been encouraged by his parents, received good medical care, and learned to be at home in the world of both short and average-sized persons, is apt to become a confident adult.[69]

A study of the psychological well-being and quality of life of persons with skeletal dysplasia was reported by Folstein et al. (1981).[70] They conducted interviews with 84 adult dwarfs between the ages of 16 and 73 at the Johns Hopkins Medical Clinic and Short Stature Symposium. The study focused on interactions among several variables: physical impairment, psychological impairment, stigmatization, and self-assessment of disability. This sample too was skewed, in that 61 percent had some college and 93 percent were employed in occupations appropriate to their education. (Persons who find their way to specialized treatment centers and symposia are likely to be better off.)

The Hopkins researchers wrestled with whether dwarfs were to be deemed handicapped (the term used in those days). Although 80 percent had little or no physical impairment, 20 percent were moderately impaired. Those with significant physical problems were apt to have had less education and were more often unemployed. They also reported the greatest number of psychiatric symptoms.

Because these categories overlapped, the investigators hesitated to draw conclusions about causality. A surprising finding was that married men and women reported more psychiatric symptoms. Only 43 percent had married, compared with 90 percent of persons with partial disabilities nationwide. The investigators raise the possibility that obstacles that dwarfs face in finding partners may have contributed in some instances to their marrying unsuitable mates, although the women, especially, tried to keep up a good front. Except for those with profound physical problems, subjects were somewhat more extroverted and no more neurotic than average, leading to the conclusion that short stature alone did not presuppose psychiatric impairment. The contribution of stigmatization to "handicap" was noted.

Group composition and research methodology are both of vital importance. One of the largest well-researched investigations is Stace and Danks's Australian study of 140 dwarfs with bone dysplasias. Their subjects were not privileged, and the results suggested that their quality of life was generally dismal.[71] The study is unique in that it attempted to assess a population—all persons with skeletal dysplasia in Victoria (about 47% were assessed)—and that it used both statistical measures and in-depth interviews. It presents a picture of great struggle: subjects described difficulties in finding secure, satisfying employment; there were fewer stable, lasting marriages than in the general population; and beginning with adulthood, friendship and intimacy seemed hard for most to achieve.

There was an unusually high incidence of medical, social, behavioral, and mental health problems among the families of dwarfed children and adults. Although thirty-four informants reported good relationships with household members, twenty-two were unhappy, frustrated by their disability and financial dependence and unable to effect change. Some had married impulsively to forestall loneliness but now regretted it.

No inquiry of this scope had previously been conducted. Earlier studies used small patient populations at a single hospital or LPA members. One might wonder whether the bleak conditions in this study were unique to Australia or representative. Australia in the early 1980s was perhaps more like the United States before the positive effects of the disability rights movement when many dwarfs had become better educated and had the support of LPA. The degree of pathology reported in the Australian families of origin is perplexing and impossible to assess from information given.

There was considerable excitement in the dwarfism community when Canadian geneticist A.G. Hunter published his dramatically different 1998 study of persons with skeletal dysplasias.[72] The contrast was particularly surprising because 136 of the 192 persons queried were Australian (among the remainder, 25 were from the United States and Canada and 24 were from the United Kingdom).

The Hunter investigation was thoughtful and far-reaching. Most subjects were identified through clinical files in the genetics departments of hospitals; a few families were identified through genetics clinics or the American and Canadian Little People's Conferences. They agreed to complete standardized and validated questionnaires designed to measure lifestyle, depression and anxiety, marital adjustment, personal support networks, and family interaction.

The central finding was that the majority of individuals with skeletal dysplasias considered their lives quite satisfying. When asked, "How satisfied are you with your life as a whole," a positive answer was expressed by 87 percent of the unmarried and 61 percent of the married subjects. (Only 52% of parents of affected individuals rated themselves as highly satisfied.) In subcategories of the lifestyle questionnaire, the answers were only slightly less positive: approximately 80 percent of subjects were satisfied with their finances; 70 percent were content with their friendships, their spare time activities, family life, and (when applicable) marriages.

Depression and anxiety scores suggest mostly favorable outcomes. Hunter found that 84.5 percent of affected adults and 92 percent of children reported little or no depression. However, although patients

under the age of 18 compare favorably with their siblings, adult patients have significantly more evidence of mild to moderate depression (18.8% vs. 7.6%). Similarly, patients' anxiety scores show some
increase in adulthood, especially for females. The investigator attributes the increase to the greater stress imposed by increased expectations of independence and social and employment concerns.

Short-statured individuals also held their own regarding self-
esteem. However, as adults, their scores were lower than those of their
unaffected siblings. There was a trend toward somewhat lower scores
among women, subjects with an average-statured parent, and those
married to an average-statured spouse. Among the study's negative
results were those relating to marital adjustment and family cohesiveness. The marital adjustment of average-statured parents seems
poorer than in the general population. Hunter hypothesizes that perhaps greater financial and medical strains, as well as restricted freedom and fears about the child's future, may interfere with the relationship. Couples in which only one member is a dwarf seem less well
off than short-statured couples.

Families seem to suffer in "mixed marriages." The short-statured
child of average-statured parents and "mixed" couples seem to have
more problems with cohesiveness and social adaptability. Integrating
differences poses a challenge. Again, it would be interesting to examine what distinguishes those who achieve a successful accommodation from those who do not.

Overall, Hunter paints a far more positive picture of the mental
health and general well-being of individuals with skeletal dysplasia
than Stace and Danks do. I asked why, and he wrote:

> I don't have any great insights into why the results differed from those
> of Dr. Danks. Certainly the methodology was different in that I was
> using standard 'instruments' that had been 'normed' on the general
> population. The data collection by Stace and Danks was more quali-
> tative.
>
> I suspect that there had been some change with time, not the least
> of which was the growing influence of support groups. I do believe

there has been a change in attitude by the general population as well as improvements in medical care and social integration. It is also possible that there was some bias of 'social correctness' in some of the responses to my questionnaires, although I don't think it was a major factor.[73]

Studies must deal with a moving target. As economic and social conditions change and medical care improves, as job opportunities and support groups appear, quality of life improves. Hunter's study records these changes while identifying trouble spots, suggesting areas for further study and intervention, such as the discord in "mixed" families.

SELF-CONCEPT AND QUALITY OF LIFE

Most self-report studies have tended to find American dwarfs reasonably content. Two of the four (the Zingaro and Griggs studies) are by persons who are themselves short statured. Gina Zingaro (1981) reported in an investigation of seventy-seven adolescent and young-adult LPA members that two-thirds considered themselves as having a better than average relationship with their families (the rest termed it average).[74] Approximately 80 percent said they made friends easily, 95 percent felt they did things well, and 87 percent felt hopeful about their futures. Among the sources of strength they valued were family support, religion, membership in LPA, development of talents, and experiencing independence. Surgery constituted their most stressful experience.

Sherrill et al. (1990) found no difference between mean self-concept scores for able-bodied youth and athletes with disabilities (including dwarfism).[75] When Mulberg (1985) investigated body image and depressive symptoms in dwarfs, diabetics, and average-statured controls, he found that dwarfs possessed the highest level of self-esteem, with a highly significant negative correlation between self-esteem and depression.[76] He concluded that self-esteem and extroversion buffered dwarfs from depression resulting from atypical body image.

Griggs (1988) found no significant differences between the self-concepts of thirty short-statured college students who were also LPA members and a comparable group of average-statured students.[77] Both groups viewed themselves more positively overall than they viewed the other population, although each group did give dwarfs a lower rating on the "physical self" scale. Griggs reported that, although short stature did not prevent individuals from developing a healthy sense of self, it was important for average-statured persons to be better educated, thereby developing a more accurate image of dwarfs. This view echoes other investigators', who have concluded that negative perceptions by average-statured persons (employers, school, and workmates) represent the greatest barrier to a normative lifestyle for dwarfs.[78]

Why should the subjects in the studies of Sherrill, Mulberg, and Griggs have as high or even higher self-esteem than comparison groups? It is hard to calculate from self-report whether subjects are overstating good self-feeling and underemphasizing problems, or reflecting genuine data. For the most part, the positive sense of self seems a true reflection. Only in the Folstein study, in which the results of the "lie" scale on the Eysenck Inventory were reported, did it appear that some (the most impaired physically) were defensively describing their condition overly positively.

The Influence of Employment Status on Personality and Mental Health

The effect of employment status on mental health and quality of life cannot be overstated. Chapter 5, Lives Today, documents the extraordinary improvement in the employment picture of dwarfs in the United States. In other countries, one of the first areas informants mention is the dire employment situation for dwarfs. In a study of twenty Chicago-area adults with achondroplasia, Roizen et al. (1990) found that education had the greatest influence on occupational level both for persons with achondroplasia and their unaffected siblings.[79] Younger individuals tended to have more education than older ones, but there was little difference in years of schooling between affected and unaffected individuals.

Notably, women with achondroplasia tended to have lower-status jobs than their unaffected sisters. The investigators hazard a guess that society's emphasis on attractiveness may be responsible for this gender-based difference. Perhaps dwarf women simply encounter the same discrimination as women in society overall. One may also wonder whether family expectations were lower for these women, as they have been for women historically, when they anticipated that families or husbands would take care of them.

Psychoanalytic Comments on Short Stature

All too often, professionals have taken it for granted that dwarfs cannot truly feel good about themselves and their lives. Some psychoanalysts base such findings on a clinical subsample of children treated with psychotherapy or psychoanalysis. Frankel (1996), for example, declared: "Recognizing their comparative smallness left them feeling vulnerable and humiliated. They responded with envy and rage toward normally endowed children and vindictively used their intellect to outwit and defeat others. They acted as if their suffering exempted them from ordinary rules and expectations. Their preoccupation also resulted in arrests in cognitive and social development. Their distrust and intention to deceive and defeat posed particular problems for treatment."[80] This account conveys more about the ignorance of the author and his colleagues than the necessary consequences of short stature. Perhaps they took for granted an inevitable "inferiority complex," such as has been held responsible for the neuroses of persons with biological or other deficits by Adlerian and like-minded analysts.

This approach can be found in articles dealing with patients whose short stature is unaccompanied by medical complications, but it has also occurred in accounts of psychosocial aspects of skeletal dysplasia. The Italian psychiatrist L. Ancona (1989) describes the birth of a child with achondroplasia, concluding that "the consternation of the medical staff and the family" is "felt by the foetus (or the newborn baby) who is hypersensitive to these primary communications."[81]

The author goes on to discuss potential sequelae such as blaming the father, scapegoating the baby's brother, the mother treating her child as a husband, familial subconscious aggressiveness directed toward the child, and families imagining "him" to be endowed with exceptional attributes. In his summary, Ancona calls the medieval jester "generally a well-adapted achondroplast" and remarks, "The problem of the achondroplast arises when his surroundings, right from the start, reject his disorder, connoting it with destructive anxiety: this seriously harms the subject's physical image, making him an outcast." He suggests that limb-lengthening surgery may repair the patient's mind-body split, but that subsequent analytic psychotherapy may be required. "Fixing" the stigmatized individual rather than mending society's attitudes becomes legitimized as the best way of avoiding society's rebuff.

This bizarre analysis was included in the respected volume *Human Achondroplasia* and was composed by the head of the Institute of Psychiatry and Psychology at Sacro Cuore University, Rome. Both the Italian emphasis on beauty and the psychoanalytic culture that emphasizes psychopathology conspire here. Fortunately, *Human Achondroplasia* also included a brief, commonsensical statement by Dr. William Shakespeare, who had achondroplasia himself, and was the father of sociologist Tom Shakespeare, who has the same condition.[82] Dr. Shakespeare recommended that new parents be told gently but firmly that their child would be mentally normal and physically fit, and would develop normally sexually, and he suggests ways of helping child and family manage life's transitions.

Short Stature and Adaptation

It is worthwhile to consider the consequences of "just being short." Although there has been less study of idiopathic short stature, D. Skuse (1987) and J. L. Ross et al. (2004) are representative of the majority of investigators, who have reported few notable adjustment problems in this group.[83] Whereas Skuse did describe some children with constitutional delay as sometimes feeling less popular and happy than their classmates—perhaps because they were less outgoing—recent studies, including Ross's, tend to find that idiopathic short stature in children does not seem to be associated with problems in psychological adaptation or self-concept. Another 2004 study of 956 public school children found no relationship between height and measures of friendship, popularity, and relationships with peers. The authors, D.D. Sandberg et al., suggest that if problems with peer relationships are identified among short or tall youths, factors other than stature should be considered as possible causes.

Nevertheless, no one reports that short children and young adults find it easy to cope with society's reaction. Martel and Biller's *Stature and Stigma* (1987) reviews the ways in which short males have often been reminded that their bodies are inferior and have developed compensatory mechanisms to shield themselves from a sense of bodily vulnerability.[84] In working-class groups, short males have sometimes become more physically aggressive; in middle-class groups, they have tended to become more cerebral in their approach to life. Most short persons sometimes resort to humor to reduce their anxiety and win others' acceptance. Martel and Biller quote short-statured actor Joel Grey, who recalls how he used humor to avoid fights with guys who were a lot bigger, but finds that in having done so, "you end up not really saying what you feel to the person because they're a danger. And you don't feel good about yourself because you've copped out, so to speak, when actually what you've done is to be practical." This quotation (which appeared originally in Keyes's *The Height of Your Life*) reflects the ambivalence that short-statured persons often feel as they develop defensive styles. Martel and Biller report conversations in which young men describe being discriminated against in sports, in attempts to date, and in other situations:

Interviewer: Did height bother you?

Subject: When you are in a crowd, at a concert, and everybody stands up and you have to stand on a chair, it's embarrassing. A thought crosses my mind that I'm standing next to someone who is 1½ feet taller than me. I'm wondering what he thinks about me being this tall, and I feel

like maybe there is an onus on me to prove that I am at least as intellectually worthy as a person.

The investigators conclude that few, if any, short men do not suffer
significant stress at various developmental stages. They do not believe, however, that feelings of self-worth are necessarily significantly
damaged.

Apart from studies of females with Turner syndrome, there have
been few similar appraisals of short stature in girls and women, although Folstein's study found women with chondrodystrophies less
outgoing and more sensitive to others' reactions in public situations.
Because this study is now two decades old, culturally defined role ex-
pectancies for women may well have altered this group.

An extremely valuable collection of studies appears in *Growth,
Stature, and Psychosocial Well-Being* (1999), a volume written by researchers from many European countries and the United States.[85]
The authors ask whether short stature is a handicap or disadvantage
for otherwise healthy children; they also explore whether there are
differences in adaptation when disorders such as Turner syndrome,
achondroplasia, or growth hormone deficiency are present. Many of
these articles present compelling evidence that short stature alone
does not lead to poor psychological adjustment or life satisfaction, in
either childhood or adulthood.

Noeker and Haverkamp grapple most effectively with the conflicting results of clinical studies, clinical experience, and population-
based studies.[86] They conclude that apparent contradictions are based
on different sources of evidence, different perspectives, and different
research approaches. (They recommend, and have developed, better
assessment devices.) They believe that clinic samples may be skewed
toward the pathological but also that short healthy children in the
general population are no more apt to be troubled, unless confounding medical or other factors exist. They conclude, "We have to ask
what specific problems, or predisposing set of circumstances have
caused a particular child to seek help in contrast to all the other children in the population that remain unaffected."[87]

Similarly, other authors in the volume focus on the question of why some adults find their situation untenable whereas others of the same height feel at ease with themselves. For dwarfs, as for the general population, "stress" is a subjective experience and the factors that provide protection against potential damage need to be further studied in the context of height, deformity, and health status.

Apart from idiopathic short stature, each separate hormonal, genetic, chromosomal, or bone disorder may bring with it its own set of stressors and adaptations. For example, Noeker et al. contrast defensive strategies observed in the families of children with achondroplasia and GHD.[88] But there are also commonalities: the personal resources necessary to develop a positive sense of self and deal with others' prejudices typically transcend diagnostic categories.

Coping Styles Associated with Particular Conditions

Earlier, it was noted that some researchers have reported that persons with achondroplasia have sunny temperaments. Little proof of this exists, although there is indication that as a group they may be somewhat extroverted. Folstein et al. did find that persons with skeletal dysplasias tended to be more outgoing than the norm. Although they did not report how diagnostic categories varied in extroversion, because forty-eight of their eighty-four subjects had achondroplasia, it is probable that this group tests as a bit more extroverted than average.

Vita Gagne, mother of Stefan, a young adult diastrophic dwarf, notes that diastrophic dwarfs are said to be determined and stubborn. Dr. Steven Kopits, her son's orthopedist, had once commented that diastrophic dwarfs had strong personalities. His view had been confirmed by her experience. Perhaps, she thought, their characters had been shaped by the fact that from early on they had had to do things differently; their joints are inflexible—a baby whose fingers don't bend at the knuckles must find original ways to obtain and grasp a pacifier.

Stefan's sister Jenny contributed, "Studies have shown that those rats who are challenged to get their own food as babies are smarter as adults." Vita agreed. She thought that their many surgeries and the stratagems they had to invent to accomplish things had caused diastrophic dwarfs to become more creative in adapting to the world.

Joan Ablon has made a similar suggestion in her study of personality in individuals with osteogenesis imperfecta.[89] One of her objectives was to see whether there was any substance to the commonly held opinion that there is an OI personality—exceptionally bright, assertive, articulate, "up" emotionally, and accomplished. Although the term *euphoric* had also often previously been applied to the group, she discovered that many participants rejected this description, feeling that it trivialized the years of painful broken bones, medical procedures, and other hardships. Ablon instead substitutes *resilient.*

She studied fifty-five adults (thirty women and twenty-five men) with OI types III and IV, using lengthy interviews and chronicling their medical, personal, and social experience. She found that her subjects displayed a variety of remarkable accomplishments. She also found that they were an irrepressible lot, determined to live life fully despite the risks. Describing their participation in adventures like going down an Amazon trail in a wheelchair, riding motorcycles or horses, or river rafting, they think, "You know what, what the hell, I might as well do it. If I'm going to get hurt at least I'll have fun doing it."

In school they had gotten good grades, led an active social life, and also had leadership positions; they now had careers as lawyers, top-level corporate and government executives, professors, artists, and writers. Those without college learned to be skilled technicians or craftsmen. They are commonly queried about both their achievements and their cheerfulness. Most credit parents and physicians with having encouraged them to aspire and try everything. Because they could not be as physically active as others, they believed, they had had time to be still and observe, and to read, reflect, and problem-solve. Some individuals with OI feel that children try to compensate for their parents' upset, trying to "make up for the fact that they are causing their family pain by keeping things light. Most people with OI end up being their family's listener and inspiration."

Is there a genetic basis for their natures? It is well known that certain conditions are associated with temperamental or behavioral patterns. Ablon discusses Williams syndrome; Klinefelter is another well-known syndrome in which affected individuals manifest similar personalities and behaviors. Ablon mentions Reite et al. (1972), who proposed a connection between the biochemistry of OI and cognitive and affective development, noting that the same "increased rate of cellular oxidation that is a component of the metabolic disturbance characterizing OI may influence central nervous system and cognitive maturational patterns."[90] They believe that the OI temperament may be rooted in this metabolic mechanism.

Whatever the origins, although most individuals admit to having some bad days, there seems to be some measure of consensus on overall philosophy. One respondent comments: "If you had to be spending all your time being bummed out that you cannot do something or you are afraid to do something, you are wasting your life. I do not know why it is, but most of the people I have met with OI have the intention of enjoying their life."

No other researcher has used Ablon's approach, assessing personality from both broad theoretical understanding and intimate personal contact. Many of the quotes in her article are quite dazzling. Although Ablon acknowledges that there might be others less well off who had little contact with doctors or others with OI, she indicates that she had endeavored to find as many as she could by various means, and that "when *anyone* spontaneously told me they knew of a person with OI they quickly described how remarkable and achieving they were, and before I talked about my findings."[91]

Persons with other skeletal dysplasias might turn out to make similar claims of resilience, and one is as apt to be as struck by the range of differences as by commonalities. Because random samples are almost impossible to obtain, and more dysfunctional individuals may be withdrawn and less accessible to investigators, it is unwise to draw more than cautious conclusions at this stage. Nevertheless, it may be that certain biological clusters characterize some diagnoses more than others and that further interdisciplinary research may reveal more about their contribution to personality.

Quality of Life with Achondroplasia

The investigation of the quality of life in achondroplasia by Gollust et al.[92] is one of the best and the most comprehensive studies of its kind. The investigators surveyed 189 individuals with achondroplasia and 136 first-degree relatives, using respected instruments in assessing sociodemographic information, subjects' perception of achondroplasia, self-esteem, and quality of life. A multiple regression analysis was performed, and a thoughtful discussion offered.

Individuals with achondroplasia (ACH) were four times as likely as first-degree relatives (FDR) to find their condition "not serious." They were more apt than their FDRs to cite different advantages in having it, most notably social interactions and friendships. Considered as a single group, the FDRs had higher quality of life, a variable that was strongly related to high self-esteem, having at least a college degree, regularly attending religious services, earning more than $50,000 a year, and viewing achondroplasia as a less serious condition. Those ACHs who had the lowest quality-of-life scores were more apt to have lower self-esteem, be unmarried, have less than a college degree, earn less than $50,000, and perceive achondroplasia as a serious or lethal illness (even though as a group, ACHs did not perceive it so). Although not *all* FDRs and ACHs were at the extremes of quality of life, there was a significant difference between the total groups.

The study certainly indicates that persons with achondroplasia have not yet caught up with their families in achieving as high a quality of life; however, it also identifies a significant ACH subgroup that is doing quite well. Approximately 30 percent of the ACHs were making at least $50,000 a year, and they were also apt to be the persons with highest self-esteem and quality of life, testament to the potential of greater economic opportunity to increase such factors. The authors also identify several implications of religious attendance, one being that community involvement is associated with greater acceptance of differences and higher quality of life.

They emphasize that persons with achondroplasia are as likely to cite disadvantages relating to social barriers as they are to cite those relating to health and functioning. All too often, the authors note, health care professionals, who tend to see disabilities as undesirable, tend to underestimate the quality of life of these individuals, attributing that reduction to medical factors alone. The investigators offer suggestions about research strategies and for clinical interventions designed to improve the life satisfaction of the group and its larger cohort in the outside community.

Depression and Anxiety in Skeletal Dysplasia

Rilke's "The Dwarf's Song," discussed earlier, highlighted the dejected state that many outsiders believe is the *natural, inevitable* condition of dwarfs. The contrasts in Stace and Danks's 1982 study and Hunter's 1998 investigation suggest that social change may have improved some of these individuals' quality of life. It is certainly true that social circumstances beyond their control can affect a whole group of individuals, causing many to become "depressed." Although there are immutable factors that will leave some better or worse off and vulnerable to depression, many aspects of individual functioning are also responsive to social change.

Depression and anxiety have always been difficult to measure. Studies that assess them via rating scales often come up with disparate findings, often because of the vagaries of self-report. In general, women are termed more subject to depression than men, but they are also more apt to acknowledge mood states and seek help, rather than deny problems and act out with alcohol or violence. To understand the multifaceted nature of depression, it is probably best to read a compelling account such as Andrew Solomon's *The Noonday Demon*, which combines a comprehensive, well-written chronicle of depression in all eras with an account of his personal experience with it.[93]

For the most part, however, when attempting to assess depression in a given community, researchers do the best they can, which means assembling relatively large groups and using inventories such as the Beck Depression Inventories used by Hunter in his assessment of 103 adults and 55 children. That study found no evidence of depression in 72 percent of children and adults, but an additional 20 percent showed mild depressive symptoms (children) or mild to mild-moderate (adults). Affected individuals are no more prone to depression in childhood than their siblings, but very slightly more so in adulthood. (The Spielberger State-Trait Anxiety Inventory was also administered, but because State-Anxiety relates to situational stress at the time the form is completed, it is difficult to assess the meaning of these scores.)

Though some dwarfism conditions are more prone to depression, persons with skeletal dysplasia generally have been found similar to average-statured individuals. Still, members of the dwarfism community have observed a good bit of depression, with some individuals doing poorly for long periods, and many others experiencing significant "ups and downs" in response to situational challenges.

Writer and LPA activist Leslye Sneider wrote about the untimely death of a longtime LP friend. Suffering from chronic pain and depressed after a divorce and the downsizing of his job, he had failed to reveal the depths of his despair to Leslye or other attendees at the annual LPA conference in 2003. After mourning his suicide, she reflected:

> We need to bring depression out of the closet and speak about it as commonly as we speak about our variety of physical problems. We need more workshops in which people can speak candidly and directly about depression and mental illness. We need to strongly encourage our peers to seek help during the week and throughout the year. We need to break down the veneer of shame that shrouds this illness. . . .

The symptoms of depression are very recognizable and we must make it our responsibility to know these signs and take appropriate action when necessary. Action can include just talking to someone or actually intervening when professional counsel appears necessary. . . . Life is not always easy, especially for those who struggle with both their difference and their inherent nature, but one thing is universal—we are all human beings and we have the capacity to take better care of each other.[94]

FUTURE RESEARCH

After all these studies, what do we still need to learn? Although some questions that have already been probed need more searching, innovative investigations, Sneider's comments remind us that we must also explore the problems that dwarfs themselves find significant. For example, in 2001, an extended discussion about ADD (attention deficit disorder) appeared on the Dwarfism List, with members wondering whether others were experiencing difficulties of this kind. Further studies might illuminate such questions and suggest interventions. Given the fact that brain research is now proceeding apace, resulting, for example, in important studies that distinguish between the brains of good and poor readers—and identifying what Dr. Sally Shaywitz and researchers at Yale call a "predominantly genetic type of dyslexia,"—it seems important to ascertain how this knowledge can prove useful to the dwarfism community.[95]

Dr. Julie Williams, a neuropsychologist who is also a diastrophic dwarf, recently spoke about some insights gleaned from her experience working with average-statured adolescents who had various brain anomalies. She had observed that social and academic dysfunction in the teen years were frequently the result of cognitive disorders, inadequately diagnosed and treated. She strongly recommended early assessment and intervention as a way of helping youngsters avoid school and personality problems later. (As indicated earlier, "experts" often overlook neurologically based symptoms and wrongly attribute life difficulties to individuals' nonacceptance of their short stature.)

At LPA conferences, there are frequent discussions of courtship, marriage, divorce, and "mixed marriages." The marriage rate among dwarfs has remained much lower than in the general population despite the desire of most to marry, and Hunter's investigations suggest that those who do marry may experience even more stress than those who remain single. A future study might clarify the reasons for both these findings and provide useful information for those seeking or entering into relationships.

Because a significant number of dwarf children have been adopted, and there are also many dwarf adults who have not resolved questions surrounding their own adoptions, there is also a need for a greater understanding of the impact of the dual combination of adoptive status and dwarfism on individuals and their families.

No issue surfaces as frequently in discussions among dwarf individuals as the problem of personal and media ridicule, yet researchers have rarely addressed the subject. Once exception is a study by Tringo (1970) who found that dwarfs and hunchbacks scored lowest in the preference hierarchy of disabilities.[96] Perhaps a similar but more nuanced study could be conducted today to see if an attitude change has occurred and to illuminate and help design ways to counter bigotry.

Not everything lends itself to formal studies. It is important to ascertain subjective factors, through discussion, that have allowed many dwarfs to create satisfying lives. It is equally important to obtain a better understanding of why other individuals surrender to despair. Both affected individuals and clinicians can then integrate these insights into their daily practice.

THE BIRTH OF A CHILD
Parent Issues and Outreach

How different it is when a dwarf child is born today from the way it was at any other moment in history. In previous generations, the family was apt to experience its shock, grief, or confusion in social isolation, without the help of anyone who had experienced bearing a dwarf child. The surrounding society might have demonstrated rejection or pity, and a family would have tended to cope with its difference stoically with little guidance. Only extraordinary parents were able to be as welcoming and appreciative of their dwarf child as of their other children.

The United States today represents a significant improvement. Suggestions of friends, social workers, or physicians or even an Internet search are apt to result in parents finding children and adults who have same condition as their child. They may contact LPA, the Magic Foundation, the Human Growth Foundation, the Turner Syndrome Society, the Osteogenesis Imperfecta Foundation, or one of the other specialized dwarfism groups that provide support and community, as well as excellent pamphlets about dwarfing conditions. Learning about their child's condition and seeing a photograph of a family like the Campbells delighting in their child encourages newcomers to this unfamiliar world (fig. 3.1).

Some parents may eventually find their way to a local, regional, or national meeting where they can converse with dwarfs, family members, and medical professionals and can meet mentors and friends with whom to share the evolving experience of raising a child who has dwarfism. It has become commonplace for a parent in rural Maine to correspond via e-mail or phone with an experienced parent in Texas who has a child with the same rare condition and obtain valuable guidance.

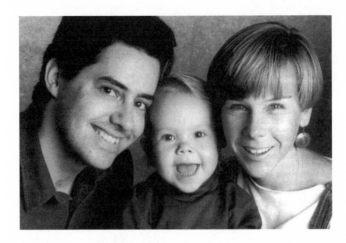

Fig. 3.1. Jim, Hannah, and Joanna Campbell. Photograph courtesy of the Campbell family; photographer: Nina Pratt.

Still, it takes great persistence to navigate the complexity of raising a dwarf child to maturity. At some point, parents might benefit from reading classic works about the impact of a child with a disability on family life, such as Helen Featherstone's *A Difference in the Family*, about a child with multiple problems, or Robert and Suzanne Massie's *Journey*, an informative memoir about their struggle with their son's hemophilia.[1] However, for those with a dwarf child, the best choices are these: Dan Kennedy's *Little People: Looking at the World through My Daughter's Eyes*, which contains a moving account of the period after her birth, as well as thoughtful reflections on dwarfism; Joan Ablon's insightful 1990 article, "Ambiguity and Difference: Families with Dwarf Children"; and her comprehensive earlier volume, *Living with Difference: Families with Dwarf Children*.[2] An increasing number of excellent documentaries about dwarfs also may serve as invaluable resources.

Ablon recounts the profound distress felt by parents. In some instances, "it affects their perception of their own identity and self worth so that they are overwhelmed by shock, anguish, and sorrow."[3] Individual reactions may vary greatly, however, and both temperament and social support can influence how quickly and optimistically the family is able to accommodate.

A recent Australian study confirms that the manner in which the news is delivered and the attitudes of the disclosing health care professionals have a significant effect on the family's coping and adaptation.[4] In most instances, the parents Ablon interviewed were informed within the first twenty-four hours: it was not uncommon for a nurse to perceive the anomaly after the doctor had proclaimed the child "normal." Rarely had the news been presented in an adequately informative and encouraging way, as this account reveals:

> The obstetrician came in first and he was very awkward and didn't say very much. He said, "She's going to be short, but it's going to be all right." He didn't tell us she was going to be a dwarf. He was very embarrassed.
>
> [You mean embarrassed that he hadn't made the correct diagnosis the first night?]
>
> He was just embarrassed that the whole thing had happened at all. The pediatrician came in a bit later. He had never seen a dwarf child. He was very blunt and businesslike. He said, "Your child is a dwarf, and the condition is called achondroplasia. She's never going to be any taller than four feet, and there will be these kinds of problems. But she'll probably be all right." Still, he was really doing his homework. By the second morning he came in with a medical book—a textbook. He turned to a page and said, "This is what she's going to look like." There was a picture of a nude, female adult dwarf with only the face and eyes blackened out. I noticed the webbed fingers and the sway back. Frankly, it was shocking to look at.[5]

In another instance, a mother had to wait more than twelve hours before her son was finally brought to her. All day, the nurses had avoided her, even neglecting her bedpan. Her requests for information about exactly what might be wrong, and for having him brought to her, were met with "I'll go see"—but the nurses never returned. Only after her husband phoned her physician that night did a pediatrician appear: He visited briefly, managed the interview with considerable unease, and departed. Once the baby was brought to her, a nurse "came tearing back," saying, "I'm not supposed to leave you alone with him." The mother thought, "What do they think: I'm going to kill him?" Despite the untoward remarks of doctor and nurses, she was finally relieved to see that the baby *did* have legs and feet, though they were turned in and crooked.[6]

In published and unpublished accounts, tales of mismanagement abound, with reports of remarks such as "You have given birth to a circus dwarf," and, in former days, suggestions that the child be institutionalized or be sent to live with a dwarf troupe in Florida. Physicians are not apt to have received training in the emotional aspects of this extremely important moment of initial revelation. Also, this dwarf infant is often the first one the obstetrician or pediatrician has ever seen, because dwarfs constitute approximately one birth in ten thousand. When a doctor *does* endeavor to become informed and is respectful and sensitive with parents, they generally recognize the effort and express their appreciation.

Cathy Holland's account is a dramatic example of a case of "breaking the news" that began extremely badly and ended well. After examining Martha at 6 weeks of age at a university medical center, doctors informed her parents that she was deaf and hydrocephalic (neither of which proved to be true) and suggested that the Hollands institutionalize her. Cathy fell apart. However, a resident who had overheard the conversation said, "Mrs. Holland, don't believe a word those people say. Martha is exhausted; they've put her through so much the last two days. You take her home and get her on her feet and she'll be fine."[7] Holland comments, "He was just a resident at the time, and he had no business saying to us what he said. But he was one of the gods of our life." Martha went on to become an outstanding high school teacher; her classroom and her courtship with husband Steve Stanley were depicted in the documentary *Dwarfs: Not a Fairy Tale.*

No matter what the first period of adjustment has been like, most parents soon become captivated by their appealing children and enjoy taking part in every experience of their young lives. What may have begun as a disappointment or seemed an insurmountable challenge is soon transformed by the parents' appreciation of this emerging and very interesting personality. For the family of Nima Ghavani

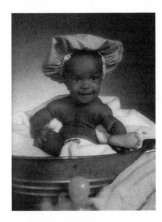

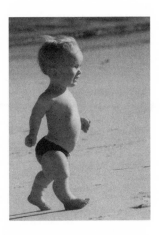

Fig. 3.2. Nima Ghavami, from the United Kingdom. Photograph courtesy of Angela Ghavami.

Fig. 3.3. Jeremy Brackenbury, from New Zealand. Photograph courtesy of James Brackenbury and Caela Kern.

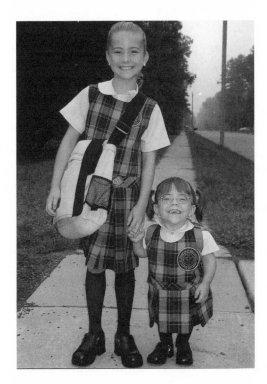

Fig. 3.4. Mackenzie Trush, age 5 years (*right*), and sister Kylie, age 8 years. Photograph courtesy of the Trush family.

in the United Kingdom, a bath is marvelous fun (fig. 3.2); for Jeremy Brackenbury's parents, seeing their son stride across the sand makes a day at the beach in New Zealand just perfect (fig. 3.3); for the Trush family in Pennsylvania, whose daughter was misdiagnosed before birth and whose early years offered anxiety-producing medical problems, watching their daughter Mackenzie and sister Kylie set out cheerfully for school is a miracle (fig. 3.4). The joy of "ordinary experiences" is heightened for parents such as these, for whom each milestone is extraordinarily meaningful.

In 1982, when my daughter Anna was 7, Joan Weiss, then the social worker at the Moore Clinic of Johns Hopkins, organized a thought-provoking training session called PACT (Parent and Communications Training) for parents willing to serve as resource persons for families of newborn dwarfs. Because of our own experiences, my husband, Saul, and I were happy to become part of this program that would help families get off to a good start. Particularly during the next decade, I served as a resource for parents of newborns and spoke to groups of residents about the experiences of families with dwarf children, including such issues as "how to deliver the news" and parental attitudes toward limb lengthening.

The second training session Saul and I attended had a combined membership of average- and short-statured adults. Many of the parents who attended the training sessions went on to assume important roles in LPA. Vita Gagne, for example, helped found and with LP Mary Carten continues to coadminister the Diastrophic Help Web page and the online Diastrophic Dynamics Newsletter; she also offers guidance on the Parents of Little People 2 (POLP2) discussion group.

Recently, LPA leadership has become more proactive, designing an ambitious outreach program, but when PACT was initiated in 1982, such programs were still uncommon. Energized after the workshops, a committee of New York parents sent materials to obstetrics and genetics departments at approximately fifty hospitals in the metropolitan New York area and to a few important agencies, such as the New York City Self-Help Clearing House, sparking many referrals. The importance of maintaining ongoing contact between local chapters and surrounding institutions cannot be overemphasized.

Although the number of calls to the New York Mets chapter waned, the original outreach had been productive. "How come it's always the mother who calls, never the father?" eleven-year-old Anna once asked. In all the years, only on three occasions has a man called—clearly, the evolving division of labor in modern family life has not altered the fact that the initial outreach in emotional crises still usually falls to the woman.

Thirty years have passed since Anna's birth, but a telephone call from the mother of a newborn still makes me relive my former confusion. I remember my urgency to know everything before I could know anything; how I yearned to prophesy a joyful future for my child, then have the power to make it come true. So I try to be a straightforward but encouraging "reader and adviser." Even though we will probably make an appointment to meet, we usually spend the better part of an hour on the telephone. I ask about her family, about how the birth went, and about how she was told about her child's condition. Sometimes the questioner is hesitant; I let it be known that even the craziest-seeming fears need to be aired and that no question is too indelicate.

"Do they all have high-pitched voices like the Munchkins?" one will ask. Most often the caller is the parent of a child with a bone deformity, and usually only those dwarfs who manifest either endocrine problems or the most profound short stature have notably reedy voices. Besides, even these do not manifest the technically altered voices in *The Wizard of Oz*. Almost everyone asks, "Do other children make fun of her all the time?," fearing their child will be the victim of incessant ridicule and abuse. I assure them that although there will be comments, especially in a new school situation, ruthless heckling occurs very rarely.

On the other hand, recognition is assured. Once the child is established in school, the physical difference dictates that almost everyone will know her by name. When Anna was in elementary school, she and I would be walking down the street, and some child would greet us with a cheerful "hello." "Who's that?" I'd ask. She didn't know the other child—but everyone recognized her, and often felt that they knew her better than they actually did. And although there were occasional rude remarks from strangers, there were also exclamations of, "Oh, how cute she is!"

The new mother, however, imagines that raising a dwarf child is mostly problematic. For most parents, the hurdle is not the need to overcome their own rejection of the child, but rather the terror that they have brought into the world a child who is doomed to unhappiness. "Do they marry?" the woman asks. (Yes, often.) "What jobs can they do?" (Almost anything, except jobs requiring great physical strength, or standing up constantly.) "Did your daughter go to a special school?" (No.)

That first contact usually moves me profoundly. How lucky it is that in this vast world of people, the caller had been able to find me. How lucky I am to have had the privilege and satisfaction of being there at that crucial, emotional moment. The confusion of the early days is inevitable and often overwhelming, but in general the less alone one is, the less dejected. If close friends and family can fuss over the baby, genuinely interested and natural much of the time, the couple is heartened. And conversely, if the couple does not go into deep mourning, others will be less apt to regard the event as tragic.

The most vital contribution to the situation is made by the parents' personalities and value systems. But other crucial assets are good family and friends, contact with a medical center that has expertise in dwarfism, and contact with at least one other set of parents who are raising and enjoying a dwarf child. For families whose child has a disability, even more than for the general population, freedom from serious financial insecurity makes a huge difference. I kept a record of families I spoke with in the early years. One of the most memorable was the very first family. This is a portion of the letter that Sue Thurman wrote us:

> David was born July 21, 1980. I feel like I am living a nightmare. Let me explain what I mean by that. We were told that David was deaf, retarded mentally, had some muscle disease, heart disease, and some kind of spine and hip disease. I've been to four pediatricians, two bone doctors, and a neurologist, who were cold, uncaring, and unhelpful in

recommending additional help. I strongly suspected David was a dwarf by the size of his arms, neck and shoulder areas. The doctors did not agree with me at all. I went to another pediatrician and told her nothing, and after examining David she told me she strongly suspected dwarfism. She later took X-rays and they confirmed her suspicions. One of my dearest friends of twelve years is a dwarf, and I contacted her, and she put me in touch with Beth [Beth Wason Loyless, an LP elementary school teacher]. She in turn contacted me and told me you were always available to any parents with this condition to help and encourage.

Right now I guess I'm still numb. I tell people of David's condition and it doesn't seem real. Other times I feel very strong and confident in our future and still other times I feel incompetent and unable to handle the situation.[8]

Parents have frequently reported misdiagnoses, attempts to treat for hydrocephalus when none was present, and distressingly vague descriptions of the child's condition. During many presentations, the physician's discomfort was manifest, and the parents were sent home with no referrals or inappropriate referrals—either to medical facilities or to support groups. When a doctor does offer accurate information and communicates it with warmth and understanding, parents recognize such efforts and are very grateful. When Dr. Steven Kopits, the prominent orthopedist to dwarf children, was introduced to a new infant, he would typically engage infant and parents and remark, "What a beautiful baby!" He would show pleasure in the encounter, and after a careful examination, would prove a gold mine of information. Now that the Academy of Pediatrics has published guidelines to help pediatricians treat children with genetic disorders, and consciousness is being raised in other ways as well, it is hoped that good experiences like these will become more commonplace.[9]

In earlier eras, that was rarely the case. Sue Thurman's letter encapsulates many of the elements that parents experience after the birth of their dwarf child—disbelief, numbness, fear of being blamed by one's child, emotional lability, and swings in self-confidence. Despite cultural and age differences, the Thurmans and we were locked together by intense feelings for our children. We visited each other several times during the first year of our acquaintance and later saw each other occasionally at meetings. I tracked them down in Sioux Falls, South Dakota, and telephoned them to ask permission to use Sue's letter.

David answered the phone, and I inquired about his current activities. He was 19 years old, working part-time as a customer-service representative for a credit card company and part-time for his church. In addition, he was an assistant director for his LPA region. When I spoke with Sue, she talked about a new mother that she had met just the week before who had a dismissive pediatrician; Sue felt very glad to be part of the "chain of help."

Sue and Ed were pleased with the young man David had become. He had been featured on a television talk show in Missouri. Sue was glad to report that after having suffered from spinal stenosis and having been unable to walk more than a block without pain, David had been operated on in 1998 by a skilled neurosurgeon in Missouri and was now transformed, physically active and pain free. But Sue could still feel her way back to those early days when, night after night, she would rock David and say, "I'm sorry, I'm sorry." (Fig. 3.5.)

I have selected a few stories to offer a sense of the wide range of persons encountered, and some of the difficulties that they have faced. I visited April and her partner, Susan, at their Chelsea apartment. Susan and April had decided to have babies close together by artificial insemination. Their firstborn, Michael, was an achondroplastic dwarf. April, a psychologist, would later write a book for lesbian families in which she would include an account of her own experiences with Michael. April and Susan visited us at home shortly after I had visited them. They had worried about the additional stigma that dwarfism might place on their son, in a family already defined by its difference; meeting Anna provided them with much reassurance and encouragement.

Sadly, four months later, April called to say that Michael had died of sudden infant death syndrome (SIDS). (Only later was it recognized

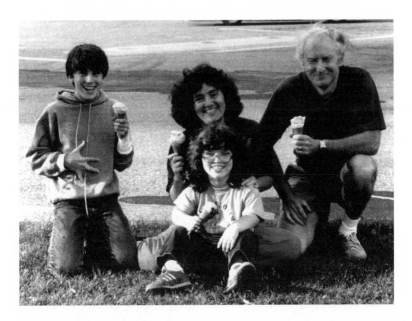

Fig. 3.5. Adelson family: (*from left*) David, Betty, and Saul; (*front*) Anna. Photograph courtesy of the Adelson family.

that achondroplastic babies with particularly narrow foramen magnums have an increased risk of sleep apnea, and therefore of crib death.) I attended Michael's funeral and was moved by the love and warmth among attendees; I communicated with April a couple of times after Michael's death—once referring a patient, and at another time complimenting her on an article she had written. I also contacted her when research about SIDS in achondroplasia began to be published, clarifying the possible cause of Michael's death. The couple has two other children, one born close to the time Michael was born, the other afterward. The year with Michael affected them profoundly, as it had propelled them briefly into the world of difference and disability, and then loss. The experience of coping with the birth of a dwarf infant, even when it is not followed by decades of caregiving, forces one to confront one's values, and find one's strength.

Those of us who have served as mentors to new parents have learned that people need to be allowed to feel whatever they are feeling rather than be counseled according to a preconceived program. Although the details vary, in most instances that I know of the adults have gone on to love each other and their children and to raise their children reasonably well despite the strains.

If family or financial problems exist, however, the birth is geometrically more difficult to deal with. Several single mothers from poor families whom I referred to Johns Hopkins or the International Center for Skeletal Dysplasia were able to manage the train trip once, but the expense of further travel soon became too much for them. Occasionally a family relocated after entering treatment and subsequently could not afford plane fare. It has not been uncommon for their local specialists to insist that they are equally competent and to disparage the renowned physicians at major dwarfism centers; sometimes the family becomes aware subsequently that their child's condition has deteriorated drastically as a result of improper care. It is difficult to find superb physicians willing to undertake surgery on these seriously compromised patients, especially if the patients are uninsured.

Fortunately, most of the families who contacted us have had happier outcomes. They confronted problems that no family is immune to—single-parenthood, job loss, family medical crises—but sought help and support, persevered, and in a majority of cases maintained some contact with LPA. It helped if they had already fought some battles. Steve and Devorah Rifkind, for instance, had been active in liberal causes. They had had to deal with their ethnic difference; Steve is Jewish, and Devorah's background is Latino and Chinese. They were somewhat less vulnerable to "what people might think."

Still, their road would not be an easy one. In the majority of dwarf births, short stature and future concerns dominate the conversation; for the Rifkinds, life-and-death questions took over. Their baby, Risa, was born with SED congenita (fig. 3.6). In the first year of her life the fact that she was a dwarf became secondary to all her other tribulations: she had had serious breathing problems, a cleft palate that caused eating difficulties, and a leg deformity that also required surgery. Keeping her alive was the overwhelming concern, as was the fear that during one of her bouts of apnea, the loss of oxygen would leave

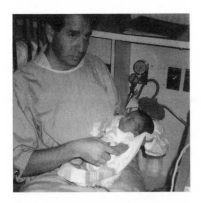

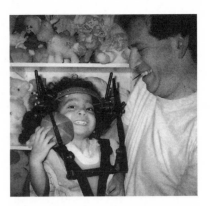

Fig. 3.6. Risa Rifkind with her father, Steven. Photograph courtesy of the Rifkind
family.

Fig. 3.7. Risa Rifkind in a stabilizing halo.
Photograph courtesy of the Rifkind family.

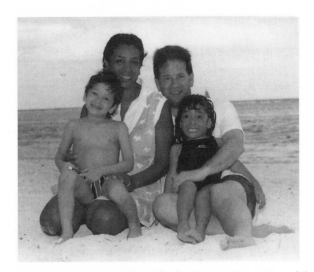

Fig. 3.8. Devorah, Steven, Julian, and Risa Rifkind. Photograph courtesy of the Rifkind
family.

her with brain damage. And so this couple was put to an extraordinary test, needing to survive at their jobs, in their marriage, and in
their individual spirits, despite Risa's repeated crises and surgeries
(fig. 3.7).

When their son Julian was born, they realized that another child in
the family helps reduce the chance of overfocusing on the affected

child; it also increases hubbub and provides a sense of normalcy (fig. 3.8). Risa has turned out to be a bright, engaging, and confident child. The family has rejoiced in her school successes and milestones, such as her bat mitzvah, which was attended by a spectacularly diverse crowd of family and friends, in religion, ethnicity, and height. Not all referrals have resulted in happy endings. Especially vivid in my mind are several brief encounters with families unable to overcome their initial anxieties about social opprobrium and the difficulties of raising a child with a disability. In one middle-class family that I met shortly after their child was born, the mother had developed postpartum depression. At their invitation, our family and an LP couple (at separate times) visited with them and offered an honest but generally sanguine picture of our lives and what their family might expect. The parents ultimately decided to give the baby up for adoption.

Several years later, the mother and I had a conversation in which she asked me if I judged her harshly for her decision. I discovered, perhaps surprisingly, that I did not. I had some concern, however, about what her other children, once grown, would make of their sibling's exile; I also anticipated that the adopted child would experience some emotional turbulence later. But I hoped that having found a home with enthusiastic, nurturing parents would prove to be the most important consideration for this child.

The availability of ultrasound and prenatal diagnosis sometimes presents even more troubling situations. On one occasion, a genetics counselor at a major teaching hospital called to tell me about a patient who had just learned that the child she was carrying was an achondroplastic dwarf: she was seven months pregnant and wanted to speak with the parent of a similar child.

I phoned her immediately, answered her many questions, and offered my view that once the initial shock was absorbed, raising a child with achondroplasia did not represent the most daunting of tasks and that most parents I knew had found it quite rewarding. She revealed that she and her husband were in their thirties, both successful professionals in a second marriage, and living in the suburbs. She was extremely happy; her wedding, her home, her marriage, all aspects of her life now seemed perfect. She introduced the subject of beauty, indicating that this area was a stumbling block for her; she and her husband were good looking, and she supposed that she might even be called vain. She had been looking forward to a good-looking child, one who could participate with them in all the athletic pursuits they both enjoyed.

Her husband was away on a business trip; she had just gotten the news about the baby and had only spoken with him on the phone. When I called back that evening to confirm the time of our meeting, she said she could not talk then but would call me the next day. When she did, it was to reveal that she and her husband had decided to terminate the pregnancy; a medical professional had referred her to a willing doctor in another state. My efforts to have her meet with us, or if not, to consider the possibility of offering the baby for adoption by one of the many prospective LP parents eager for a child, were unavailing. I left the phone shaken.

Of course, that the woman was pregnant with a dwarf child like my own had a significant impact. It is clear that in this brave new medical world the polarized ideological stances of pro-choice and anti-choice advocates require revisiting. A great deal of discussion among persons with disabilities and their families, geneticists, and hospital ethicists will be necessary if individuals and institutions are to deal with these issues reflectively and wisely.

Whether parents are told about their dwarf child before or after the birth, they often experience conflicted feelings, the most common of which Ablon identifies as initial stunned associations to the word dwarf (e.g., to leprechauns or circuses); openly emotional reactions of mothers and stoic stances of fathers; varied styles of informing families and friends, and those recipients' varied reactions; and significant effects of the birth on marital relationships. Though the situation has improved somewhat with the advent of documentaries and other positive representations of dwarfs in the media, the mystique of dwarfism and its countless associations still figure into many parents' reactions. Because most have known few, if any, dwarfs previously, they tend to be vulnerable to negative mythic stereotypes and to feel totally in the dark about what kind of real future they dare hope for: "The problem is, we wanted to know too much. When you have a normal kid, you don't sit and anticipate everything that's going to happen to him for the next 18 years. You don't say, 'He's going to get busted for smoking pot, and he's going to misuse the car, and he's going to have problems dating!' You don't worry about all that ahead. But that was our problem after Sid was born. We were worried about everything. We anticipated all the problems and all the agonies, and everything he was going to have in his life."[10]

A second ambiguity involves the parents' uncertainty about their relationship with the child's dwarf identity as the child develops. On the one hand, they sometimes insist they treated this child no differently from their other children; in the next breath, they say they had a constant or recurrent awareness of the fact of the difference caused by the child's dwarfism. Some parents would go for a time without such consciousness; and suddenly, a specific encounter, or just catching sight of their son or daughter with taller friends, would bring it home to them.

A similar sort of commuting between points of view occurs with respect to disability status. Although most dwarfs are not significantly impaired most of the time, there are those who experience several surgeries or require walkers or scooters. A good many go back and forth between able and less able status. Contradictions abound. Although many dwarf children or adults may take advantage of a handicapped sticker in some situations, they may still not acknowledge themselves as having a disability.

Ablon concludes that parents who are able to accomplish the tasks of normalization and demythologization can experience considerable relief. Their task has been made somewhat easier, now that dwarfs are no longer presented only as elves, space creatures, and purveyors of magic. The recent wave of more realistic presentations in documentaries, television talk shows, and sitcoms has somewhat penetrated public consciousness.

The Discovery Channel's *Dwarfs: Standing Tall* is repeated regularly, and many viewers praise it. Will the parents of a newborn dwarf daughter, who have regularly enjoyed watching dwarf actress Mere- dith Eaton in a starring role as an attractive, capable attorney on *Fam- ily Law*, view their her own daughter's prospects more optimistically than previous generations did? One might guess that they would not experience the same confusion or negative charge as parents whose only previous associations with dwarfs were elves and circus clowns.

It helps immeasurably to have one of the booklets and brochures published by dwarfism groups and specialized centers. Thirty years ago, parents had to visit medical libraries, often trying to decipher frightening and unintelligible technical accounts, to gain even mini- mal understanding of their child's condition. Now, every organiza- tion has detailed, wonderfully produced literature. Among the best are the publications of the Midwest Regional Bone Dysplasia Clinic, which has produced several booklets about both common and rare skeletal dysplasia conditions. Each booklet includes the "natural his- tory" of the condition (what developments and medical problems may be anticipated at various stages), discusses how to monitor them, and tells what therapies are available. It also advises parents what spe- cial considerations should be taken into account in a school setting.

The pamphlet on achondroplasia is particularly useful. Parents previously would visit their pediatricians, who consulted their height charts, and unhelpfully told the parents that their children were at the second percentile of the normal population. They were not apt to have a clue as to the range of when various milestones might be ex- pected, what hazards to watch out for, or what was "normal" for this child. Only doctors who in their training had somehow luckily be- come knowledgeable, or those willing now to make the extra effort to educate themselves, were able to answer the questions parents had. Nor can they be expected to be conversant with the quotidian aspects of each condition.

For this reason, it is wonderful that a parent can now acquire liter- ature that cautions about what problems to look out for and famil- iarizes the reader with the range of time when various milestones can be anticipated (table 3.1). The graphic representation of the many ways an achondroplastic baby "gets around" (fig. 3.9) is marvelous: it

TABLE 3.1.

When can I expect my child to . . .?

Skill	Range (in months) for children with achondroplasia (25th–90th percentile)	Average age (in months) for average-statured children
Sit, without support*	9–20.5	5.5
Pull to stand	12–20	7.5
Stand alone	16–29	11.5
Walk	14–27	12
Reach	6–15	3.5
Pass object	8.5–14	6
Bang two objects	9–14	8.5
Scribble	15–30	13.5

Source: Pauli, R. M., P. Modaff, E. Fowler, and C. A. Reiser, *To Celebrate: Understanding Developmental Differences in Young Children with Achondroplasia* (Madison: University of Wisconsin, Midwestern Bone Dysplasia Clinic, 1997). See Appendix 2 for further information.

Note: Principally because of various physical features, children with achondroplasia not only have some unusual adaptive ways to perform motor tasks but also show delays in attaining many developmental skills. Such delays usually do not reflect cognitive limits. If your child's development is substantially outside of the ranges given, you should talk with your child's physician.

*We actively discourage unsupported sitting before 12 months of age for babies with achondroplasia.

reassures parents that behaviors that may seem quite strange to outsiders are normal and adaptive for their child. As Pauli et al. note, "Many children with achondroplasia do not pass through the customary stages of ambulatory development that lead to learning how to walk. . . . Only about twenty percent of children with achondroplasia ever crawl in the traditional way. Because of their short arms and legs, those who try to do so find their plump bellies dragging on the floor; because of their large and heavy heads, as well as hypotonia and neck instability, holding the head up for an extended period while crawling is difficult."[11]

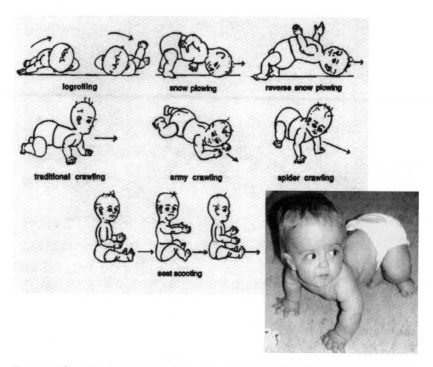

Fig. 3.9. Schematic drawing showing achondroplastic babies learning to get around. Photo demonstrating spider crawling. R. M. Pauli, P. Modaff, E. Fowler, and C. A. Reiser, *To Celebrate: Understanding Developmental Differences in Young Children with Achondroplasia* (Madison: University of Wisconsin, Midwestern Bone Dysplasia Clinic, 1997).

Writing about the early efforts of programs such as PACT brought home to me once again the enormity of the changes that have taken place in the past two decades. These days, it is more common for parents to avidly pursue avenues for assistance than simply wait for mentors to find them. The truly transformational Internet has made networking an option for many.

New parents these days are usually referred first to chapter presidents. Families with specific rare conditions most often contact organizations associated with the condition that they have found on the Web. Online discussion forums, such as the Parents of Little People site (http://groups.yahoo.com/group/parentsoflittlepeople2) are particularly helpful to parents whose children have a form of dwarfism.

Although most parents who post are average-statured, some are LPs, and LPs who are not parents are invited to offer the group the benefit of their experiences. Parents discuss a variety of salient issues—how doctors presented the news; the difficulty establishing accurate diagnoses; the dilemma of how to handle the destructive comments of relatives; the difficulty locating the best information, ongoing medical care, and surgeons for a child's condition; questions relating to interactions with schools and peers, and teenage social problems. In the following quotations, names have been changed or omitted.

Here is the response of one parent to another's concern:

> I was in your place back in Feb. We went to visit Dr. Scott in duPont. What a terrific experience! We just had our second visit on 7/2 and came back with a sense of relief. We are relieved that Paul is being seen by someone who deals with hundreds of children with all kinds of dwarfism. They know exactly when to intervene and when to let it take its course. Dr. Mackenzie acted immediately on getting a brace for Paul. The kyphosis was really worrying us. I didn't know how much until we were driving home, my heart felt so much lighter.
>
> I know you are nervous but I can assure you that it is going to be a great visit. Please e-mail me privately. I have something else I want to forward to you.

Parents can provide each other with a wealth of information. Answering a query posted about hydrocephalus in hypochondroplasia, another parent indicates that she does not know it to be a concern in that condition, but that it occurs in achondroplasia:

> Doctors have now decided that they only be treated for hydrocephalus *if* they become symptomatic to it. Too many babies have been shunted by physicians who see a scan and jump the gun, assuming that they have full-blown hydrocephalus. . . . It is interesting that some patients can have foramen compression, be decompressed and not develop full-blown hydrocephalus *but* then there are others who can have the compression, be decompressed and then have to be shunted a week or two later. No rhyme or reason as to why. I have asked the leading experts about this, they just answer 'We don't know.'

The writer recommends having a baseline computed tomographic (CT) scan or magnetic resonance imaging (MRI) done of the foramen area of the brain to assess fluid on the brain, and then keeping watch. If the child becomes symptomatic to either one, she says, the parent should proceed with a neurosurgeon who is experienced and knowledgeable in treating achondroplasia or hypochondroplasia.

Parents are often better informed about their child's condition than anyone except physicians who specialize in the area. Some may worry about parents offering advice, but in general, they do not overreach. The rare ill-informed posting is apt to be corrected, and respondents are also quick to recommend the specialists with the greatest expertise. Parent mentor Vita Gagne often functions as a consultant on the Parents of Little People site; the mother of Stefan, an adult diastrophic, she is knowledgeable about other conditions as well (fig. 3.10). Vita responded to query I sent her:

> Yes, these Yahoo clubs are *wonderful* and something that has opened up a whole new world for the parents involved. One mom, for instance, said that she wished she lived next door to me, but then I reminded her that I do sort of live right in her house—in her PC—and was willing to answer any questions. . . . The only reason I stay in these clubs is for the same reason we all did the PACT thing years ago—parents of young LPs want and need the advice and info that only parents of older LPs can tell them. What they choose to do with that advice and info is, as always, their choice, but at least they have it with just a few keystrokes.[12]

Vita's response to one parent who had recently received a confirmation of her daughter's diagnosis captures the essence of the situation:

> Nancy, I'm glad that you finally have a diagnosis for Joia. Now you can deal with the practical aspects of this type of short stature, whatever they are. As for pediatricians who overreact, the best thing you can do is provide them with information about Joia's type of dwarfism, or perhaps direct them to a reference in a medical journal article that describes the ins and outs. You will always be the expert on this compared to any pediatrician, though, so get used to it! By becoming the expert,

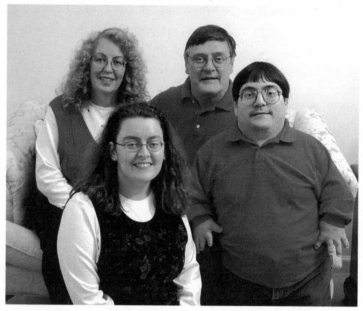

Fig. 3.10. Gagne family: (*back*) Vita and Bob; (*front*) Jenny and Stefan. Photograph courtesy of the Gagne family.

however, you are actually doing yourself and Joia a favor because you'll know when to ignore any pediatrician's overreaction.

Raising a dwarf child has become a collaborative effort between doctors, patients, families, schools, and society overall. Parents on the Parents of Little People Web site have proved especially helpful to each other in preparing the family for their Individualized Educational Planning (IEP) session. These days, the family of a child with any kind of disability is invited to meet with school representatives, including regular and special education teachers, to discuss what accommodations may be necessary for the child's schooling. The family is also entitled to a representative who has special expertise about the child's condition.

Here is a sample of online advice concerning an IEP:

Hi Louise,

A couple of other things to consider are the bathroom (can he use the stalls, reach the faucet, etc.?); will he take the regular bus or a special van, etc.; playground equipment (are there any restrictions on what he can do, i.e. monkey bars and trampolines are usually no-nos).

A good idea is to see if you can bring him into the classroom he'll be in next year. Have him sit in the chairs; are they comfortable? Can he reach the table or desk? The coat rack? Take him into the bathroom and do a "dry" run. By being in the school you'll be able to see for yourself what he might need. Make a list while you're there and bring it with you to the IEP meeting. It's amazing how fast this stuff just flies out of your head when faced with all those official looking people! Good Luck.

For those of us who reached maturity in a previous era, when the educational system either excluded or quarantined children with disparate disabilities in a single stigmatized group, it is wondrous to discover that an effort is now being made to create an environment designed to accommodate each individual's needs. Institutionalized prejudice has become unlawful and often has been replaced by true concern.

The POLP Web site deals with other practical matters, from toy recommendations to musical instruments, and parents share experiences and advice about health insurance and SSI (Supplemental Security Income). But beyond the practical, probably the most moving postings have to do with helping individuals in some sort of emotional distress. Here is one particularly poignant message:

> Ever since we found out about Lauren's diagnosis (Achon.), my mother-in-law has never missed an opportunity to be completely nasty to me and treats Lauren like she has a disease. She has even told me that I am lucky (my husband) hasn't left. According to her it is somehow my fault that Lauren has Achon. (I must have done something while I was pregnant, like stand in front of a microwave, took drugs, etc.) We have tried to teach her about Lauren's condition by taking literature and articles and videos for her to see and her only response was, "Lauren's not going to look like *that* is she?" The rest of my husband's family (including my husband) tolerate her behavior. . . . My own family has been very loving and supportive. Has any-

one ever had to deal with this sort of problem? How did you handle it?

This inquiry elicited many shared experiences and suggestions. One begins:

Hi Joan,

I am sorry that your Mother in Law is behaving so badly. I guess I am fortunate that my M_I_L is very accepting and has so much un-conditional love. Paul's dwarfism is not an issue for her. My parents on the other hand took a bit of time to understand the whole thing. They were in denial for a long time. They would say stuff like, "pull on his arms and legs when you feed him." The ignorance is sometimes real funny. Paul is almost one and they are coming around little by little in accepting that he will be small and have a regular life. I am lucky that most of these conversations are in another language that hubby does not understand. . . .

My father-in-law is another ignoramus. After a very peaceful din-ner last Thanksgiving, hubby put on the Discover video, "Dwarfs: Walking Tall." My father-in-law almost refused to watch it and said, he is not going to be like *that*. "You'll see, he is going to be taller than all of ya! The doctors will fix him." Well, I went off screaming at the top of my lungs (with Paul in my arms) how I do not want him to be in Paul's life if he cannot accept his dwarfism. . . . I might have been a lit-tle emotional but I think I was right in speaking up and letting him know where I stand. . . . [Now] my in-laws babysit every day while we work full-time. My father-in-law is head-over-heels in love with him. We never discussed his acceptance anymore. In time, I hope that he understands that the dwarfism is as much a part of Paul as his sunny smile.

The writer concludes with some suggestions about encouraging communication between the husband and wife that will dispel any hidden animosity or guilt. "Lauren's dwarfism is no one's fault," she writes. "You have been *chosen* to be Lauren's mom. . . . It is an honor. In time the dwarfism will fade in comparison to everything else about her. *Good luck* in your waiting and dealing with this adversity. It will get better!"

A new problem that has arisen since the advent of prenatal screening is the number of dire but incorrect predictions made about the babies evaluated. One mother writes in that she has just been checking the POLP Web site and has been surprised at how many parents had been given wrong diagnoses:

> at 34 weeks we were told our unborn daughter had thanatophoric dysplasia also [a lethal condition]. We too were shown the "Big Red Book" and we were told we could go to Kansas, the only state to perform late term abortions. We went for a second and third opinion and were told the baby had achondroplasia. As of now we have a healthy, beautiful, strong-willed little girl who is undiagnosed but doctors feel she has hypochondroplasia.

It is hoped that growing awareness of the potential for error in prenatal screening will promote further discussion about when to use it and great care in arriving at diagnostic conclusions and presenting the results.

Although more than 80 percent of children born with dwarfing conditions are born to average-statured parents, in an increasing number of families at least one of the parents is a dwarf—or both are, as in the Trombino family. Anu and her husband Mark found an obstetrician, an expert in high-risk pregnancy, to ensure the happy birth of their daughter Priya (fig. 3.11). Concerns of dwarf parents often overlap with those of the average statured, but dwarf individuals may encounter some other problems. They must figure out the logistics of managing the physical demands of caring for a child, including one who may be average statured and heavy to carry. In addition, there may be times when politics comes to the fore, as in a court case, when an average-statured and a short-statured parent are negotiating a divorce, and the dwarf parent's ability to gain custody is threatened by the court's assumption that her size makes her less fit. In response to these types of ever-more-frequent situations, LPA has recently

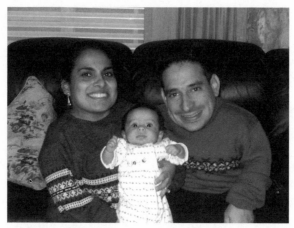

Fig. 3.11. Anu and Mark Trombino with daughter, Priya. Photograph courtesy of the Trombino family.

drafted a position paper entitled, "The Individual with Dwarfism as Parent."[13]

The article makes the competency of dwarf parents clear. It quotes Meg Gil, wife of Arturo Gil, who appeared in the Discovery Health Channel program entitled *Medical Mysteries: Little People, Big Lives:* "We don't parent using our bodies or physical force. . . . It's out of respect and compassion that we parent." Their average-statured daughter Lily tells her friends, "These are my parents, and they can do everything your parents can do, they're just little. . . . I think my parents are good and I like their being little."

Cara Egan, LPA Health Care Policy Advisor, indicated that the group needed to accumulate statistics about the number of dwarf couples with children, as well as the number of single parents in LPA, so that in the case of a court challenge, a dwarf individual's case could be bolstered by the compelling evidence that being short statured does not compromise one's ability to parent, and that many individuals are doing the job very well. To assist dwarf parents expecting a child, Ellen Highland Fernandez, a dwarf parent herself, has written a valuable work.[14]

Whether short or average in height, in most instances, parents of dwarfs who leap into the struggle do find support and discover ways to overcome physical and social obstacles. Often the most stressful occasions occur when a child is experiencing a new phase—joining a playgroup, entering preschool, elementary school, or intermediate school, or feeling left out when friends begin to date. At such times parents commonly need more than ordinary reassurance. Old-timers suggest that parents learn to accept that emotional valleys are as inevitable as peaks, and that, recognizing that they will have some "down days," they should try not to be overly hard on themselves.

Raising one's children as members of various communities makes a world of difference—an extended family, the dwarfism community, a religious community, a hospitable neighborhood, or a political or other interest group. Feeling known and at home in many milieus is especially important to persons with visible differences. How the hazards and benefits of increased scientific knowledge will unfold is uncertain. What is certain is that dwarf children are being born at what seems to be a remarkably great rate. Our most urgent concern, then, is to offer the best information and emotional understanding possible to assure a proper welcome for this latest important child.

4 ~

ORGANIZATIONS
From Self-Help to Advocacy

Dwarfism organizations provide assistance to families from the moment a child is born. Although members may join or leave during various periods, the knowledge that the organization is always available gives them a sense of security. Because they share profound medical and personal events in their lives, many of them come to perceive each other as extended family.

By creating organizations whose primary goal is to provide support and advocacy for affected individuals, members have unleashed a powerful, collaborative effort that has also transformed the medical establishment and promoted social change. Dwarfism groups afford physicians the members' perspectives on ethical issues and patient care; they provide subjects for research; they sometimes offer grants or financial support for medical studies. In return, physicians offer invaluable guidance and caring treatment.

Most often, dwarfism groups were formed by a few determined individuals who found a few like-minded others and partnered with a medical institution. Advocacy goals evolved as the groups pushed for research activity to meet their medical needs and asserted their demands for physical and social accommodation. Although neither patients nor physicians have achieved their goal of assuring health care to all in the United States, they have succeeded in creating a sense of community unprecedented in previous eras.

Early organizations of short-statured persons were generally frivolous enterprises rather than bastions of support or advocacy. The *Guardian* for 25 June 1713 describes the formation of the first recorded association of short-statured persons—a fancy club for little men. On December 10, the shortest day of the year, the main dish at the first meeting at the Little Piazza was shrimp. Members had to be less than five feet. The group put forth the following manifesto: "It is the unanimous opinion of our society that since the race of mankind is granted to have decreased in stature from the beginning to the present, it is the intent of nature itself that men should be little; and we believe that all human kind shall at last grow down to perfection, that is to say, be reduced to our measure."[1]

They were derided by the Tall Club, which "threatened to bring these self-important little persons away in a pair of panniers, and imprison them in a cupboard till they apologized." More than two centuries would pass before substantial groups of short-statured individuals would again organize, but with very different objectives in mind.

LITTLE PEOPLE OF AMERICA

The small cadre who created Little People of America (then called Midgets of America) in 1957 was not completely clear about the group's reason for being. Although most dwarfism groups grew out of the concern of parents about their affected children, this organization was formed by adults. In 1998, I spoke to founder Billy Barty about the group's inception; he described the events with considerable animation.[2]

He had been performing with Spike Jones in Reno, when Nick Bourne, of the Riverside Hotel, spoke to him about organizing a convention of little people. "What do you have in mind?" Barty had asked. Apparently, Bourne had a publicity stunt in mind. To advertise Reno as "the biggest little city in the world," he proposed inviting a group of dwarfs to the hotel and providing free rooms and inexpensive meals. At Barty's invitation, twenty-one persons convened, forming the nucleus of an organization of dwarfs. After the gathering, the attendees contacted hospitals, schools, fraternal organizations, and even prisons to find potential new members.

When the group met in Las Vegas in 1960, it was able to attract 100

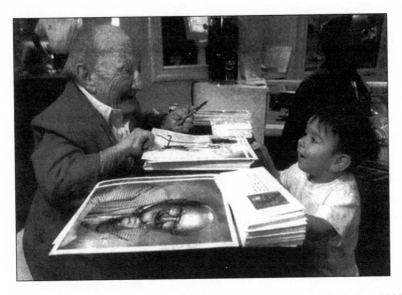

Fig. 4.1. Billy Barty meets with 2-year-old DJ Holland at an autograph signing, 1999. Photograph courtesy of Associated Press

persons; by 2004, it had grown to more than 8,000 members (fig. 4.1). Fewer than half of these are LPs; the rest are family members, medical professionals, and a few others. Given that only about 2,000 of the 8,000 members of LPA are adult LPs, the organization has been remarkably effective, in service to its own members, and in attracting attention in the media and inspiring the creation of groups in other nations.

According to Barty, his original objective was to hold a national convention that "showed to the world that little people aren't just in services, but are capable of doing professional jobs." Later the organization defined its goals more broadly: "The purpose of LPA is to assist its members in adjusting to the social and physical problems of life caused by their small stature through mutual assistance and the personal examples of each of its members."[3] The bylaws recognize the group's deep commitment to the fundamental need "for people of small stature to become useful members of society through education, employment, and social adjustment, and to focus public attention to the fact that the magnitude of any physical limitation is a function of attitude of both the small and average-size person."

Martin Weinberg's influential article and two comprehensive works by Joan Ablon highlight the advantages of LPA membership and the difficulties members are trying to overcome.[4] The significant concerns that Weinberg's informants mentioned in 1968—employment, romance, medical problems, and friendship—have remained compelling. When he queried persons about why they felt good about their experience in LPA, the respondents cited these reasons: "A feeling of security, friendship and fraternalism. Knowing I am not alone and able to talk freely without shyness and embarrassment gives me a sense of security and comfort. I have gained an improved outlook toward myself, my condition and the world in general. I no longer feel sorry for myself."[5] For some persons, a single goal, such as finding a mate, may be the reason for joining. Others may have more radical goals, such as changing the status of dwarfs in society (fig. 4.2).

Individual groups vary, and their ambience has also changed through the years. When my family and I joined LPA in 1974, we were disappointed to find little content at local meetings beyond announcements of the next regional or national convention and the sale of raffle tickets, and we rarely saw more than a handful of attendees. Perhaps the heterogeneity of New York, the quickness of its pace, and the fact that people have busy, complicated lives with many cultural events and distractions had made them less apt to attend meetings. No single explanation can probably account for the differences between the groups that prosper and those that do not. Vigorous personal leadership, especially by short-statured chapter presidents, and physical proximity to a center with medical expertise in dwarfism contribute to a group's vitality, such as those in Texas, Florida, and California.

The Los Angeles group has the additional advantage of a built-in community of entertainment industry professionals, and, until his death in 2000, the energizing presence of Billy Barty. Its members also have access to Cedars-Sinai, a medical center with significant dwarfism expertise that also houses the Skeletal Dysplasia Registry. San Francisco has long had a successful group with monthly business meetings, holiday parties, and summer picnics. Charismatic LP Harriet Stickney, after retiring from teaching, devoted boundless energy

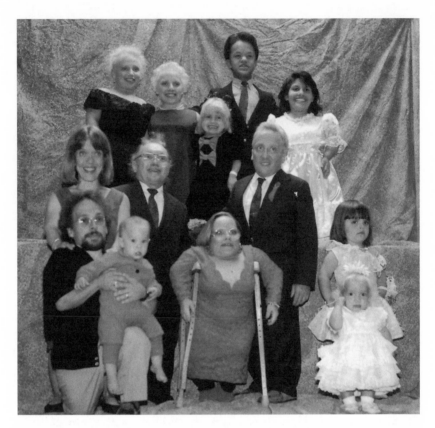

Fig. 4.2. Members of LPA at the 1992 National Conference in San Francisco; Photographer: Gary Parker.

to members and to encouraging average-statured parents of dwarf children. Such devotion of time and energy is rare. In 2003 she and her husband moved back to Wisconsin. The chapter has continued to flourish, with younger activist members and their proximity to helpful medical centers. Two significant presences are Ericka Peasley, clinic coordinator for the Skeletal Dysplasia Center of Kaiser Permanente, and Ginny Foos, clinic coordinator at the Children's Hospital in Oakland; these two institutions constitute the Northern California Skeletal Dysplasia Clinic. In addition, the chapter benefits from the expertise in growth hormone disorders available at University of California, San Francisco and from the talents of orthopedists at Stanford University.

The New York Mets chapter gathered strength in the 1990s under the leadership of energetic presidents Devorah Rifkind and Barbara Brullo (now Spiegel). The four New York area chapters (Mets, Long Islanders, Mid-Hudson, and New Jersey) have recently begun having successful shared activities. In 2003 they were delighted by the creation of the Center for Skeletal Dysplasias at the Hospital for Special Surgery in Manhattan, for which chapter members had long campaigned. Previously, most New Yorkers had to travel to duPont in Delaware, Johns Hopkins, or the International Center for Skeletal Dysplasia in Maryland for treatment.

One problem that LPA and many other voluntary organizations face is the difficulty in attracting minorities. Although dwarfism is equally distributed among all groups, membership tends to be white and middle class. Part of the reason may be that poorer, working-class individuals face more problems and have little time and energy left over after work, parenting, and sometimes church attendance, and that dwarfism is approached differently in their communities. Also, if they attend a small group meeting and find "nobody like me," they are unlikely to return. The next month, another minority family attends and, despite members' efforts, feels alienated by the group's composition. Great efforts must be made to connect people informally, arrange transportation, and encourage personal friendships. Special efforts are currently being made to reach out to the Spanish-speaking community.

Because the fourteen districts and sixty local chapters of LPA are geographically diverse, members look forward to semiannual regional meetings, and especially to annual conferences. No longer called *conventions,* both to reflect their serious purpose and to make attendance tax- deductible, the national conferences are events where short-statured individuals can feel relaxed and, for a change, be a visible critical mass. In addition to nonstop informal socializing, there are also tours of local attractions, talent and fashion shows, a dwarf artists' exhibit and reception, an international reception, and a dance and a banquet. There are also important group presentations and workshops.

Individuals savor the freedom of uninhibited movement in this welcoming, better-fitting world. Hotels make an effort to retrofit rooms for shorter visitors and provide stools at registration desks and reaching sticks for elevator buttons. Attendees' enthusiasm is palpable. Until the bylaws were changed in the 1980s, average-statured members (then known as parents' auxiliary) could not vote. Their enfranchisement, spearheaded by a new generation of activists, represented a leap of faith. The tensions addressed paralleled the ones confronted by other minorities, such as blacks and whites in civil rights groups in the 1960s. The leadership of LPA explained that it was not reasonable to expect rapprochement with the greater society if a trusting working relationship was not forged among LP and average-statured members (usually parents, as 85% of dwarf children are born to individuals of average height). Paul Hagen is budget advisor; Dan Kennedy is LPA Online editor, and others play helpful roles in local chapters. Often an average and a short-statured member will collaborate, such as Vita Gagne and Mary Carten, who run the Diastrophic Web page together. Short-statured adults also serve as role models for average-statured parents and their LP children. Almost all national offices continue to be held by LPs, by general agreement.

In public or political situations a dwarf must represent the group. When LP Angela Van Etten and others fought to institute new access regulations for ATMs, their argument could be made much more effectively because agencies could observe directly that small persons have different size and reach requirements. Cara Egan, former Vice President for Public Relations, made a conscious decision to arrive just a bit late to a meeting in Washington, D.C., where she was representing LPA. She did not hesitate to "make an entrance" and allow the door to shut noisily; she felt it might be important and useful to attract notice visually before verbally promoting her cause.

Through the years, the mission of the group has broadened. In 1986, Len Sawich and several other members formed the Dwarf Athletic Association of America (DAAA). Entrants now compete in boccie ball, power lifting, track and field, basketball, and volleyball. In some instances, courts are modified; for example, a short court design enables players to achieve the feel of full court basketball without the stress of full court running.[6] Dwarfs also compete in World Championship Paralympics. As a result of strong lobbying efforts by DAAA President Pamela Danberg, they have gained the right to compete only against other dwarf athletes in a category such as track and field.

The second International World Dwarf Games were held in Peterboro, England, in 1997; the third in Cologne, Germany, in 2001. At the Peterboro games 200 dwarf athletes competed, including 21 from the United States. The standout of the event was 46-year-old Peter Conico, 4'6", who won six gold medals in swimming, two gold and one silver medal in track and field, and three gold medals in basketball as a member of the U.S. team. Erin Popovich, a 4 foot 2 inch dwarf from Montana, set four world records and won three gold and four silver medals for the United States at the 2000 World Paralympics; she was chosen from among 400 U.S. athletes as flag bearer in closing ceremonies, and, after recovering from osteotomies to relieve knee pain in October 2001, she went on to carry the torch for the Winter Olympic Games in 2002.

In just over a decade, the idea that dwarfs could make athletic participation a significant part of their lives has been realized beyond the originators' wildest dreams. Not only "stars" benefit. The DAAA aims to instill fitness and health as a lifelong process for dwarfs. Pam Prentice's exercise video, *The Perfect Little Body Workout,* represents one important way of encouraging individuals to practice physical-conditioning habits appropriate to them at home.

The adoption committee has also flourished. Many dwarfs are physically unable to have children; others for various reasons prefer to adopt dwarf children who lack loving homes and families. Nancy Rockwood (who died in 2004) headed the Adoption Committee from 1987 to 1999. She helped place children from the United States and, more often today, from countries as far-flung as South Korea, Russia, Bulgaria, India, Colombia, and the Philippines.[7] Maintaining ongoing contact with adoptive families through LPA conferences, she reported that almost all families had been pleased with the outcomes. Later coordinators, such as Joy Wyler, Ruth Stratton, and Kimberly

Ayers, have continued in Rockwood's tradition, communicating that the service's goal is to find a loving home for every dwarf child, whether with LP or average-statured parents. These children sometimes have rare syndromes or medical complications.

Advocacy is one of LPA's most vital functions. In two major battles, the fight to ban dwarf tossing and the campaign to have dwarfs and wheelchair users taken into account when agencies establish access regulations, activist lawyer Angela Van Etten has led the charge. These matters, media issues, and the achievements of members are often addressed in *LPA Today,* an increasingly well-written and professionally produced publication.

In 2002 LPA published its first annual report, describing its programs, including a health advocacy fund, travel fund, artist coalition, educational scholarships, adoption programs, public access initiatives, and community outreach. Its multistep membership data analysis was deemed essential to the medical, health advocacy, and social programs contemplated. For the first time, a director of development was appointed to raise funds to support these programs. Billy Barty's 1957 Reno stunt has led to a successful support group fast becoming a full-fledged member of the activist disability community.

THE HUMAN GROWTH FOUNDATION

The Human Growth Foundation (HGF), a group that originated from the need for treatment of growth hormone deficiency, has 30 chapters and 1,000 members and has published important booklets on growth disorders. Although it has offered assistance to persons whose growth has been restricted for a variety of reasons, its major efforts have involved persons with hypopituitary disorders. HGF also educates people about other growth problems, notably Russell-Silver syndrome, Turner syndrome, and Prader-Willi syndrome, and it has published an excellent booklet about achondroplasia. Its quarterly newsletter, *Fourth Friday,* offers up-to-date research information about such issues as delayed male puberty, intrauterine growth problems, and the effects of growth hormone on cystic fibrosis. It also notes the "starter grants" that it has supported.

Lois Warshauer of Long Island, New York, a prominent figure in HGF through much of its history, joined when her son was four—part of what she called "the second wave." The first wave was the core group that included Barbara and Al Balaban. Committed to finding a solution to their children's growth problems, the parents helped found HGF. They had been willing to mortgage their homes to get the group off the ground and had indefatigably collected the pituitary glands that might make the difference between a child remaining tiny or growing to somewhere between 5'0" and 5'7".

Warshauer speaks movingly of her twenty years as an active member, manning the parent hotline, fund-raising, and coordinating events with doctors. Having done this also helped prepare her for her later administrative positions. "In Human Growth I learned to administer, to speak to groups, and to walk into a hospital like I belonged," she says. "Who was I?—a little housewife—but I put on a blue suit, introduced doctors and parents, and made things happen."

She remembers the difficult times when her son, now 5'1" and married with a child, was getting shots of growth hormone and longed only to "be regular." In those days, one had to find a hospital that had protocols to administer hormones in a research study. After a bad experience at one hospital, the Warshauers went to North Shore where Dr. Fima Lifshitz treated their son. They then served as a referral source for other applicants, often participating in grand rounds.

One difficulty was that final height was unpredictable. Although doctors might mention a figure such as 5'6", for many children achieving that was impossible. Some were not helped at all; those families were apt to become secretive and disappear. An occasional member would continue working for Human Growth even though her child had not benefited. In addition to the distasteful task of imposing a regimen of three injections a week on their child, families had to deal with uncertainty and possible disappointment. How long should treatment be maintained? How tall was tall enough?

Sadly, in later years, she heard from a few former members that they had contracted Creutzfeldt-Jakob syndrome, the debilitating disease that afflicted some patients injected with human pituitary hormone before synthetic hormone became available. And, since the arrival of managed care, another problem that concerned her was that HGH was not available to all who might benefit. Finally, for Lois and others, participation had been a rewarding, almost full-time job. Now, many women are working full-time and their necessary energies have been lost to support groups. A decade ago, unable to attract new members, the New York-Long Island chapter of HGH became inactive.

In 1963, Barbara Balaban's son Jeff received a diagnosis of a hypopituitary deficiency (fig. 4.3). The pediatric endocrinologist told Barbara they had no store but would administer treatment if the Balabans could obtain the glands. She remembered, "We sat and cried for three days. We then proceeded to write a letter to everyone we knew— everyone Al knew at medical school, the parents of our children's friends, neighbors, everyone—asking them to help. We started in October. We went to visit a friend at Christmas and returned to find on our doorstep a container with four glands, making a total of one hundred."

Once they realized that they had more than they currently needed, they agreed to give some away on loan to another child. Persevering in their challenging task, they were tracked down by Gene Latimer, who explained that the government was starting the National Pituitary Agency to collect glands from all contributors. "He told us the top collector had been NIH, the second the VA, and the third was something called Balaban! Would we be willing to join?" says Barbara. "At this point we had years of glands stored. We said that we would turn over our sources and our glands, as long as we were assured that we would always have enough for our child."

The Balabans recognized that collecting pituitary glands could not remain a cottage industry. Under the aegis of Jim Brathovde, five families met at Johns Hopkins, where Dr. Robert Blizzard, then head of pediatric endocrinology, had treated Brathovde's son. Each family

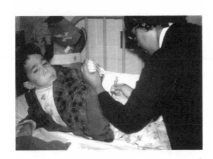

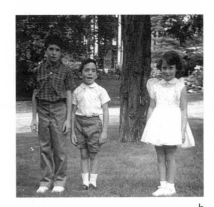

a

b

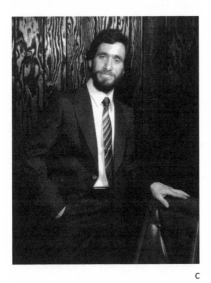

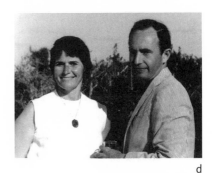

c

d

Fig. 4.3. Human Growth Foundation. (a) Jeff Balaban receiving human growth hormone injection, 1961. (b) Jeff Balaban with older brother, Rob, and younger sister, Julie,
1961. (c) Jeff Balaban as an adult. (d) Barbara and Al Balaban, 1965. Photographs courtesy of Barbara and Al Balaban.

agreed to start a chapter of the organization that would become the
Human Growth Foundation in 1965. Blizzard put members in touch
with physicians and encouraged physicians to offer the names of families to help. The group's mettle was immediately tested when NIH
found it would have to delay a collaborative health study that would

treat 100 children until funding began six months later; the fledgling HGF initiated its organization $25,000 in debt to help.

Help came from many directions. Gwen and Fred Mahler from Texas had a child with a hypopituitary disorder, and Fred, a pilot for TWA, organized other pilots to transport glands to the Hypopituitary Agency. Gwen Mahler, a former stewardess, got Clipped Wings, the airlines' philanthropic group, to raise funds for HGF. Balaban reported that although some treated children grew and others did not, the atmosphere among families was respectful; they felt they were all in it together. Jeff Balaban continued receiving the painful shots three times a week for eight years, between age 8 and 16 years, attaining a final height of 5'5". Finally, unable to stand it, he protested. He stopped treatment although he understood that had he continued, he might have grown a bit more. Barbara remained an HGF member, but passed the torch on to "the second wave," later using her skills on behalf of a breast cancer organization.

Now that synthetic hormone is available and familiar routines in place, the remaining battles of patients with growth hormone deficiency are more likely to be fought against recalcitrant insurance companies. Nevertheless, the memories of the early years remain vivid for Barbara and others. She speaks of her undying gratitude to Dr. Blizzard, declaring that doctors like him "redefined the nature of medical care."

Although HGF has provided literature and seed money for research into a variety of dwarfing conditions, it tends to be identified with pituitary deficiency disorders. There has been some membership overlap between HGF and LPA, but a significant divide remains between persons who are dwarfs and those who seek to graduate out of that group, although both sets of individuals may genuinely understand the problems the other group faces.

THE MAGIC FOUNDATION

Organizations tend to wax and wane as their missions and leadership change. Only a persistent investigator could ferret out the reasons that the Magic Foundation, which covers much of the same diagnostic territory as HGF, was established in 1989, and by now has become another major force in the dwarfism community. In any event, the Magic Foundation (the acronym stands for Major Aspects of Growth in Children) is an important national organization devoted to providing support and education, focusing on growth hormone deficiency, adult growth hormone deficiency, congenital adrenal hyperplasia, precocious puberty, Russell-Silver syndrome, Turner syndrome, and others—approximately 100 conditions altogether. Most members, however, have a child or adult in the family who is affected by growth hormone deficiency or a thyroid or other glandular disorder.

Five families of children confronting growth disorders formed the Magic Foundation. The group's Web site describes how the Chicago-based foundation grew from a kitchen-table project grounded in the women's common concern about their children into a major national organization. It expanded from twenty members in 1989 to more than 6,000 in a dozen years; it has published many brochures, established a variety of divisions, and responded to callers' concerns.

THE NATIONAL MUCOPOLYSACCHARIDOSIS SOCIETY

Members of the National Mucopolysaccharidosis (MPS) Society confront a situation that differs from that of most other dwarfing conditions. The mucopolysaccharidoses (MPS) and mucolipidoses (ML) are genetic lysosomal storage disorders caused by the body's inability to produce certain enzymes that normally break down dead cells, often causing damage to the heart, bones, joints, respiratory system, and central nervous system. Although the diseases may not be noticeable at birth, the signs and symptoms develop with age as more cells become damaged by accumulated deposits.[8]

Although children with mucopolysaccharidosis or mucolipidosis are short statured, this is not their greatest problem. Although these children are affected to different degrees, the conditions tend to be more severe and are often life threatening. Among the MPS syndromes discussed in greater detail on the Web site are Hurler, Scheie, Hurler Scheie, Hunter, Sanfillipo, Morquio, Maroteaux-Lamy, and Sly syndromes; I-cell disease and pseudo-Hurler polydystrophy are also discussed.

Despite its difference from various other dwarfism groups, the essential function of the National MPS Society is the same: to help families cope as they wend their way through the maze of informational and emotional trials. When I called Marie Capobianco, the organization's fourth president, she was retiring after twenty years.[9] She was still answering the hotline at her Long Island home, however, offering help to anxious callers and putting out a newsletter.

She had had three children: a son, born in 1974, a daughter, born in 1976, and another daughter, born in 1978. The first two children had Hurler syndrome and eventually died of it. Her youngest daughter does not have it but is a carrier. Significant personality change as well as physical change accompanies this condition. Capobianco spoke with emotion about the difficulties of her years raising "two wild kids"—dealing with the extraordinary physical demands of the earlier period and the grief of caring for them in a vegetative state in the later period. Although eventually she prayed for God to take them, in the meantime she had focused on tasks such as finding good schools and other accommodations.

The organization's origins resemble the other groups'. In 1975 three or four mothers met at Johns Hopkins with social workers Jill Sugar and Joan Weiss and Dr. Irene Maumenee and created the organization. Through the years, they worked at finding affected families, making referrals, and encouraging research. Sometimes, when their children died the families left the group; in Capobianco's case that did not happen. Currently the group has 700 members. I spoke with Linda Shine, then the new president of the MPS society, about the outlook for treatment breakthroughs. All too often there had been encouraging news and disappointing outcomes.[10] An encouraging development had occurred through clinical trials of a chemically reproduced enzyme for Hurler and Hurler/Scheie syndromes that could not ameliorate retardation but did affect bone quality. One boy experienced a dramatic change in facial structure, and his headaches were helped. The real change, she anticipated, would ultimately come through gene transplants. Shine emphasized the urgent need for research for MPS/ML conditions.

In January 2003, the FDA Endocrinologic and Metabolic Disease Committee voted unanimously that Aldurazyme (laronidase), an enzyme replacement for the treatment of MPS I, would be made available to patients as soon as possible.[11] The medication had been shown to increase pulmonary capacity and endurance.

No effective treatment yet exists for pseudo-Hurler syndrome (ML III), a condition that affects Tetsuya, Sally and Yuki Motomura's 20-year-old son.[12] Their family, which includes two older sons, Jun and Kazuma, has led a peripatetic existence because of Yuki's position as a diplomat (fig. 4.4). Sally is a talented artist from Rhodesia (now Zimbabwe). When Tetsuya was born in Paris, nothing had seemed unusual, but he stopped growing by the age of 2. When he was evaluated at 1½, the first physician incorrectly recommended surgical intervention; later evaluations in France, England, and Japan, however, confirmed that Tetsuya had pseudo-Hurler dystrophy. Language problems in France had made it difficult to communicate the nature of the condition.

The Japanese doctor recommended a support group in England, where through a "weird coincidence," Sally encountered a woman, whom she had once met briefly at a party in Japan, whose child had Hunter syndrome—and whose handling of her child Sally had admired. That MPS connection proved invaluable; the MPS societies active in many countries and the international symposia are useful for researchers and for family support. The following years were filled with searching for good medical advice and appropriate schools as the family relocated; Tetsuya's happiest time was in Austria, where he was mainstreamed at a small K–12 school, with the assistance of Sally's visiting niece, who served as his aide.

Both medical and schooling issues needed increased attention as tissue became denser and Tetsuya was less supple and required a wheelchair. The greatest medical assistance was offered by a New York

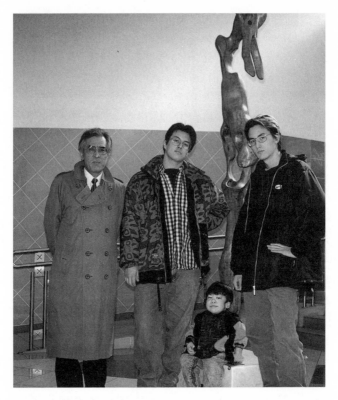

Fig. 4.4. Tetsuya Motomura with father, Yuki, and brothers, Jun (*left*) and Kazuma (*right*). Photograph courtesy of the Motomura family.

pulmonologist who recommended a CPAP device. Tetsuya had been suffering from puffiness, enormous fatigue, and bad night sweats and other symptoms; with the device, his quality of life improved enormously.

The course of each condition differs. The nature of each condition may be understood not only by reading about studies or details in the group's excellent pamphlets, but sometimes in photographs. Sally showed me a compelling photograph of two brothers with Hunter syndrome (at different stages of their disease's progress). The lively expressiveness in the face of the younger brother had disappeared from the face of the older one, and the sense of loss was palpable.

The "search for a cure" remains a central focus for members of the

MPS society, who keep tuned in for the latest studies.[13] As soon as results are available, they are posted on the National MPS Society Web site. Although it had been a relatively small and undercapitalized group, this organization and its Canadian counterpart have recently embarked on serious fund-raising efforts, while continuing their valuable support work. Because of the enormous demands presented by caring for their children, they have a harder time finding members with energy for volunteerism. Still, with the help of unaffected friends, they have initiated "walk and run" fund-raisers, and in 2003 awarded seven grants of $30,000 each for research. The experiences of families with MPS/ML can be found on the organization's Web site, and posts of those with Morquio syndrome, a serious but less extreme form of MPS, can be found through links on LPA Online.[14]

THE TURNER SYNDROME SOCIETY

Turner syndrome is a chromosomal condition that occurs when one of the two X chromosomes normally found in females is missing or incomplete. It is one of the most common chromosomal abnormalities, occurring in about 1 of 2,500 live female births. Approximately 50,000 girls and women are affected in the United States, with approximately 800 babies with Turner syndrome being born each year. The most common characteristics of this syndrome are short stature and lack of ovarian development, sometimes accompanied by kidney, thyroid, cardiovascular, skeletal, or hearing problems.[15]

Among the treatments that have been of enormous importance to members are growth hormone treatment, estrogen replacement therapy, and reproductive technology allowing those who choose to be able to bear their husbands' children by using implanted embryos. Through the use of growth hormone, many girls with Turner syndrome are able to gain two to four inches more than their expected height. The society is of great assistance to families throughout their lives: when the diagnosis is presented to parents, when preadolescent and adolescent girls are coming to terms with their feminine identities and fertility concerns, and in adulthood, when they are confronted with the realities of marriage and the possibility of childbearing. The society also regularly provides members with updates on a variety of health matters.

The Turner's Syndrome Society of Canada was formed in 1981 and included some participants from other countries. In 1987 two women, Lynn Tesch and Julia Rickert, founded the Turner Syndrome Society of the United States. Feeling strongly that they wanted to make a vital difference for future generations of girls and women, they reached out for funding, notably to pharmaceutical groups. An ongoing relationship was initiated, prompted in part because affected persons use growth hormone, estrogens, and other medications. The Society has fulfilled a pressing need and has grown rapidly. By 2004, it had fifty-five chapters and support groups, with 2,350 members and 11,000 individuals on its mailing list (fig. 4.5).

Lexi Krell from Alaska and Emily Pawlowski from New Hampshire, two 14-year-old girls with Turner syndrome, and Rebecca, Emily's unaffected 12-year-old sister, attended the society's 2004 convention in St. Louis. Even more than for most adolescents, the teenage years are a crucial period for young women with Turner syndrome.

Lori-Ann Pawlowski, Emily and Rebecca's mother, is president of the Northern New England Turner Society. Both she and Lexi's mother, Kathy Krell, who is a nurse, emphasize the importance of ongoing contact. Kathy feels that the group opened her eyes to how important it is to network and do one's homework, at both early and later stages as new information appears. Because Emily was diagnosed at birth and Lexi's condition was first recognized when her growth dropped off at 18 months, they were able to begin growth hormone treatment early. Emily is now 5'1½" and Lexi is 5'2". Before the advent of growth hormone and sophisticated diagnostic procedures, their final height would have been closer to 4'8"—the average for untreated Turner girls.

Passing on information about the help that is available is a vital function of this organization. It also has assembled an impressive packet of informational materials, including newsletters, fact sheets, a medical bibliography, and a personal article by Lynn-Georgia Tesch,

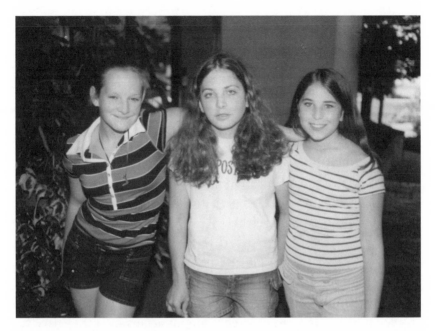

Fig. 4.5. Lexi Knell and Emily Pawlowski, 14-year-old teenagers with Turner syndrome, and Rebecca Pawlowski, Emily's unaffected 12-year-old sister, attending a Turner Syndrome Society convention in 2004. Photograph courtesy of the Turner Syndrome Society.

its executive director from 1987 to 2000, when Merriott J. Terry succeeded her. In her account, Tesch expresses what the group has meant to her and may mean to others: "The chance to know others like yourself is one of, if not the greatest, aid in making the best of a poor situation. To know and talk to another who has had similar experiences is immeasurably helpful. It softens the pain of feeling like a stranger in one's own land. I know my confidence and self-esteem have increased in direct proportion to the strength and number of friendships I have made, particularly in the past year or two, with other Turner syndrome women."[16]

THE OSTEOGENESIS IMPERFECTA FOUNDATION

Osteogenesis imperfecta (OI), sometimes called brittle-bone disease, is a genetic disorder of imperfectly formed bone collagen, characterized by bones that break with little or no apparent cause.[17] It is classified in five types, ranging in severity. Persons may have a normal appearance with only occasional fractures or severe growth retardation and as many as 200 fractures in a lifetime. Only about half of those with OI are short statured. Especially when a child is seriously affected, medical and caregiving problems can be formidable. For parents, the emotional concerns are substantial. Balancing the need for physical protection with the task of encouraging autonomy in children is no simple feat, and dealing with the round of unpredictable calamities and pain presents a perpetual problem for parents and the affected individuals themselves.

Many readers responded to articles by Gemma Geisman published in *Redbook Magazine* in 1968 and 1970. About ten or twelve families got together to form the foundation in the Chicago area where several of the families had gone for treatment at Shriners Hospital, and in 1972 the first medical conference for physicians and geneticists was held.[18] Once again, the enterprise of a single person, and the eagerness of a few others, led to a enormously productive collaboration between families and the medical establishment. The group now has more than 1,000 members: most either have OI or are family members of persons with OI; some are physicians and other medical staff. Unlike some other groups, the OI Foundation does not have chapters, but twenty support groups do exist, and referrals are made to them through a central office in Gaithersville, Maryland.

Especially when a child is seriously affected, medical and caregiving problems can be formidable. Interventions have included splinting the fractures or surgically implanting metal rods. Bracing is often needed to reduce scoliosis. Some types include dental and hearing problems and diaphoresis (excessive perspiration). Pain control is an ongoing concern, especially in the most severe cases.

Many of the personal stories of parents who are raising a child with OI describe an unending and often fruitless search for significant amelioration of symptoms. Interesting accounts of families' efforts to find solutions are often posted.[19] Finally, there seems to be real progress. In 1998 an encouraging study at Montreal Hospital for Children reported that the drug pamidromate caused a reduction of bone loss and significant increases in bone mineral content.[20] Chronic pain was reduced, and the children became more mobile. Further studies have substantiated the results, and suggested that bisphosphonates facilitated early surgical intervention in young children. Articles about treatment with neridronate (administered intravenously) and alendronate and risedronate (given orally) also reported positive findings. At the same time, mouse model investigations have identified worrisome questions as well as reasons for optimism. The OI Foundation's Medical Advisory Council, in an excellent article in 2004, attempted to put research and clinical data into perspective, recommending caution. They noted that despite beneficial increases in bone density, there was some concern that there might also be a detrimental increase in bone stiffness and brittleness after prolonged treatment. They suggested further controlled studies and made recommendations about timing and dosage.

During ongoing scientific conferences such as the annual meetings entitled New Research Strategies in Osteogenesis Imperfecta, first held in 1999, positive and negative results are exchanged. Among the developments discussed by the 27 presenters at the group's 2003 meeting at the Hospital for Special Surgery in New York were studies of collagen structure and formation, mouse models, stem-cell transplantation, and gene suppression, as well as the more specific results of treatment with bisphosphonates and improved surgical techniques.[21] The strengthened partnership between the research community and the Children's Brittle Bone Foundation was also noted. Despite the serious obstacles persons with OI face, their personality profiles suggest that they often exhibit significant talent, positive temperaments, and resiliency.[22]

DWARFISM GROUPS ALTERED IN FUNCTION OR NO LONGER ACTIVE

Other groups, even some that no longer exist, have had significant roles. In 1975 Billy Barty established the Billy Barty Foundation, designed to provide scholarships and offer employment opportunities, adaptive aids, and information to persons who asked for help. Because it did its own fund-raising, mainly through a celebrity golf tournament, and had a small Board of Directors, it allowed Barty to cut through red tape in making philanthropic disbursements. Between 1997 and 1999, the foundation dispensed $48,000 in scholarships to fourteen students. After his death in 2000, the group reduced activities, but it raises funds for scholarships and financial aid at two golf outings a year, in Los Angeles and Cincinnati.

New groups form constantly. Often, they are not distinct, tax-exempt entities, but a Web page designed to offer support and communication to others with the same diagnosis. There are several Web sites for skeletal dysplasia conditions. Morquio syndrome is different enough from some other conditions to have led families to establish a separate group. The Jeune Syndrome's Information/Support Network, with approximately eighty families, is another such resource. Many of these groups' Web sites are overseen by only a single member and have very few active leaders.

The Short Stature Foundation

In her suicide note, Richard Crandall's daughter had written, "I can not handle the life God gave me as a short-statured person." The Short Stature Foundation, flourishing between 1984 and 1998, was Crandall's living memorial to her. With the help of McDonnell Douglas, he developed an adaptive device catalog; the Dole Foundation offered a telemarketing job-training program for dwarfs; and other employers were encouraged to develop job opportunities. The group's greatest achievement was the publication of *Dwarfism: the Family and Professional Guide,* a volume written with the assistance of Dr. Charles I. Scott and others. It explained some of the major diagnostic categories and offered other information and helpful advice.[23] When Crandall died, this group too became inactive. Gracie Oliver Crandall, his life partner of fifteen years, and his son Mykell asked that donations be made to the Little People's Research Fund.

The Little People's Research Fund

The Little People's Research Fund (LPRF, discussed in chapter 1, Medical Aspects) has limited its scope. It no longer subsidizes treatment or helps sustain Pierre House, a residence for patients' families. But despite setbacks, executive director, Charles E. McElwee, and his associates remain hopeful that after a review now underway, at least some of Dr. Kopits's vital research findings will appear in journal or book form.

THE INTERNET REVOLUTION

Perhaps no development, apart from disability rights legislation, has had so profound an effect on advancing the cause of persons with dwarfism as the Internet revolution. A recent article commented on "the power of the Internet to organize isolated, information-starved people into a community." Journalist Dan Kennedy has been a major force ensuring that relevant Internet news will reach the dwarfism community. Kennedy's daughter, Rebecca, was born with achondroplasia in 1992. Because their physician had not told the parents about potential respiratory problems in achondroplasia, a bad cold was transformed into a life-threatening emergency, and Becky nearly died. She had an emergency tracheotomy and required supplemental oxygen for the next two years: "Eventually Becky outgrew her problems and today she's a happy, healthy 5-year old. But my wife, Barbara, and I resolved that no parent—or, at least, no parent with a computer and modem—should have to go through what we went through alone."[24]

Kennedy describes this situation more fully in his 2003 volume *Little People: Through My Daughter's Eyes*. With the encouragement of Ruth Ricker, then president of LPA, in early 1995 he set up a site that included "Frequently Asked Questions"; eventually he was asked also to manage the Dwarfism List bulletin board.[25] He redesigned and expanded the site, and, with the help of others, includ-

ing David Bradford, created a rich resource for the dwarfism community. "The List keeps me from feeling as if I live under a rock somewhere," Patty Abrams, an average-statured Long Island mother, commented.[26]

The Dwarfism List is the largest discussion group, but more specialized ones exist as well (e.g., for Christians, parents, teenagers, and
LP actors). There are also several chat rooms. The List has more than
a thousand members, who alert each other to dwarfism-related films
or television shows and express views about life experiences and controversial issues. Sometimes average-statured students ask for help in
writing papers about dwarfism.

The destruction of the World Trade Center on September 11, 2001,
led members to discuss how to plan for emergency evacuation from
work or school. A person with a given medical problem may ask what
others' experiences have been with surgery, physical therapy, exercise,
or chiropractic care; someone might recommend methods of pain relief. Participants sometimes also offer helpful hints about products—
clothing, cabinetry, bicycles—and strategies for dealing with grocery
carts and supermarket personnel.

Some postings have been criticized as needlessly argumentative
or petty—the Internet seems to have a way of disinhibiting individuals—but overall, the List is valuable as a source of information
and a forum for expression. Even occasional wrong-headedness
seems like an improvement over the isolation of the past!

THE NATIONAL MARFAN FOUNDATION

Interesting comparisons may be made between the conditions of
short-statured individuals and persons with Marfan syndrome, a
connective tissue disorder seen among persons who tend to be unusually tall. This syndrome is associated with life-threatening heart
conditions and serious eye problems, among other symptoms. Because persons with Marfan syndrome appear tall and "normal," in the
past most of those affected did not realize that they had the condi-

tion; as recently as twenty years ago it was not widely known. However, the National Marfan Foundation's campaign to spread the word to physicians and affected individuals has been effective, and with the group's financial support of research activities, great advances have been made in diagnosis, drug therapy, and surgery. Patients with Marfan syndrome now are much healthier than in the past and most achieve close to normal longevity—a development that has been called one of medicine's greatest success stories.

Families of the very short and very tall turn out to have a great deal in common, as well as some differences. I have had the opportunity to explore these with Priscilla Ciccariello, now president emerita of the National Marfan Foundation, who was responsible for spearheading its growth. Priscilla is the mother of seven sons; three them were affected by the condition. Her husband, Charlie, her son, Steven, and her grandson, Oakley, have all died of heart problems associated with Marfan syndrome. But hundreds, perhaps thousands, are alive today because of the work that she and her associates have done. She has received many awards in recognition of her remarkable efforts.

Through Priscilla I came to recognize the importance of the various "umbrella groups" that allow the voices of persons with one of the more than five thousand genetic conditions to be raised and heard. Among these organizations are the Genetic Alliance (formerly called the Alliance of Genetic Support Groups), which focuses on conditions genetic in origin, and NORD, the National Organization for Rare Disorders, which deals with a variety of uncommon conditions and diseases, helping groups develop organizational and fund-raising strategies. Both groups include Marfan syndrome and several types of dwarfism among the syndromes they address.

Of particular relevance for individuals with bone conditions are NIAMS (the National Institute of Arthritis and Musculoskeletal and Skin Diseases) and the Coalition for Heritable Disorders of Connective Tissue. Priscilla is currently copresident of the CHDCT, which deals with the dystrophies of both tall and short persons. She is also one of the few nonscientist participants at the conferences of the American Society for Matrix Biology, a group whose members are engaged in ground-breaking research, much of it relevant to skeletal disorders. Her varied experiences have intensified her feeling that organizations should not simply compete with each other for private and public funds for medical goals, but collaborate—lobbying for legislation and promoting research and other mutually beneficial goals.

In addition to their many other functions, umbrella groups also promote the understanding of difference. Priscilla and I had both observed the ways in which height affected social distance—with the twelve inches that separate a very short from an average-sized person seeming to create far more social distance than the twelve inches that separate an average-sized from a very tall individual. At times complex reactions may result from encounters between persons at the extreme ends of the spectrum.

Priscilla describes one "umbrella group" meeting at which a variety of conditions were represented. She and two of her young adult sons with Marfan syndrome, Peter and John, had joined the group while the others were already seated and engaged in enjoyable conversation. The discussion continued, and when everyone got up to leave, Peter's extreme tallness became very noticeable, and he suddenly realized that several of the others were "little people." Standing, he felt different, as if he had suddenly become older than the others. After the initial shock of cognitive dissonance faded, he once again took note of the LPs' greater age and maturity, recapturing his previous sense of who they were as more senior individuals. But the encounter made a permanent impression, causing Peter to reflect even more on the impact of height on relationships.

SMALL DIFFERENCES

Keen awareness of height differences exists between persons with Marfan syndrome and dwarfism, and even between tall, affected members with Marfan syndrome and shorter members of the National Marfan Foundation. However, this awareness has been still greater in LPA, where members have had to come to grips with not only the differences *between* dwarfs and nondwarfs, but also the wide range of diagnoses and heights *within* the group. Persons with achondroplasia, the tallest of whom are about 4'6", are in the majority. Those with a variety of other diagnoses may be at least a foot shorter. Sometimes tensions and social distance have been experienced between taller and shorter members of the group, or between members more and less affected by disabilities. In recent years, however, the membership has become increasingly aware of inequities, and individuals have made greater efforts to learn more about everyone's situation, thereby creating greater comfort for all.

Just how far consciousness has been raised was apparent a few years ago when a member suggested a "king" and "queen" contest at the national conference, an event that had been a regular feature in early years. Very quickly, members of the Dwarfism List sent postings indicating that they would veto any such event. They did not want to ape society's misplaced exaltation of traditional beauty, a standard that might lead to shorter or different-looking members being seen as less valuable.

Each of the 5,000 known genetic disorders presents striking variability and poses enormous challenges. In all disability groups, conscious efforts are required to overcome any internal, potentially divisive bias. No longer can supposed "normates" be viewed as the gold standard for human appearance or behavior; what organizations like those discussed here hope to provide is an appreciation of difference that will foster a new ethical humanism.

5 ～
LIVES TODAY

This is a historic moment for dwarfs. As a result of the social changes of the past several decades, this "people who were not a people" have now joined other minorities, identity groups, and disability groups in demanding "a seat at the table." In the court era, dwarfs by and large existed at the whim of their rulers and owners. Beginning in the eighteenth century, many exhibited themselves and became entertainers for want of other employment. Their difference marginalized them and frequently occasioned ridicule. Only a few individuals, through exceptional talent or family connections, were able to achieve eminence. During the past thirty years, dramatic changes have occurred, both in the numbers of persons who have access to educational and vocational opportunities and in individuals' positive sense of self. At least in Western nations, dwarfs are now employed in almost every occupation that does not require hard physical labor.

What has brought about such revolutionary changes? Medical advances have played a crucial role in making dwarfs healthy, active participants in society. But social and economic forces have made even greater contributions. World War II represented a turning point, allowing male dwarfs to find employment as mechanics in the airline industry and other related fields. Even more important, when great numbers of disabled veterans returned to college under the G.I. Bill, appreciation of their contribution led to the creation of ramps and other physical accommodations. This trend persisted after the Korean and Vietnam wars. Resulting changes have enabled even the smallest dwarfs to attend colleges that would have been out of reach in earlier decades.

The achievements of the civil rights movement of the 1960s helped stir the consciousness that led to disability rights legislation.[1] Individuals with disabilities were acutely aware that the Civil Rights Act of 1964 did not include them; they and their supporters helped enact the Rehabilitation Act of 1973, in which the needs of the "handicapped" first began to be addressed.[2] This act prohibited any federally funded agency from discriminating against persons with disabilities, thereby laying the foundation for making equal access for this group a civil right. The Individuals with Disabilities Act of 1975 ensured that every child would be granted the right to a free and appropriate education in the least restricted environment.

Not until 26 July 1990, however, when the Americans with Disabilities Act (ADA) was signed, was really effective legal ammunition provided. The ADA essentially bars physical and social barriers that keep persons with disabilities from full access to schools, jobs, and public places, requiring institutions to make necessary accommodations. Children and adults with disabilities are now mainstreamed as never before, and they finally have recourse to fight discrimination. Angela Van Etten has reviewed the implications of disability legislation for LPs, and further information and legal assistance is available elsewhere.[3]

Angel Shields, current president of the Central Florida Chapter of LPA, has an accounting degree. She also earned an additional certificate from a one-year program in computer-aided drafting and design at Valencia Community College: at her graduation in 1998 she received its prestigious Beverly Chapman award. Back in 1965 when Angel, a diastrophic dwarf, was growing up in Pennsylvania, her talents were disregarded.

Her school board insisted that she go to a special school for persons with disabilities forty miles away.[4] When her mother, Eileen, took her there, she found a small, isolated group of children of all ages with varied disabilities, including retardation. Eileen appealed the decision from principal to school board to the governor's office, and in a highly publicized ceremony, Governor Scranton granted Angel permission to go to her local school. Today, families like the Shieldses need not battle for inclusion. Instead, they are invited to consult with schools about what accommodations might be necessary for their child. Before the ADA, only 61 percent of persons with disabilities graduated from high school; now 80 percent do.[5]

Technological developments have also contributed. Scooters and Access-a-Ride systems have ensured that persons with limited mobility need not be shut out of educational opportunities or gainful employment. Increased air travel has facilitated close relationships across continents and oceans, and relocation for personal or economic reasons. The Internet has caused an explosion in the transmission of medical information about dwarfing conditions, enhanced dwarfs' knowledge of their history, and increased their sense of community.

THE INTERNATIONAL SITUATION

Bethany Jewett-Stark's Travel Fellowship

Awareness of the situation of dwarfs in other nations was first raised in the United States in 1987, through the pioneering work of Bethany Jewett, a young anthropologist who was awarded a Watson travel fellowship when she graduated from Swarthmore. Her venture was symbolic of a new generation of dwarfs, who had begun to explore and define their identities.[6]

The combination of her condition, pseudoachondroplasia, and her professional background made her uniquely tuned in to the nuances associated with dwarfism in various cultures. More than a decade later, she still felt some nostalgia for the excitement of that year.[7] However, she found herself oddly distanced from the urgent youthful drive for self-discovery that had inspired her study. In the intervening years, life experience granted her a secure identity. After receiving her master's from NYU, she had worked for Simon and Schuster, Frommer's *Travel Guides*, and *Discovery* magazine. Now married to Adam Stark, a visual artist in the film industry, Bethany was taking a hiatus from professional activity: much of their energy

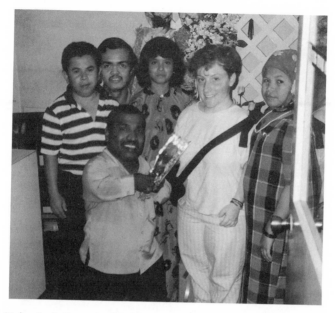

Fig. 5.1. Malaysia: Bethany Jewett-Stark, Watson Fellowship recipient, with LP friends in Malaysia. Photograph courtesy of Bethany Jewett-Stark.

was used in caring for their young twin sons, who had been born prematurely with significant health problems (fig. 5.1).

Her recollections of her travels remain sharp. Jewett had spent most of her time in New Zealand, Sweden, England, and Australia. She also traveled briefly to Malaysia, China, Nepal, India, Italy, France, Spain, Tahiti, New Caledonia, Singapore, Hong Kong, and Holland, seeking out informants who had contacted LPA at some point. In general, she found that organizations existed in countries in which dwarfs were best off. (At that time they existed only in Western Europe, Australia, and New Zealand.) Asians spoke about their isolation, families that had hidden them away because of shame, and the absence of governmental assistance, but also interdependence:

> [One Malaysian] could not understand why buildings should be specially adapted for people when there were always many people around to help him reach something. I was getting into a taxi with another lit-

tle person there and he called a man over from the street to help him; neither he nor the man were surprised, and the little person almost acted as if it was his right to be helped. I soon got the feeling that independence had a different definition for people there. Somehow people are all part of a big interconnected network or family and perhaps do achieve an interdependence to such an extent that they don't feel as though they are burdening others or are subservient to others by asking for help.[8]

The issues that elicited most comment were labeling, medical concerns (including limb lengthening), social issues, and identity formation.

LABELING PREFERENCE

The issues that Jewett identified remain salient. Individuals still argue about preferences for terminology such as *dwarf, little person, LP, short-statured individual,* and *person with restricted growth;* almost anything but *midget* has its advocates. Jewett found that many persons in England, Sweden, and New Zealand felt discomfort about using the term *dwarf* because it carried negative mythological associations; the British group calls itself the Restricted Growth Association. One New Zealand geneticist remarked that dwarf conjures up images of evil mystical characters and should not be used for real people. Other New Zealanders felt that it pushed persons already on the periphery of normalcy further toward abnormality and considered it an insult.

Swedish respondents also rejected dwarf (*dvarg*) as a condescending term with fairy tale associations. Short-statured members preferred *kortvuxna,* which means short grownup, but many average-statured parents preferred *kortvaxta,* which means short-grown, noting that their children were not grownups. Some adult LPs objected to that designation, viewing *kortvaxta* as signifying small things, not humans—and so it went, with strong feelings on all sides.

As Jewett notes, in the United States *dwarf* is commonly used merely as a descriptive, accurate medical term and, relieved of its mythological load, has increasingly gained acceptance. Members also use the terms *little people, LPs,* and *short statured,* while objecting to *midget.* The need to distinguish proportionate persons from those with skeletal dysplasias seldom arises, but when it does, *pituitary dwarf, endocrine dwarf,* or *growth hormone–deficient person* is used. To confuse matters still further, *midget*—the "m word," derived from midge, an insect—is still used as a descriptive term by midget wrestlers and some others.

In the nineteenth century, Barnum referred to Tom Thumb as a *dwarf; midget* was later used to refer to small performers. By the time *The Wizard of Oz* was made, a hierarchy had emerged, with proportionate short-statured persons regarded as the more desirable category (only they were chosen as actors for the film). Disproportionate dwarfs were more common in circus and sci-fi roles. Only gradually did *midget* acquire its current negative loading.

In the United States, many individuals dislike *little people* because it suggests fairies and children. (I know at least one short-statured person who will not join Little People of America while it keeps that name.) The community accepts *LP*—the neologism carries no historic baggage—but the public is mostly unaware of it and does not use it. Some organizations have adopted *short statured,* such as the Short-Statured People of Australia or the Association Belge des Personnes de Petite Taille; *restricted growth,* used in England and Denmark, is considered cumbersome and formal by others. These changing appellations and discontents parallel the evolution from *colored* and *Negro* to *people of color, black,* and *African American,* but nothing satisfies everyone. Identity is not a simple business.

PERSPECTIVES ON DWARFS IDENTIFYING AS DISABLED

Jewett also addressed the question of why some dwarfs willingly identify as persons with disabilities and others reject the term. The United

States, Scandinavia, and England have taken the lead in disability rights legislation and issues. England's 1995 Disability Discrimination Act requires employers to make reasonable adjustments to the premises for persons with disabilities and to modify equipment, alter working hours, and reallocate unsuitable duties.[9] Also, those who are registered with the Employment service may be eligible for support under the Access to Work system. It pays most of the cost of transportation and furniture such as computer chairs, etc., with employers making an average contribution of 20 percent. The Access to Work scheme uses central government funds to enable the individuals with the greatest disabilities to earn a full wage in an environment in which their needs can be met.[10] Sweden and Denmark, which have very advanced social service systems, are also generous to persons with disabilities. In the United States, LPA joins with disability rights groups to address specific issues, such as correcting physical barriers, but many members choose not to identify as disabled, as a sense of being unimpaired is vital to their self-image.

Lawyer Angela Van Etten, LPA disability rights activist, has written an article emphasizing that a person may be both disabled and independent.[11] In fact, most dwarfs gain independence through a lifelong process of adaptation, using stools, reachers, walkers, and scooters, and sliding and wheeling heavy items: "the bottom line is that we don't let the limitations incapacitate us; we just find another way of accomplishing our goal." Van Etten firmly believes that it is possible to affirm the disability label while rejecting the patronizing attitudes and "pity party" that have often accompanied it. In doing so, one may reap both legal and health benefits.

When health problems become chronic, many little people, after exploring alternatives, find it necessary to avail themselves of the disability benefits that the U.S. government provides—a modest living allowance and health insurance. Fewer than 5 percent of the membership of LPA currently list themselves as recipients of disability payments, but probably a greater number have received them at some periods of their lives. Less impaired individuals come to terms with the "disability" label when it allows them to take advantage of such benefits as parking stickers or workplace accommodations.

In her Johns Hopkins University master's thesis, Cara Egan, LPA's National Health Policy Advisor, traced the growing willingness of LPA members to identify with the disability movement and make use of advocacy.[12] Several issues have been particularly prominent: the campaign against "dwarf tossing," where average-statured individuals compete in bars to see how far they can hurl a dwarf; the need to make ATMs and gas pumps accessible; concerns about airbag safety; and, most urgently, the need for LPs to exert influence in genetic decision making and health care. In 2001, Jenny Clark, the mother of a 15-year-old son with diastrophic dwarfism, wrote a trenchant article entitled "Battling Your HMO: Your Second Job."[13]

Egan has often joined with other groups that share a similar agenda. In June 2001, she and other LPs took part in the People's Genome Celebration. EEOC (Equal Employment Opportunity Commission) commissioner and LPA member Paul Miller led sessions on genetic discrimination and privacy. Several photographs of dwarfs were included in the Positive Exposure exhibit, designed to break down stereotypes of persons with genetic conditions. Events of this kind, becoming common in the United States, are unimaginable in most nations.

THE HISTORY OF INTERNATIONAL
DWARFISM ORGANIZATIONS

For the most part, countries that have formed organizations for dwarfs are nations where a measure of affluence and a democratic government facilitate the formation of self-help groups and pay significant attention to the needs of persons with disabilities. The formation of the group originally called Midgets of America under Billy Barty's aegis in 1957 was followed by the burgeoning of dwarfism organizations in approximately thirty countries during the next half-century. Usually, one or two individuals sparked a group's creation.

The second group to appear, for instance, was initiated in 1962, when actor George Whitaker married Rosemary Gribble, an LP who had seen him perform in Australia. The two traveled to New Zealand where they helped form the Little People of Australia. Within a year, the two groups reorganized themselves into separate New Zealand and Australian associations.

The British group was formed in 1968 when orthopedist Martin Nelson returned to England after studying at Johns Hopkins. With Charles Pocock, an LP who was head of the Disabled Drivers Association, he established the Association for Research into Restricted Growth (now the Restricted Growth Association [RGA]). The RGA had 500 paid short and average-statured members in 2000, with an additional 800 on their list of contacts. According to Honor Rawlings, because of the national health service, medical care is free and quite good; nevertheless persons must often educate professionals, many of whom have not encountered someone with a dwarfing condition. In an increasingly enlightened world, RGA members entertain greater aspirations.[14]

Not every country that attempted to start an organization was successful at the outset. Sometimes negative attitudes were overwhelming. In 1977 Martin Monestier wrote in *Les Nains:* "There are five to six thousand dwarfs in France. They live in retreat, hidden, without relations among them, the butt of derision. Prisoners of an invisible ghetto, one sees them on sidewalks, public places, subways and stores."[15]

At an organizing meeting in 1976, forty journalists appeared, but only twenty potential members—"most of them already part of the world of spectacle." Notary Brissé-St. Macary, in his opening address, called for individuals not to allow themselves to be hidden any longer, but admitted, "When I pass before a shop window that reflects my image, I find myself ugly and hate myself." His words raised a furor; if a man who was ostensibly presenting himself as a model to other French dwarfs could speak of hating himself, how could he expect others to aspire to self-acceptance? The group elected Madame Priatel, the average-statured mother of a 9-year-old dwarf, as president, supposedly because she was better suited to appear before the public.

In 2001, I communicated with Natalie Pretou, a diastrophic dwarf, and her average-statured husband, Fabien, about the French association and the overall climate for dwarfs. They indicated that there are about 10,000 short-statured persons in France, one-third of whom are children. Personnes de Petite Taille currently has 500 members; it holds an annual meeting in the spring and sponsors occasional telethons.

The Pretous viewed the situation for dwarfs as unfortunate. Only the most aggressive find work; the rest manage on social assistance. Public places make no provision for persons with disabilities. The Pretous find some persons curious and others mocking, or even wicked. Whereas most simply do not notice, others stare and then are dismissive. Fabien feels that southern European countries are especially bad, and that a country such as Romania is worst of all because of the legacy of Ceausescu, who confined ill children and those with disabilities in orphanages. Natalie thinks about living in the United States, where she would not have to be subjected to the "cons" of the French.

The situation is much better in northern Europe. In 1973 Gunilla Elinder, the average-statured mother of a one-year-old LP, started a parent group in Sweden after attending an LPA convention. In 1982, through a psychology magazine, she was able to locate an adult LP, Britt-Inger Bowman. Bowman followed up on Elinder's suggestion that she attend the first International Conference for Little People in Washington, D.C., and upon her return, she established the Föreningen For Körtvuxna (the Association for People of Short Stature).

Belangenvereniging van Kleine Mensen was established in Holland in 1975. Margreet Jonge Poerink communicated with me from Holland in January 2000, noting that the group currently had 280 members, 90 of them parents. Meetings were held several times a year, with parents' meetings particularly well attended, and average-statured parents and children were benefiting from meeting adult little people and hearing about their experiences. Nuria De Oro Bertran of Spain organized the CRERER (Associación Nacional para Problemas de Crecimiento), also known as the European Growth Association. Another Spanish group is Associacion ADAC (Associación para las Deficiencias que Afectan al Crecimiento y al Descarrollo). In April 1988 in Madrid, the group hosted an international meeting attended by members of thirty-six organizations that had some vested interest.

In recent years some inroads have finally been made in the Balkans, South America, and Asia. George Sofkin of Bulgaria first visited the United States in 1995 to attend the LPA convention in Denver. He was astounded by the contrast between his experience in Bulgaria and what he observed at the Denver event. In a February 2000 e-mail, he remarked, "The tolerance . . . of people here is lower, much lower than in the States or Western Europe—I mean tolerance toward persons with disabilities, mostly dwarfs. . . . Here the government behaves as if there are no persons with disabilities. . . . [There are] many problems with human rights, unemployment, and very low standard of living."[16]

Sofkin helped form the Little People of Bulgaria in 1996—the first such group in any of the nations previously "behind the Iron Curtain" and one of the first among Balkan nations. Sofkin is proud of his group, whose 200 members represent a high percentage of Bulgaria's dwarfs, but he is unhappy that the Western LP organizations do not help economically. Outward appearances of comfort can mask for persons in poorer nations the fact that most LPs in the United States also have difficulty financing their lives and their medical care. There is little largesse to share—although helping struggling groups abroad may be a future goal.

In extreme distress and requiring surgery, Sofkin could not find anyone with sufficient expertise in Holland. After appealing to physicians in the United States and Western Europe, he had surgery in Holland: his health improved, despite lingering problems. By 2004 the situation for Bulgarian dwarfs overall had also become somewhat better. As a result of media coverage, public tolerance increased and, despite what Sofkin characterizes as continuing "government discrimination," members of LPB can now receive free care at the best hospital in Bulgaria. The group's economic enterprises and some private and government assistance from the United States have also helped.

The Little People of Kosovo was formed in 2002; a predecessor, Little People of Yugoslavia, had been formed in 1994, but ceased to exist because of the destruction caused by the war in Kosovo. The present group has 700 members; it is unique in that it must try to appeal to previously warring Albanian and Serbian communities and also in that it is officially part of an umbrella group of persons with disabilities. Its president, Hiljmnijmnijeta Apuk, who has economics and bachelor of law degrees, works as a District Financial Officer.

By May 2003, the first group in Africa, the Dwarfs Association of Nigeria (DAN), had been formed. Founded by Uche Onuha, DAN vowed to fight discrimination. Many in that country view seeing dwarfs as a bad omen, even running away from them on the street; at the same time, some have become active in the film industry and in home videos, often playing comic roles.[17]

In December 2003, the first group in Eastern Europe, Little People of Poland, provided contact information to LPA Online. No information is available, however, about the situation of dwarfs in Russia today. Monestier reported in *Les Nains* that in 1961, the Supreme Soviet ruled that "struggling Soviet comrade dwarfs have a right to retire at 45 years instead of 65, and female comrade dwarfs at 40 instead of 55 if they have been employed at least 15 years."[18] If this is accurate, it is interesting that the group was singled out—perhaps a nod to the special role of court dwarfs in Russian history. Given the economic strains in Russia in the 1960s and subsequently, it seems unlikely that dwarfs enjoy comfortable circumstances there.

At present there are groups in Argentina, Australia, Belgium, Bulgaria, Canada, Chile, Colombia, Denmark, England, France, Germany, Holland, Ireland, Israel, Italy, Finland, Korea, Kosovo, Japan, Malaysia, Mexico, New Zealand, Nigeria, Norway, Poland, Scotland, Slovenia, Spain, and Switzerland. Among the most active are those in England, Germany, and Canada. (Canada, which, like the United States, is so widespread, has groups in Quebec, Ontario, British Columbia [fig. 5.2], and Manitoba.) Although formal international meetings have occasionally been organized, they have tended to be poorly attended and poorly represented.[19] However, each year there is an international meeting at the LPA conference.

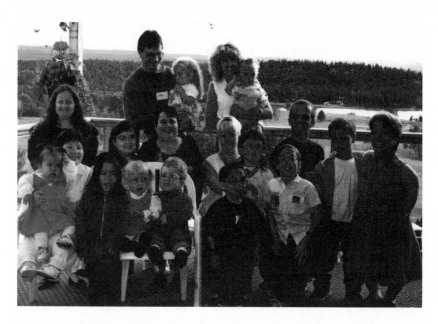

Fig. 5.2. Little People of British Columbia Society for Short Stature Awareness. Photograph courtesy of Little People of British Columbia Society for Short Stature Awareness.

Most countries have no organizations, and those who do attract only a small percentage of the nation's dwarfs. Sometimes, groups that sound as though they are counterparts to dwarfism groups turn out to be quite different. When physical education teacher Chi Hua created an organization in China to combat discrimination and low self-esteem, he was overwhelmed by requests for membership, and forced to lower his height requirements.[20] The height levels had been set at 5'7" for men and 5'3" for women—average or above average for Chinese persons—and even the lowered level was just an inch shorter. Hardly a Little People of China yet!

In fact, a chilling report in *TIMEasia* in December 2001 noted that thousands of young Chinese women and a few men (70% of them college educated) are spending great sums for cosmetic limb-lengthening surgery to enhance their chances for good positions. Competition for professional positions has led to height being used to disqualify applicants. A would-be diplomat, for example, was told by a top Beijing university that she was not tall enough to qualify for the English department. "They told me that Chinese diplomats have to be tall," says Xiaowei, "because foreigners are tall and we don't want to look too short next to them."[21]

China does not have self-help and advocacy organizations such as those in the West. The nation's discrimination toward the short statured is consistent with its attitudes toward others with disabilities. A *New York Times* article highlighted the rampant discrimination against highly qualified persons, even those with minor defects. Liu Wenxiu, who had a slight limp, had among the best entrance exam records in her province but was denied admission to Nanjing University and all the other schools to which she applied. "There is severe discrimination against disabled persons," said Ms. Liu through tears, at the technical school where she later enrolled with help from the Hunan Province Disabled Persons Federation. "And I feel that I have been refused not just by the school but by society as well. Before this I felt quite positive about myself; everyone has imperfections, right? Now I have lost all self-confidence."[22] Colleges justify rejecting applicants because they are judged on their ability to place graduates in jobs, and they know that persons with disabilities will have difficulty whatever their credentials.

Tao Jie, professor of English at Beijing University, indicates that all is not bleak—that, in fact, China has made important strides through the efforts of Deng Xao Ping's son, himself with a disability. One significant cause of the prejudice against persons with disabilities, Tao suggests, is a legacy of belief that a congenital defect is a shame, or punishment for an ancestor's wrongdoing. In the past, individuals have been hidden in the home. Since 1949, welfare institutions have been established to care for individuals given up by parents. Of course, Professor Tao indicates, there have always been enlightened persons who did take better care of their children.

In 1989 a 30-year-old dwarf named Li Gnoli sued his mother for neglect.[23] His parents divorced shortly after his birth, and the court had granted custody to his mother, who instead left him with an aunt. Although he was returned to her when he was in the third grade, she neglected him and did not allow him to attend school. The neighborhood committee later found him factory work, but after he fell ill and was hospitalized, his mother neither visited nor allowed him to return. The factory paid his hospital bills and gave him food coupons and pocket money. He took his mother to court to obtain food coupons and publicize the fact that society had treated him better than his own mother.

Another 1989 news item criticized a restaurant in Fuchien that had employed only dwarfs as waiters to attract patrons and increase profits.[24] A 1992 positively toned article highlighted two talented dwarf friends—a painter named Cai Lequn and a calligrapher named Yang Xiaoju—who had apprenticed in an arts and handicrafts factory and lived together. Both had presented exhibitions and were highly acclaimed. The article notes that former Defense Minister Zhang Aiping had written to them, expressing admiration for their spirit.

In China, as in most countries—even the United States—achievement by a person with a disability is still greeted as a remarkable display of courage, a triumph over anticipated obscurity and failure. Such reactions represent a middle ground between true acceptance and outcast status. That outcasts are still common in other Asian countries, however, was revealed in a 1996 *New York Times* article about the persons with disabilities in Japan. Journalist Nicholas Kristof presented a moving account of how entrenched rejection of persons with disabilities has been until recently.[25]

Osamu Takahashi, 49 at the time, reveals that his crippled body and deformed hands were less of a burden in childhood than his sense that his father felt not love but embarrassment for him. He felt his entire family regarded him as a monster; his siblings made him disappear when their friends visited; he was served food alone in his room; he was not sent to school and was allowed out of the house only once a year, at night.

Although Mr. Takahashi's situation may have been extreme, shame was a characteristic Japanese response to disabilities, in part because the society is so homogeneous, in part because of its emphasis on conformity. One man in a wheelchair described being regarded as a troublemaker, just for being in a coffee shop. A young woman using a wheelchair was not allowed to take entrance exams by many universities. After she finally found acceptance at one and graduated, she was told repeatedly by employers that they would not employ a person with disabilities; she was forced to accept a job at a center for persons with disabilities in Tokyo.

Recently there has been some progress in eliminating physical barriers and some talk of disability legislation. Akiko Saito, who volunteers with individuals who have physical and mental disabilities, concludes that things are better in the United States because it is "accustomed to different people, different ethnic backgrounds, different religions and so on. Japan is not like that, and in Japan the disabled have long been isolated."[26] Remarkably, just five years after that article appeared, another announced: "Social Warming: Japan's Disabled Gain New Status."[27] It reported the appointment of Satoshi Fukushima, a deaf and blind associate professor, who would be designing a curriculum focused on eliminating social, psychological, and physical barriers.

Several factors are mentioned as encouraging change: because of economic turbulence Japanese society is now less socially cohesive; barrier improvements originally designed for the elderly serve the persons with disabilities as well; the availability of the Internet has improved knowledge and communication. *No One's Perfect,* describing Hirotada Ototake, a man without arms and legs, has become a best seller, and persons with disabilities have become more commonplace on popular television shows and city streets; Hajimi Sen, a man with cerebral palsy, has been elected to the Kamakura City Assembly.

In this improved climate, a Little People of Japan organization had been formed. In 2001, average-statured photographer Etsuko Enami Nomachi, who has photographed several LPA conferences, responded to my query about the group: "Last week I met the President of Japan Little People. We have two groups. One is JLP, the other is Tsukushi-no-kai. JLP has about 20 members. Very little group, because many Japanese little people don't like to go outside."[28] I later

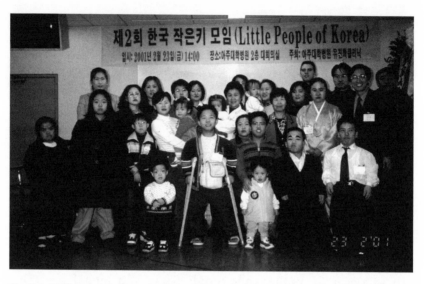

Fig. 5.3. Little People of Korea. Photograph courtesy of Little People of Korea and Dr. Hae-Ryong Song.

learned that the impetus for creating JLP had come from John Lusk, a Christian missionary to Japan, who knew LPA vice president Lee Kitchens. That relationship led to an invitation for three Japanese dwarfs to a 1998 LPA conference. They returned home and started a group.

Hae-Ryong Song, a pediatric orthopedic surgeon in Korea, had studied in the United States and knew Dr. Michael Ain. Song spearheaded the formation of the Little People of Korea (LPK) in 2000, with the cooperation of the Whang family, a father and four brothers with achondroplasia, and Dr. Hyun-Ju Kim, a geneticist and pediatrician at Aju University hospital (fig. 5.3). Hoi-Dong Whang, the eldest brother, became its first president.

Their goal had been helped immeasurably by the efforts of the Korean Broadcasting Company (KBC). At the July 2000 LPA conference, Korean filmmakers collected footage aimed at demonstrating for the Korean public that dwarfs could live a fulfilling life. In 2000 and 2001, KBC presented a fifteen-episode documentary about the Song family and LPK. More than 5 million viewers in this nation of 45 million watched the series. Also, Seoul Broadcast System helped LPK with several documentaries. Under the leadership of Dr. Kim, the LPK Foundation was formed to help provide medical treatment, scholarships, brochures, and Web page management.

The media campaign touched viewers, changed attitudes, and led to donations. Most importantly, it created a viable organization with amazing speed; LPK now has 150 registered members with dwarfing conditions. Dr. Kim, along with dwarf and average-statured college students, traveled to Australia and met with members of the Short Statured People of Australia, resulting in yet another documentary. Several books have also been published in Korean about dwarfism and the LPK.

Israel, a modern Western society in most ways, offers good medical care and educational funding to persons with dwarfism. Its short stature group, Amutat Nemuchei Koma, has seventy-five families. However, as a 1993 film *You Just Can't Hide It* reveals, the mood of many individuals is not as positive and upbeat as in many Western nations. Several persons in the film describe difficulties with acceptance and self-acceptance. Some, such as Talya Hahn, a microbiologist in charge of a laboratory at the renowned Weitzman Institute, have eventually found good positions despite significant employment discrimination. Others have faced social barriers: one woman's family told her she would have to leave home if she continued dating a dwarf computer engineer. Although this computer engineer feels good about having "made it" professionally, he worries about having a child like himself because he believes that 90 percent of dwarfs are not as fortunate as he. The film is enlivened by the spirited humor of dwarf comedian Aharon Zilberg, but the overall tone is anxious. An Israeli friend commented that persons with disabilities, unless they are military heroes, are sometimes looked at askance. She noted that the Israeli-made 2000 film *Liebe Perla*, however, had been very well received and seemed to be part of a trend toward greater enlightenment.

Even now, there are many areas as yet untouched by the urge to form organizations. Two sisters from Kenya who attended the 2000 LPA conference were excited about meeting American LPs, because there was no dwarfism organization in Kenya, and they had never encountered others like themselves. They conjectured that most were encouraged to be cared for at home and not venture out. Difference tended to be denied, or at least not discussed. Short persons regularly strained to reach a counter at work but did not think about requesting adaptations to make life easier, nor did their employers suggest any. At the conference the sisters were delighted to discover pedal extenders that would enable them to drive a car and purchased a set.

Still, Kenya had some advantages. One could not be turned away for lack of insurance in an emergency room. Although people like herself who were employed and had insurance had some advantage, medical fees were generally low. When a person could not afford care, friends and relatives typically chipped in. Discrimination was less overt in Kenya, they believed, than in some countries. Once, applying for a position in the United Arab Emirates, one sister had submitted a resume and been complimented on her excellent qualifications. However, when she arrived for her interview, the receptionist looked at her and said that her prospective employer would be unavailable. Although such encounters have been reported in all nations, they are reportedly particularly common in North Africa and Asia.

There are some countries where one can find even more extreme examples of attitudinal "arrested development." At a fertility festival in Bhutan in 1999, to which infertile couples from the West came in hope of finding a spiritual path toward conceiving a child, a jester sashayed around, swinging a wooden phallus. Behind him four dwarfs in puffy skirts and two dancers dressed as cows feinted and boxed.[29] Those of us fortunate enough to be part of this recent golden age of opportunity would do well not to forget that all stages of the history of dwarfs continue to be represented throughout the world.

Nothing has been said so far about South America. Although Monestier had commented on an earlier effort to start a group in Brazil, little had been heard again about that nation or others. Therefore, I was particularly excited that a group had formed in Chile. I met Marcello Reyes at the LPA conference in Portland in 1999 and again at the

2000 conference with his wife, Antoinetta. The couple was accompanied by their dwarf toddler son Federico, and two average-statured children. Medical consultations found Federico to be in good health, and Reyes was pleased also to encounter many thriving LPs.

Between the two conferences Reyes attended, an excellent television show in Chile had highlighted the lives of dwarfs and spurred interest in Fundacion Pequenas Grandes Personas of Chile. Many respondents were isolated and poor and had had little medical attention. The group welcomed them, referring them for treatment to geneticist Gabriela Reppeto, who had trained at Johns Hopkins. The Chilean organization now has 400 members; 100 of them are short statured.

In 2002, Matias Ezequeiel Sierra posted on the Dwarfism List the news that an organization Zoe del Griego (Full of Life) had been formed in Argentina for people of short stature, aimed at mutual support, social change, and integration. By its second year, the group had grown from eight to twenty members. Colombia has also recently formed a group.

Of all the nations mentioned, Denmark must be judged the most progressive, leveling high taxes to pursue a benevolent social policy. Erik and Hanne Eriksen, two parents who were among the seven Danes attending the LPA 2000 conference, noted that the government not only provided free surgical care, but also paid for family or other caregivers to stay home and attend to patients. It offered subsidies to those able to work only part-time and provided necessary home improvements and assistive devices. Perhaps in part because of governmental financial assistance, five or six members had elected to have limb lengthening.

Denmark's Landsforeningen for Væksthæmede (Organization for Restricted Growth) began as a parents group in 1988 (fig. 5.4). One of its roles is to help members deal with the bureaucratic maze they need to negotiate. Because the government has cut back its assistance somewhat as costs escalated, needs must be substantiated. The group has 150 dwarf members (50 of them adults), and a greater number of

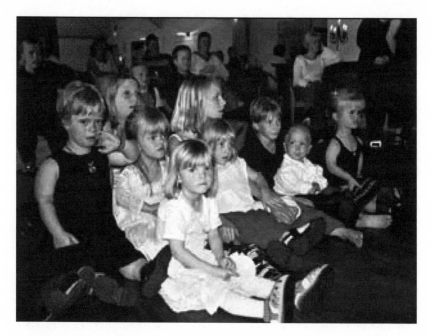

Fig. 5.4. Little People of Denmark. Photograph courtesy of Little People of Denmark.

average-statured members. More than half the dwarf members are single, and those who are married are more apt to have average-statured partners.

LIFE STAGES

The Early Years

Births are always great dramas, defining moments that intensify all the previous history of family, friends, and community. Anxiety during the early period sends parents' minds on a speeded-up trajectory, but ruminating on the future only distracts from immediate concerns, obtaining good medical advice, breast-feeding, toilet training, schooling, etc. The wisest ones learn that if they provide a loving, accepting household, this child, like others, can be expected to thrive.

A critical issue in early childhood is the "loss of innocence" moment, when the child asks his parents why he is so short, commonly by age three or four. A 5-year-old may say: "I don't want to be a dwarf! I want to be big like you! (or grandma)." If the parent is also a dwarf, the child may wonder why both are short.

Fred Short queried other members on the Dwarfism List about the best way to answer questions of this kind. Wanting to inculcate pride in a child, he is impatient with answers that say, "Yes, you are small, and you will always be small, but . . ." He believes in using the word, but suggests that the respondent's assertion may be "fine, *but* it is not the whole truth!" One respondent, Helene Whitaker, declares that she has never found the right answer either; however, she rejects the wrong ones:

> I don't subscribe to the "God made you special" thing at all. Special implies "better than" and any five year-old worth her salt will know it's not better to be small. My mother tried that one on me and I never bought it and I told her so . . . Also I don't think it's particularly help-ful to tell kids that because they are little they help others understand difference and teach others tolerance. My Mother also tried that one (when I was exactly five years old) and all I could think was what a "bummer" (though that word wasn't around back then), I have to suf-fer so others can learn from me? That sucks and even a kid knows that. The worst one was when my mother said, "God has a plan for you and we don't know what that plan is but you'll have a special place in heaven!" So great, terrific, "I have to live out an unknown plan so af-ter I live I'll be 'special'". Geez. Looking back on it, I'm not sure what she should have said and I often ponder this question but perhaps some honesty about how we really don't know why you're different, life isn't fair and that sucks, and it probably won't be very easy but I think things will turn out all right and we're going to be here for you and work on it together.[30]

The first such inquiry or protest by a dwarf child is often remem-bered as a defining existential moment by the parent, if not by the child. But it must be dealt with time and again on different levels, and must not be brushed aside or trivialized. Beth Wason Loyless, an elementary school teacher who now has children of her own, once spoke at a Johns Hopkins symposium about the positive things her family had done in rearing her. They had loved her, treated her according to her age, and given her the privileges and responsibilities of an eldest child. But one mistake they did make, she said, was, subtly or not, discouraging her from talking about the difficult parts. One ought not pretend, she concluded, that life for dwarfs is the same as for everybody else. The differences need to be given their due without allowing them to cast a constant shadow.

Good parents naturally communicate that they find their child appealing and competent; they encourage interests and efforts that they hope will lead to accomplishments. Although it is fine to mold good values and battle bureaucracies, they also must learn to intervene *only* when necessary, demonstrating their trust in the child's own growing resources.

The Teen Years

After the initial shock has been absorbed, childhood is often a cheerful time, especially for those children lucky enough not to have overwhelming medical problems. They may have to learn to cope with teasing, but that is not the end of the world for most. However, in their teens and young adulthood, as individuals date, pair off, and later seek a wonderful life partner, they may face formidable obstacles. Parents cannot serve up any simple happy solution. Often young people hide such dilemmas from their families.

Because a notable part of forging an identity during this period seems to revolve around personal appearance, dwarfs may struggle with self-acceptance even more than others. Teenagers relate success to being able to attract good-looking partners and often do not consider dating someone who departs drastically from society's norm and risking a "courtesy stigma"—stigma through association. This fear is less present in friendship, particularly when relationships have existed since childhood. Making new friends may be harder, espe-

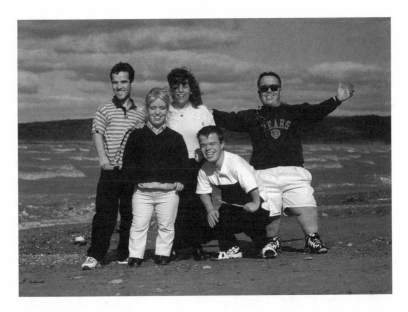

Fig. 5.5. Young adults of the Restricted Growth Association, England. Photograph courtesy of the Wellcome Trust.

cially for the introverted. It helps to have diverse skills, including the
ability to drive and access a car to increase mobility.

England's RGA has published a pamphlet addressing some of these
issues.[31] It discusses the importance to adolescents of thinking about
a career, becoming absorbed in interests (e.g., sports, drama, dancing,
or computers), and just going out and having a good time. The authors recommend that teenagers not dwell on their restrictions but
rather become passionately involved with life, seeking support and
friendship in and outside dwarfism groups (fig. 5.5). They also caution that one is a representative and has a responsibility to other
short-statured individuals not to act irresponsibly.

The pamphlet recognizes the importance of sexuality and, noting
the influence of both hormones and attitudes, discusses responsible .
sex and contraception. The authors also recognize that some individuals may find that they are homosexual and must come to terms
with yet another difference—but one that may provide potential for

emotional growth. One gay young man comments: "When I finally realised—or at least admitted to myself—that I fancied other blokes, I thought to myself, 'Trust me—not just a dwarf, but a gay dwarf!' Actually, what I've found is that my gay friends just accept me for who I am. Being gay, they're all different too, so me being small isn't such a big deal."[32] The pamphlet also discusses limb lengthening, a controversial procedure confronting teens.

Some young people first join LPA during adolescence, looking for friends among whom they can find understanding. Other teens, brought to the group as children, now leave, wanting to explore their identity outside it. Some return in adulthood. Those who do remain throughout adolescence frequently enjoy good times and deeper discussions of difference that they experience as life giving.

Few escape the "popularity contests" of adolescence. Experiencing rejection among one's dwarf peers can be particularly painful, because one cannot blame the benighted attitudes of the outside world. But most find at least some acceptance in the organization. Adolescents who do not join can still get through these years without crises, through their studies, hobbies, and enjoyable time with family and friends. Some brooding is apt to occur, but isolation is less common these days.

Just how important the teen years are to future success is indicated by a recent finding that adult males in their thirties, now the same age and height, who had differed in height as teenagers, were experiencing different levels of success in the labor market. The worker who had been taller when a teen now earned a "wage premium" of as much as 15 percent.[33] The study suggests that because children who are short as teenagers are more apt to be teased or excluded, they may experience diminished interpersonal skills or self-esteem.

This finding may be viewed as a call to arms. Adolescents must find satisfying outlets during these years to enhance self-esteem and develop talents and leadership abilities. It has been reported that shorter kids tend to avoid extracurricular activities and that participation is associated with success in later life.[34] They must be encouraged to stay in the game.

Romance, Sexuality, and Marriage

The information about love and marriage in earlier eras is limited. Art and literature contain only rare representations of couples. In the courts, marriages between two dwarfs were more the rule. One of the most famous pairs was celebrated in this Edmund Waller poem written for the wedding of seventeenth-century court dwarf painter Richard Gibson and his bride, Anne Shepherd:

> Design, or chance, make others wive,
> But Nature did this match contrive;
> Eve might as well have Adam fled,
> As she denied her little bed
> To him, for whom heaven seemed to frame
> And measure out this only dame.

In the nineteenth century, the public continued to delight in the spectacle of dwarfs marrying each other: all of New York turned out for the wedding of Tom Thumb and Lavinia Warren Bump, and Abraham Lincoln welcomed them on their honeymoon. Both these marriages seem to have been love matches. Although in the courts and the entertainment world, opportunities for dwarfs to meet prospective partners were greater, nevertheless the pool of possibilities was limited. Most probably did not marry.

Journalists Walter Bodin and Bernet Hershey, in *It's a Small World* (1934), estimate that perhaps 22 percent of "midgets" marry, though it is unclear whether these persons are proportionate or disproportionate. Sensationalistic and patronizing though it can be, theirs is one of the few early surveys of marriage statistics.

These findings are echoed by the even smaller total percentage reported by Mörch, the respected scientist who published a 1941 work about chondrodystrophic dwarfs in Denmark.[35] He found that thirteen of thirty-nine men in the group he studied had married, and only one of thirty-eight women had married. (There had been some births without wedlock, however, and it was not clear how many persons had had relationships.)

Although reported results do not always agree, the situation seems to have improved somewhat, at least in the United States. Dr. Judith Hall, in a 1974–75 survey of 150 LPA members with achondroplasia, reported the highest marriage rate of any study: 75 percent of the women and 60 percent of the men had been married.[36] A 1981 study at Johns Hopkins found that 43 percent of seventy-four persons with skeletal dysplasia who were over the age of 20 had been married and that it was not merely the degree of physical impairment that determined whether or not they found mates.[37]

Alasdair Hunter's investigation of more than a hundred mostly Australian subjects also reported that 43 percent of LP adults were married. It is unclear whether Hall's discrepant result had to do with the fact that all these individuals had achondroplasia, rather than a broader spectrum of conditions, or the fact that respondents were a specific, self-selected group. However, all other surveys, even the most recent, find marriage rates of less than 50 percent.

The total LPA database of 25,000 persons—both active members and others who have contacted LPA through the years—offers further data. In April 2000, there were 5,508 adult LPs listed, 3,198 single and 1,288 married. After adding persons living together, widowed, or divorced (though these are vague category headings, to be sure), the total number known to have been in committed marital or cohabiting relationships reaches 1,624, or approximately 30 percent of the members. It seems reasonable to assume that the marriage rate of nonmembers is also apt to fall well below the national average. Because marriage is generally a desideratum among LPs, some may find it discouraging to discover the rate is not higher. However, the database does not note the many individuals in relationships who are not living together, and it is silent about how many persons are in homosexual relationships. It does not breathe a word about whether individuals are single by choice or, if married, content or discontent. Finally, it cannot prognosticate the future for the very different generation of young adults now coming of age. A more ambitious investigation is needed.

What is known is that finding a partner has never been a simple matter for persons with dwarfism, probably more so in the past. Older members Ellie Ostrom and Robert Spector tell the story of how some persons had met. Ellie's mother put an ad in the Jewish newspaper *The Forward* that began "Short girl looking for companionship." It was spotted by Robert's aunt, who urged her nephew to answer it, and so Ellie and Robert arranged to meet. Although they both became members of LPA, even named king and queen at one convention, they did not marry each other. Robert met his wife Joyce at the 1971 convention.

In former days, prospective partners tended to be introduced on the basis of stature alone. Two persons might still be brought together because they were the only dwarfs their age known to family or friends: I once met an Orthodox Jewish couple, born in different countries, who had been brought together by their religious communities—the only dwarfs known to each.

Bill Roberts spoke of his own experience of isolation to *Newsday* in 1989: "I was living totally in the average world back then. All my friends were big and we used to go to parties and drink beer and I was one of them. But when we got older, I saw that the girls wouldn't look at me the same way they looked at my friends. I asked my older sister if there was something wrong with me and she said, 'Ask a girl out.' So I asked out ten and they all said no."[38] Roberts joined LPA and found a girlfriend there. There are more women than men among the young adults in LPA, in part, people conjecture, because men are less apt to admit openly that they are encountering difficulty in the greater world.

Two journalists wrote articles in the 1990s highlighting the courtship process today. Both were reporting on their reactions to their first LPA conventions. In "Dwarfs: A Love Story," average-statured John H. Richardson of *Esquire* offered an outsider's view of the dating scene.[39] In "Dwarf Like Me," John Wolin, a 4 foot 7 inch journalist and editor for the *Miami Herald,* described his turbulent feelings during this first encounter with a large assemblage of other dwarfs.[40]

Richardson interwove three major narratives, including one about a couple who met at the conference. Reading Richardson's uncomplimentary description of their romance, one might not expect them to end up together. But in fact, they did and are still happily married. Their admirable qualities were not seen through Richardson's distorted prism. He later published *In the Little World*, an expansion of the *Esquire* article.[41] His work, which contains significant factual errors, often seems like a modern version of earlier voyeurism and opportunism—a gossipy, self-important account. He writes, for example, "Evidently flatchestedness is rare among dwarf women—their big behinds and big breasts make them almost a parody of the *Playboy* ideal. Or a rebuke."

Although Richardson does capture some significant aspects of the courting life at an LPA convention—notably, the excessive urgency that a compressed week of activities imposes—that aspect is dealt with far more intelligently and sympathetically in Dan Kennedy's memoir, *Little People: Through My Daughter's Eyes*.[42] Kennedy's searching account probes deeply into his own and others' attitudes about the conference experience.

The 45-year-old John Wolin reflected on the emotional aspects of his convention experience in 1993, describing his discomfort at being "a stranger among my own people," having previously avoided all but minimal contact with others like himself. The reader is drawn into Wolin's tale of personal soul-searching and journalistic information gathering. For the first time in his life, he finds himself at 4'7" towering over many others. His guide at the conference, attractive, short-statured trainer Pam Prentice, mentions Wolin's tallness and good looks, and he feels more embarrassed than pleased. At the same time, he finds himself envying those who can compete in Dwarf Athletic Association games. Wolin, who walked with canes because he had minimal strength in his legs, was a sports writer, but surprised himself by not attending any sports events at the conference.

He did attend the meeting called "Is There a Sexual Problem? An Open Forum about LP Sex." He quotes Beth Tatman, the Florida chapter member who led his group, as she recalled a seminar for dwarf women given at Johns Hopkins in the mid-1970s, led by a male pediatrician: "He passed out a vibrator and other goodies and we passed them around like hot potatoes, everyone was so afraid to hold them. . . . He showed slides of people getting into every position in the world. I raised my hand and said, 'I have six steel rods in my body. If I got into one of these positions, we'd need a blowtorch to get me out. That doctor's slides do not apply to us.'"[43]

Very likely only a few audience members had osteogenesis imperfecta, Tatman's condition. But all of them shared the reality of bodily difference and its attendant social experiences. They benefited from having a guide such as Tatman, who, as Wolin reflected, "cannot just roll in and out of the hay without effort, someone who will never, ever, under any circumstances, be able to do it in an airplane restroom and then write Penthouse about the experience. Many of us have trouble coupling. We may not fit together. Our limbs may be too short or too rigid to bend around our partner's. We may not be able to reach."

Tatman captures the essence of several possible sources of little people's difficulty in becoming expert lovers: "Much of the dwarf population missed the years the basic ground rules were learned. . . . We're naïve. We never leaned over in a movie and gently let a hand fall onto a breast. First, we likely don't have the date. Second, our arms aren't long enough.[44] Because of the spinal cord damage many of us suffer, we may have trouble with erections, or having achieved one may find orgasm a guest with a mind of its own, appearing rarely, if ever, when desired."[45]

At a meeting such as this, persons openly discuss the joys and problems of sexual encounters. They benefit not only from "helpful hints," but also from knowing they are in good company in their determination to pursue sexual satisfaction in whatever way is uniquely right for them. In this atmosphere, persons may be inspired to reflect and reexamine their own history. Wolin is generously candid:

> I lost my virginity the summer after graduating from high school in a whorehouse in Guatemala City. And as a young working man, would

satisfy my needs through the "day rate" offered by the hookers down the hall in my apartment building. My only other choice was unleavened frustration and loneliness. I never truly made love until I got married. . . . .

For much of my life I feared—and *fear* doesn't really do justice to the brutal emotion I felt—that I would never be married. Lack of a mate, lack of a partner in life, can make other problems seem trivial by comparison. Loneliness can be the most chilling prospect of all, the one that challenges even our will to live.[46]

Wolin understands (as Richardson does not) what drives a young couple to become quickly infatuated with each other at a convention and perhaps even leads them to make ill-advised marriage decisions. For many there are painful moments when the likelihood of finding a compatible partner can seem like an unreachable dream.

The outlook is brighter today than it was when either Tatman or Wolin was growing up. Young adults have higher self-esteem and are increasingly comfortable with their sexuality. Almost every edition of *LPA Today* contains pictures of a bride and groom smiling out at the reader (fig 5.6). Although statistics on this generation will not be available for some time, the marriage rate will likely increase, because short-statured persons have more opportunity to meet others through dwarfism groups and to encounter average-statured partners at college and work. But the road is still not easy, and whenever this milestone occurs, it is apt to represent a peak experience for the couple, and a happy ending for families that have balanced anxiety with high hopes.

Many persons do not marry. Particularly today, this by no means signifies that they have not been in relationships or been sexually active; most dwarf adults are apt to have had some measure of romantic and/or sexual experience. Despite how self-evident this may seem, many single dwarfs report that often they, like other persons with disabilities, are assumed to be celibate or asexual by "normates," unless contradicted by open conversations. One must also remember that lack of marriage does not mean lack of happiness. In fact, the study

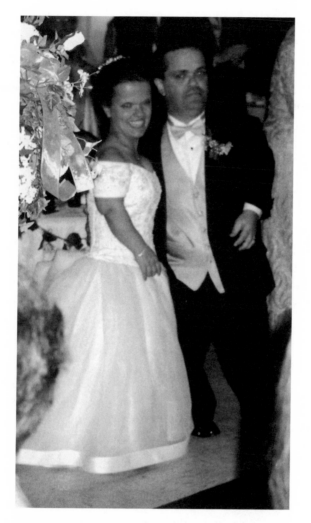

Fig. 5.6. Marriage of Barbara and Rick Spiegel. Photograph courtesy of Bette Sitzwater.

by Alasdair Hunter mentioned in chapter 2, Psychological Aspects, finds singles expressing greater life satisfaction than married individuals.

Despite all the information that is still missing in the area of sexuality and romance, we have progressed well beyond the wild surmises of many early commentators. Bodin and Hershey claim that proportionate dwarfs are very sexually active: "'Making' a woman of normal size is ordinarily no problem to a young attractive midget," they report, because through maternal solicitude or curiosity, women are frequently eager to experience sex with midget partners.[47] Midget women, they declare, are at a disadvantage because the dangers of childbirth often led them to avoid sex altogether—though occasionally they became prostitutes. Bodin and Hershey portray females as flirtatious and males as possessed of a Napoleonic need to prove an impossible manliness. Their evidence on many issues was not challenged until cultural anthropologist Elsa Davidson wrote her recent insightful critique.[48]

In 1968, sociologist Marcello Truzzi noted "numerous cases which have been reported of midget females who have been employed in prostitution, posing in some cases as children for Humbert Humberts' jaded appetites." Truzzi also asserts that male homosexuality "would be blatantly in conflict with the ultramasculine projection of most midget males." He cites as evidence the fact that Bodin and Hershey's 233 informants report no such cases—"the midget has quite enough trouble by just being a midget."[49]

In fact, there is no evidence of a high incidence of prostitution among dwarf women any more than there is evidence of homosexuality's absence. Enough dwarfs have spoken about their bisexual and homosexual orientations to suggest they are as prevalent in this group as elsewhere in society. The French writer Monestier also mentions female prostitutes, a male prostitute who boasts, "women of the best class had recourse to his services," and Scandinavian pornographic reviews that have erotic scenes with dwarfs and animals.[50] Accounts such as these, as well as libidinous court scenes, have been used as "proof" of dwarfs' lasciviousness. Such material actually only demonstrates that financial and emotional circumstance can lead to exploitation. Still, similar proclamations about dwarf or "midget" sexuality persist in various venues. The making of *The Wizard of Oz* was inaccurately portrayed in the media as a cauldron of alcoholic and sexual activity. Advertisements offering persons opportunities to sign on to pornographic Web sites featuring dwarfs are common.

Most laypersons would probably assume that short-statured individuals are apt to marry each other. Like Waller's seventeenth-century wedding ode quoted above, an eighteenth-century epigram to "a short and handsome lady" affirms the notion that such a choice is ordained:

> If little things with little folk agree
>> As little Bett allows
> O, then may little Bett at last decree
>> And wed a little spouse.[51]

But short-statured persons are motivated by other reasons. Some may feel that another dwarf will be more apt to understand them. Acceptance may seem to flow more naturally—one need not prove the worthiness of one's body, and the "fit" may also be easier. Finally, because of the existence of an organization such as LPA, the opportunity to find someone is now greater. One can meet many others looking for a partner who does not communicate the message that this difference bespeaks inferiority.

Of course, the couple must discover that they have more in common than size if their marriage is to succeed. Only one study has investigated this question. Dr. Alasdair Hunter has found that the level of marital satisfaction is higher among couples where both are short.[52]

A perhaps surprising LPA statistic is that in 2001, among 804 married LPs, 418 were married to another LP and 386 to average-height partners—not a great difference. Among nonmembers, it is even more likely that the short-statured individual will have married an average-statured mate. Whatever the statistical averages, many mixed-height couples declare that they are happily married. They denounce or ignore the prejudice they sometimes encounter. Occasionally, it has even been expressed in legal rulings; a couple in Brazil had difficulty obtaining a marriage license because of their great disparity in height. Even respected literary critic Leslie Fiedler made this assertion in the much-praised *Freaks:* "My own limited observation suggests that though Dwarfs occasionally achieve peaceful and enduring marriages with non-Dwarfs, such relations more typically conceal a desire to exploit the Freak partner either economically, as in Todd Browning's fictional case, or sexually, as in Victor Hugo's *L'Homme qui rit*."[53] Fiedler's undocumented "typical desire to exploit," like so much written in the past, reflects the author's often unconscious prejudice. All kinds of couples who depart from the norm are apt to elicit stares and comments. Like poet John Donne, they may be moved to declare, "For God's sake, hold your tongue and let us love!"

Even in LPA, such persons sometimes encounter prejudice—the inference being that by "marrying out" they demonstrate that they do not accept themselves as dwarfs. LP lawyer and author Angela Van Etten tells the story of Adrian, who was talking to a group of other short-statured persons; they behaved warmly until she pointed out her average-statured husband, Derek; they then gave her the cold shoulder. Adrian wondered, "Did they think I had married above my station, or was I seen as a traitor?"[54] Van Etten believes that the relationships between short and tall are based on the same principles of attraction that affect everyone. Ruefully, she recounts other instances of bias and rude remarks toward persons who, before hearing them, had been unaware that they had a "mixed marriage." about here.

Monica Pratt, former LPA administrator, is a 2 foot 8 inch woman married to Neil, a chemist, who is average statured. Several dwarf women have told her that her marriage to Neil indicates that she is not accepting of her stature and is clear evidence that she needs someone to take care of her. "*I* don't want a father-daughter relationship," one woman scoffed. Monica has also taken flak for having Neil carry her on occasions when a scooter is unavailable (fig. 5.7).

Nevertheless, they have learned to cope with the prejudices of prospective employers, the stares of strangers, and the vocal qualms of family members. They met in college and were friends for six months before they became aware that their intimate, trusting relationship had developed into a romantic one. Their family had mixed reactions; it turned out that Monica's mother had never expected her to marry,

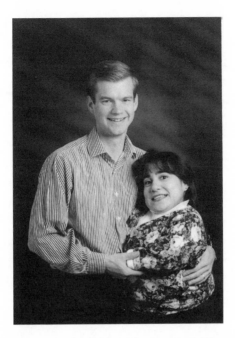

Fig. 5.7. Monica and Neil Pratt. Photograph courtesy of Monica and Neil Pratt.

and Neil's mother had trouble viewing her as a real person. The fathers turned out to be more accepting. Neil describes his father as sensitive and loving toward all kinds of people, irrespective of race or nationality.

Their history has helped make them understanding leaders of "interspatial" workshops at LPA Conferences. One short-statured woman observed that the tall partner is apt to be regarded as a saint, as having a screw loose, or as having a "little person fetish." Some participants discussed problems such as affairs or mistreatment; others affirmed their happiness in their relationships and offered advice. One woman, a dwarf, did not want to appear prematurely at the office where her husband had recently become employed lest he encounter prejudice. He put a picture of her on his desk, thereby tactfully "breaking in" his workmates.

There are many more mixed-height couples listed as members than ever appear at LPA conferences. Some dwarf partners arrive without their average-statured mates and need to be encouraged that the mates are welcome. Sometimes dwarf husbands stay away, feeling it is enough to have "made it" in the average-statured world.

Through the ages neither stigma nor troubles have prevented some short and average-statured persons from falling in love. Seneb, an important member of a royal Egyptian household, was married to an average-statured woman; eighteenth-century court dwarf Boruwlaski wrote moving letters that successfully importuned his future wife to accept his proposal; and Christopher Smart, a popular eighteenth-century poet, wrote a poem for a taller woman whom he advised not to judge "your lover's quality by quantity or weight." Promising her both fame and tenderness, he tried to charm her into acquiescing.[55] History does not tell us whether the lady was won over by Smart's passionately reasonable argument, but many have echoed his sentiments.

Choosing Whether to Have Children

What used to be a given, that marriage would be followed soon afterward by children, can no longer be assumed even in the average-statured population. In the case of little people, the choice of whether to have children is even more complex. One young adult dwarf decided to have surgery that would make it impossible for her to bear children. She was quite certain she would never want the responsibility of bringing into the world someone who would have to cope with the medical and social problems she had known.

There are couples who decide not to bear or adopt children because they feel that they can just about manage their own lives and significant health problems. They may also have resolved to use their available energies for a more global sort of generativity, engaging in social advocacy or nurturing others who are not their own children.

At one case conference in the 1970s at the Johns Hopkins Moore Clinic, Dr. Victor McKusick was asked what he felt about dwarfs having children: he hesitated a bit, and then offered the opinion that he thought a couple might do well to decide to have just one child—or at least to limit the number of children in the family. McKusick appreciated the wish to have children, but his experience had made him aware of the difficulties they might encounter.

Although not all dwarfs would agree with this approach, it is extremely rare in LPA to see a family in which dwarf parents have more than two children. Matt and Amy Roloff are among the few couples that are the parents of four; as it turned out, three of their children are average statured and only one is a dwarf. The lively world they have created for their family has been featured in many articles, as well as in Matt's thoughtful autobiography, *Against Tall Odds*.[56] Still, this trend toward smaller families exists in the greater society: Accounts of families with six or more children were common in past centuries, but parents of this large a family today may be subject to amazed, sometimes unfriendly questioning.

Whether a child will be a dwarf or average statured is unpredictable. The genetic odds in individual situations are generally known, and often depend on whether the conditions of each affected partner are dominant or recessive. However, these are only odds, and each birth represents a separate toss of the coin. For each couple that decides to have a child, the decision is an affirmation of their own lives, and a leap of faith about the lives they may expect for their children. Pregnant LP women are not uncommon in LPA these days. (See Ginny Foos, clinic coordinator of Medical Genetics at Children's Hospital in San Francisco, who is shown in fig. 5.8 with her husband, Joe, computer salesperson and interim president of the LPA San Francisco chapter.) By now there is a growing community of LPs who have given birth to or adopted children. New babies are regarded as a cause for a celebration, and there are always many pairs of arms eager to receive them.

One cannot always predict, however, what the attitudes of new or prospective parents will be. On a Phil Donahue show in the 1980s, two couples described their very different attitudes. Leonard Sawich, a psychologist and humorist who had written an excellent article about the ironies of life as a dwarf, discussed the evolution of his own thinking about having a child. Although his wife, Lenette, also a

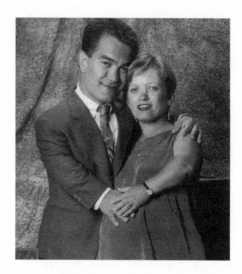

Fig. 5.8. Joe and Ginny Foos. Photographer: Gary Parker.

dwarf, did not care whether their children were short or average statured, Len expressed a preference for a dwarf. But he had not always felt this way: "When I was a young kid, I had vowed that if there was a chance that my children would be like me then I would never have children. Then I went through a whole coming out process where I began to ask myself well, what's wrong with being a dwarf. Then after I began to realize that there was nothing wrong with being a dwarf, then why wouldn't I want to have children like me?"[57]

Harry McDonald, an engineer, married to Carol, an average-statured woman, described his reaction to his son's birth: "When Brendan was born I saw him coming out of the delivery room and my first reaction was like father like son—I went home and was really depressed because of the fact that I knew what life was—I've lived it. I've gone through the name-calling, the prejudices so to speak, and it was depressing to know that I did this to him." Harry's worst fears were realized. Brendan became paralyzed and died tragically in his twenties. Harry himself, who had held leadership positions and had appeared on television as a goodwill ambassador for the dwarfism community, died in his fifties, not long after. These events, while quite rare, cannot be factored out as impossible.

Sometimes a mildly affected individual elects to have children, and they turn out to be more seriously compromised. That was the experience of Mark Andrew Berseth, who has osteogenesis imperfecta. His wife, Lorraine, gave birth to a son and a daughter with the condition; the son suffered a fractured clavicle at birth and exhibited other signs of a more serious form than his father's. Nevertheless, Berseth attempted to remain optimistic: "But as Lorraine and I surrender any plans for his life we may have had and accept God's plan, we'll come to experience that blessing in our lives. We love our children and cherish the privilege and shoulder the responsibility of parenting them. . . . Together Lorraine and I will experience the joys and the heartaches that come when an O.I.'er begets an O.I.'er."[58]

Every story is different and every outcome unpredictable, but the question of whether to have children is one that many LPs grapple with. Shortly after Watergate, one young woman mentioned to an older member of the dwarfism community her quandary about whether it was morally responsible for her to bring a child like herself into the world. Her friend responded that she found it ironic that rarely did anyone question the right of someone with Nixon's moral character to have children, but people did question whether persons with physical disabilities like dwarfism should do so. Several years later, the young woman married happily and had two children—one a dwarf and the other average statured.

Sometimes persons from different nations have dissimilar views. British LP Simon Minty attended an international dwarfism conference at which several German LPs mentioned that they did not intend to have children.

They said they felt a "pressure" not to have children who were short-statured. When I tried to find out why they felt this pressure it was hard to establish; possibly internalized oppression but they did mention government and public perceptions and attitudes too. It was almost (and I am buying into a stereotype here) that short statured people might be seen as a burden, as not an "efficient" member of society. I also know of a German geneticist in Toronto who expressed the same feeling. The contradiction for me is that these people seemed very secure in themselves, (at least on the outside) were successful and intelligent, yet still held this point of view.[59]

Minty did not believe these attitudes might be linked to the influence of earlier German eugenic thinking. He mentioned Tom Shakespeare's study of U.K. RGA members that found that more short-statured couples said that they would not choose to have dwarf children than did average-statured parents of dwarfs.

Because some short-statured persons in both countries expressed qualifications about childbearing, and because the young Germans had been embarrassed by their Nazi forbears' ideology, Minty felt that other factors must be at work, among them the experiences that they had had as children. Also, he volunteered, their attitudes may not be representative of short-statured persons who do not attend conventions.

Adoption

Some couples prefer to adopt a dwarf child who has been given up by his or her own birth parents. Adoption is also a major concern in LPA because childbearing is often medically difficult for dwarfs. Sometimes, as in achondroplasia, a couple has experienced the tragedy of bearing a "double-dominant" child, one that cannot survive. Even more than in society overall, many couples are eager to adopt a child, preferably an infant, but few babies in the United States are available for adoption. Children with disabilities, including dwarfism, can sometimes be located. The LPA adoption committee is helpful in connecting prospective parents and children and in advising couples how to negotiate the process. These days, foreign adoptions are most common, with pictures of children in need of parents appearing in almost every issue of *LPA Today.*

There is a higher percentage of adopted persons in LPA than in the society in general. In the past, it was far more common than now for American parents to relinquish their dwarf children for adoption. Although no formal survey has ever been conducted, it seems that the numbers of older members of LPA who are adoptees is substantial. At the 1999 LPA convention, a workshop was held for persons considering a search for their birth parents.

I spoke to Cathy Sarino, who had initiated and run the "adoption reunions" workshop. Professionally, she coordinates an adoption program for children with special needs in British Columbia; she is also the mother of a young-adult LP daughter. Although adoption is often discussed in LPA, she said, the focus is usually on how to adopt and not on the issues surrounding adoption. Dwarf adoptees may fear they were surrendered because of their dwarfism. After Sarino heard two young people discuss their concerns about having been adopted, Sarino had concluded that there was an unrecognized need for a venue for discussion.

Sarino felt that adoptive parents could easily underestimate the importance of adoption in their child's mind. Especially as the young people approached adolescence, their parents needed to take the time to deal with questions relating to the adoption, whether the child was asked to draw a family tree at school, or identity issues were surfacing in adolescence or young adulthood.

Among adoptees Sarino has spoken with, approximately half have expressed interest in searching for birth parents. They hope for a good outcome, but express fears. In February 2003, with the help of Dr. Song, Mary Beth Ely and her daughter Katy found Katy's birth family in Korea, brother, sister, and cousins, and attended and enjoyed the LPK convention. "I loved them," Mary Beth wrote to the Dwarfism List, "I feel as if I have gained two other children."

Occasionally, an adolescent LP becomes pregnant and gives up the child to an LPA couple, and the two families continue to know each other. Continued association occurs naturally when all parties remain active in the organization, a unique situation. Sarino also mentioned that prospective adoptive parents are forced to deal with their differences again, as they are evaluated by an adoption agency. They have to convince a sometimes skeptical social worker that short-statured, sometimes physically compromised persons can be good parents.

Peter Valuckas, father of two adopted children, is a diastrophic
dwarf who has worked as an adoption professional. He has many interesting stories about the vagaries of adoption. He himself turned
down the possibility of adopting the very desirable child of a professional couple because he feared that complications might ensue
because the family lived nearby. Indeed, a year later the birth father
regretted that he had given his child up and sought to reverse the decision.

Patty Bowers, whose daughter Amy has Kniest syndrome, believes
the demand for dwarf babies among little people is growing because
of an increasing marriage rate and awareness of potential birth problems. Sometimes eagerness to adopt can lead to awkward situations.

When Amy was born, medical personnel handled "breaking the
news" to her parents very badly. "There's your baby!" they said with
obvious discomfort. The next morning, Patty's husband Grant told
her that something was wrong with their daughter, a cleft palate. "Is
that all?" she said. The baby was handed to her to hold while, sur-
rounded by ten doctors and nurses, Patty was told that Amy had
Kniest syndrome. They said that she would be blind, deaf, and crippled like a pretzel. Tears rolled down Patty's cheeks, but she could not
wipe them because Amy was in her arms. "Get me out of here!" she
said, and Grant wheeled her from the room.

Outside, some LPs waited, having somehow been told that there
might be a dwarf baby available for adoption. But Patty and Grant
had no intention of giving Amy up. Instead, they found her good
medical care and joined LPA. Although Amy did have some medical
complications, they were not nearly as dire as those predicted. At her
high school graduation in 2002, her parents rejoiced to see her heading for the platform as she received one honor after another.

Fortunately, "breaking the news" scenes like the one described are
increasingly rare; so are prospective parents "waiting in the wings."
Usually, adoptions are arranged formally, and prospective parents are
helped through the maze. Although most are dwarfs, average-
statured parents are also invited to inquire about adopting children
listed in the committee's files.

More and more, dwarf parents are bringing home foreign-born children. One such mother is Ruth Ricker, former president of LPA, who adopted 6-year-old Michael Janis Zutis Ricker in Latvia in 1997.[60] In an LPA article, she reported that Jani (pronounced Yanni) was a wonderful kid, happy, thoughtful, and comical, and occasionally mischievous. She noted that he adored his grandparents, his cousin, and Ruth's roommate. For a while, Ricker reduced her work and extracurricular schedule to help him acclimate to his new world, but she has since returned to a full schedule. An Equal Opportunity Specialist with the U.S. Department of Education Office of Civil Rights, Ricker is a disability activist in many arenas and a participant in the church where Yanni has attended Sunday school. But whatever the differences among the many narratives of adoptive parents the essential similarity reverberates—the profoundly gratifying experience of finding a child to nurture and love.

Deciding to bear children and deciding to adopt are not mutually exclusive choices. Brian Morris, recently retired as president of a certified public accounting firm, and his wife Linda, who became a dietician after being rejected by college nursing programs in a discriminatory era, are the parents of four children, two of whom are adopted. The Morrises are one of a growing number of three-generation families: they have a granddaughter, Alicia, who is also a dwarf.[61]

The Mature Years

During their mature years dwarfs, like most others, focus on building careers, achieving financial security, and enjoying their homes, families, and friendship networks. For those who are still single, finding a partner often remains a goal; work and friendship assume increased importance, as does extended family. Most leadership positions in LPA are held by members between thirty and seventy, most in the forties, but some older.

Often individuals delight in customizing their homes to accommodate their short stature. Many also find themselves dealing with physical, especially orthopedic, problems. Surgery for persons with skeletal dysplasia is not uncommon: spinal stenosis problems increase in achondroplasia, and arthritic joints deteriorate in a number of other conditions. Much energy goes into making decisions about surgery, and, if impairment is present, figuring out ways to sustain independence. Reduced energy is also a significant factor for persons with adult growth hormone deficiency, and others. Although most persons try not to retire early from the world of work and prefer not to ask for disability payments (both ego and the size of payments militate against this path) serious impairments may allow individuals no alternative. For the vast majority, work remains a central, defining part of their lives and a source of pride.

The challenges of the physical world, substantial for short-statured persons in youth, become even more daunting for most dwarfs with each passing year. The venerable Fred Short, an English contributor to the LPA Dwarfism List, is now sixty. A retired teacher, he also paints and gardens and is quite sociable. In one post, he describes a struggle to manage two home repair chores. Usually, he explains, he and his wife Linda rely on hiring plumbers, electricians, landscapers, etc., to do any specialized heavy work. But on this occasion no one seemed to be available. "We said, 'Sod it! We'll do it ourselves.' I tell you, the seven dwarfs have nothing on our labor ability and determination when the two of us set our minds to it! Bring in the ladders!"

Short continues with a graphic description of the couple's successful removal, repair, and remounting of a door. Rehanging a wall clock, however, defeated them. While he was able easily to drill and plug the holes on the wall, he could not remount it; ultimately, he recognized that short of rigging up some form of complex scaffolding system, there was no way that they were going to get the clock back up. "It was at this point, we realized Time was going to stop us Dwarfs! Time in fact to eat humble pie, put lashings of salve on our pride, and ask our Norwegian Hunk of a physiotherapist if he could possibly assist us in our plight. *This,* this folks is where life just ain't fair! He walks in (making sure he didn't bump his head on our low ceilings), said, "Is

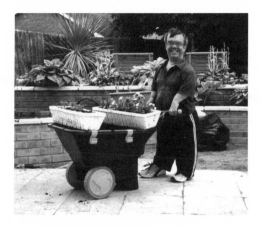

Fig. 5.9. Fred Short, retired teacher, in his garden. Photograph courtesy of Fred Short.

this the clock?," then with absolutely *no* effort, lifted it, walked to the wall, and placed it on the fixings! *He didn't even need the ladders!"* Short praises the virtues of patience and resolves to leave such jobs to the able bodied, at least till the next time. He concludes, "Fred, chuffed with his door, frustrated with his clock!"

Short's essay renders admirably the problems dwarfs face, especially as they age. It also captures the spirited determination to keep active and stretch limits. That the Shorts have been successful is apparent in an article that they have written about the garden they planned and had installed (fig. 5.9). It took into account their different bodies and their increasing years as well as their passion for gardening and their aesthetics. They have described their project in *Carryongardening,* the online magazine of Thrive, the British horticultural society whose mission is to enable disadvantaged, disabled, and older people to participate fully in the life of the community.[62]

Not everyone is as fortunate in having the health, imagination, and economic means to ensure comfort in the later years. To enhance that possibility, many persons who have been able to function independently with minimal assistance decide in their fifties or sixties to move closer to family, continuing their active participation in others' lives, but beginning to lead more interdependent ones.

VOCATIONS

> What are they to do with their lives? Their choice is decidedly limited. Unlike normal children, they cannot plan careers at will. Innumerable doors are closed to them. They cannot be aviators, policemen, engineers, electricians, chefs, laborers, bus drivers, clerks. The professions are closed to them. A doctor, a lawyer, a school teacher no taller than a small child, not only would be laughed out of countenance, but would probably starve to death.
>
> It is because of this drastically limited selection that so many midgets turn to the theatre, the carnival, the circus for a livelihood.[63]

The authors of *It's a Small World* (1934) go on to mention shopkeepers, jewelry makers, salespeople, and an architect, but the contradictions elude them. Bodin and Hershey's work was relied on as an authoritative investigation long afterward; in 1968, sociologist Marcello Truzzi, relying heavily on its data, calls it a "somewhat sensational but nevertheless valuable journalistic report."[64]

There is one respected early source for statistical vocational information, Ernst Mörch's 1941 report about dwarfs in Denmark.[65] He studied thirty-nine men and thirty-eight women. Among the men he found twenty-one artisans, three tradespeople, four clerks, one musician, one circus clown, one souffleur, and eight unskilled laborers. Among the women, there were nine seamstresses, one married woman, one owner of an embroidery shop, one teacher of housekeeping, one music student, one music hall performer, one farm owner, two housemaids, and seventeen untrained women.

Reading this list reminds us how dramatically the world has changed for dwarfs. Industrialization is partially responsible for the differences, and social changes have led to the near disappearance of "untrained women." Dwarfs, who previously were at the lowest rungs of the economic ladder, if employed at all, have become better educated and entered most professions, businesses, and service occupations.

These changes happened relatively recently. Only 6 of the 143 persons attending the 1960 convention of LPA were professionals. Most of the rest were unemployed or underemployed.[66] A 1977 survey revealed a modest improvement: approximately 18 percent of respondents were employed in professional and managerial positions, 27 percent in clerical, 12 percent in skilled work, and 18 percent in semiskilled or unskilled. One-fourth were unemployed. Income figures revealed that 60 percent had incomes of less than $10,000 a year, and none made more than $20,000 a year.[67] (In today's terms, most would make under $30,000, with the highest under $60,000.)

Only one recent investigation (Gollust et al.) reports income levels of persons with dwarfism.[68] Studying 189 persons with achondroplasia and 136 of their first-degree relatives, it finds that 31 percent of the ACH group and 73 percent of the FDR group make more than $50,000 a year. Although 46 percent of the ACH group has completed college or graduate school, and a slightly higher figure of 59 percent of the FDR group has done so, the difference in their educational levels does not fully explain the greater discrepancy in incomes. Nonetheless, that even one third of the individuals with achondroplasia in the study are now making a decent income is encouraging, compared with past statistics. One ought not to draw unwarranted conclusions about the U.S. dwarf population overall from this sample, but the study does suggest that the educational and economic situations of at least a substantial percentage have improved.

One can get some sense of the changes that have occurred by looking at the resumes of some of the older members. It is not uncommon to find someone who has made a transition from a physically demanding job to another that requires intellectual or interpersonal skills, or exchanged a position in entertainment for another in the "straight" world. One such example is the career trajectory of 74-year-old Joe White, who left Harvard University at 18 to become a clown for the Barnum and Bailey circus. White subsequently had a job as Little Oscar for the Oscar Meyer Wiener company, acted in *Over the Rainbow,* and wrote five books about magic. Late in life White held a very different position as an officer of the senior citizens commission for the city of Cypress.

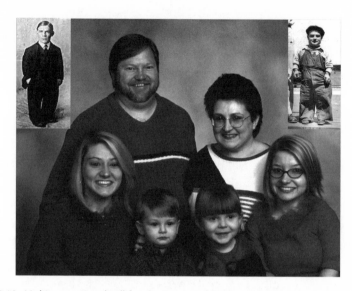

Fig. 5.10. Multigenerational Hill family: Dean and Reba with children, Candace, Chandler, Charity, and Kendra. Reba Hill's grandfather, William S. Cawthon c.1880 (*inset left*) and father, William P. Cawthon c. 1960 (*inset right*). Photograph courtesy of Reba Hill.

Another talented individual from an even earlier generation was William Cawthon. His daughter, Reba Hill, admires her father, who married at 47 and died of septicemia in 1976 at the age of 65. Cawthon, who had average-statured sisters, had been employed in carnivals as a young man and subsequently worked for NASA (National Aeronautics and Space Administration) for twenty-five years fabricating minute missile instrument parts; after that, he owned a watch shop and was very popular in his community.

The Hill family is also an example of a multigenerational family with dwarfism (fig. 5.10). Three of the four children of Reba and her average-statured husband Dean have pseudoachondroplasia. Reba's grandfather, a telegraph operator of English, Dutch, and Irish ancestry, was one of three brothers with dwarfism; her great-grandfather had the condition as well (although it had not yet been named). Their original family had been quite well off, living in huge houses with servants in Tennessee. However, despite this prosperity, her grandfather had committed suicide: in great pain from his condition, he did not want to burden his family. The care that later generations had access to was unavailable to him.

Like Cawthon, many persons in previous generations had careers that included traditional jobs and intervals as performers; now, these latter occupations tend to be less prominent. Nevertheless, many persons, for instance, still take time off from regular employment to act in Radio City's Christmas pageant, securing nest eggs to cover education, home, or medical expenses.

The 2001 LPA database reveals how dramatically the employment picture has changed. Many more individuals are employed in positions that require a college education. Approximately 26.3 percent of respondents are professionals. The categories include 100 teachers, 17 social workers, 15 lawyers, 10 clergy, 6 doctors, 4 psychologists, and a psychiatrist. There are sixteen persons who are computer specialists. Several others have occupations in the sciences, including nurses, engineers, biologists, an astrophysicist, an archaeologist, and a chemist. There are twenty-four artists, including fine artists, graphic artists, and designers; there are also architects, and ten persons who are writers, journalists, or editors.

The managerial and business owner category constitutes about 15.6 percent of the total, including fifty-eight accountants, some bankers, human resources directors, vice presidents, systems administrators, and a range of persons described as administrators, managers, coordinators, executives, and various business owners.

Approximately 45.9 percent are employed in various service, administrative, office work, and sales occupations. Approximately 10.8 percent are employed in craft, operator, or farm occupations, including factory workers, laborers, maintenance workers, fast-food workers, and housekeepers, as well as skilled workers: a commercial fisherman, a farmer, mechanics, and plumbers. An additional 1.1 percent are "self-employed."

Acting and entertainment is a significant category for this group. There are approximately a hundred actors or entertainers of various kinds, with twice as many male as female actors. There are also musicians, drama teachers, and comedians, and several television, radio, and music producers and promoters. Because actors and entertainers have been so prominent in the history of the group and have always been quite visible in LPA, the size of their representation is surprising. However, it is well known that there are many persons with other primary jobs who shuttle in and out of the entertainment fields; only the first choice has been registered as the person's occupation.

Only two persons list as clowns, another as a rodeo clown, and another as a ringmaster assistant. The stereotype of dwarfs as circus clowns seems no longer to apply. Their numbers are significantly reduced even among non-LPA members. Although they never constituted more than a small percentage of dwarfs, they somehow became engraved in the public consciousness as representative or even sole examples.

I wondered how the profile of the LPA database compared with that of the country overall. The results revealed that the two groups did not differ in most respects. The general population in the 2000 census had 33.1 percent in management, professional, and related occupations; LPA had 41.9 percent. The general population had 41.7 percent in service, office, and sales; LPA had 45.9 percent. The only categories that were substantially different were construction, production, farming, and maintenance occupations, where the general population totaled 24.1 percent and LPA 10.8 percent.

Probably the most astounding statistic of all is the percentage listing themselves as unemployed—1.4 percent as compared with the 25 percent unemployment rate that Scott found in 1977; an additional 2.7 percent are on disability. Among others not currently on the employment rolls, or having some part-time work, are 135 homemakers, 352 college students, and 144 retired persons. The unemployment and disability statistics should be approached with considerable caution, however. Many individuals did not fill in the employment category at all. There is no way of knowing whether they simply overlooked it, or chose not to answer the question, and so we cannot determine whether they are employed or unemployed. Also, non-LPA populations are apt to contain greater numbers of persons who are more profoundly disabled, mentally retarded, or socially isolated. But even as compared with Scott's group (individuals in touch with dwarfism centers) the contrast is great.

The growing number of college students suggests a future that should at least be as promising as the present. Despite the fact that I obtained guidance in establishing categories and assessing these statistics, I am inexperienced in this area, and so I recommend treating the results as suggestive rather than definitive.[69] Further evaluations by professional demographers are recommended. Also, one cannot extrapolate to the much larger numbers of persons with dwarfism who are not in LPA and perhaps may not be as well off. All that said, it is still evident that a great transformation has taken place, and the curve is heading upward. Many members recall "how things used to be." Paul Miller, now in his early forties, is a law professor at the University of Washington, and a former Economic Employment Opportunity Commissioner. During his early years in LPA, the only professionals that he was aware of were schoolteachers; they were seen as special and were highly respected. When he was growing up, many dwarfs were glad to have any jobs at all. He finds it particularly exciting to witness the tremendous difference in the younger generation's self-esteem and life expectations.

INDIVIDUALS IN SEVERAL SELECTED OCCUPATIONS

Brief descriptions and photographs of a number of individuals are included here to communicate graphically some of the diverse vocational choices of the past two generations of dwarfs. Corresponding as they sometimes do with the list of occupations that Bodin and Hershey asserted that dwarfs could never attain, they serve as a visual disclaimer. Perhaps their presence may imprint in the reader's consciousness a truer reality than that provided by the flood of media images, common even today, of dwarfs as fantasy figures or clowns.

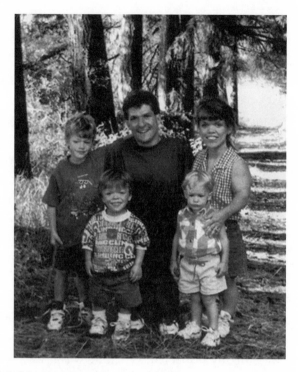

Fig. 5.11. Roloff family: Matt and Amy with children Jeremy, Zachary, and Molly.
Photograph courtesy of Matt Roloff.

Matt Roloff

To capture the enthusiasm and spirit of this new era for dwarfs, there
is probably no better short route than reading Matt Roloff's autobiography, *Against Tall Odds*.[70] Roloff's energy, creativity, and determination, the leitmotif of his original family, are characteristics that rarely
occur in the same measure elsewhere. He has managed to perform admirably as a software sales executive, maintain a happy marriage and
raise four children, construct a 34-acre farm where fantasy structures
abound, and undertake the presidency of LPA (2002–2004) (fig. 5.11).

Roloff's book offers some clues to his vitality in its description of
his parents, who faced extraordinary obstacles. They too had four
children; two sons were diastrophic dwarfs and another had a life-
threatening heart ailment; only their average-statured eldest child, a
5 foot 10 inch daughter, had no disability. *Against Tall Odds* describes

how his parents raised him with loving discipline and good sense, encouraging him to be both hard working and fun loving. Such values made a deep impression on him. Although in young adulthood he had a brief bout with addiction, he was able to surmount it; it helped to make him understanding of others' issues.

Roloff also portrays the often-muddled world of Shriner's hospital, where he spent a good portion of his youth. Because little was known about his type of dwarfism, much of the surgery performed on him was experimental, and a significant portion may have been neither successful nor necessary. But he had the parental support that few others confined in those hospital walls received.

His coming of age corresponded with the computer revolution in Silicon Valley. Although he had been an average student, he proved to be extremely diligent and sociable from an early age as well as instinctively entrepreneurial. A designer at Altos Computer Systems, he worked on several projects that continued to be used in years to come, and he quickly rose within his company. A risk taker, he went on to become a sales executive for some of the largest software companies in the world, playing a key management role in helping one organization move from its status as a $100 million company to a $2 billion company in four years. He mastered this new field, unbound by "the tyranny of the credential," without college coursework. In 2002 Roloff decided that he wanted to use his experience to benefit LPA and set the group on an ambitious course. With the initiative of the groups' first director of development, Leslye Sneider, a fund-raising plan was established; other programs were also designed. In 2004, Rick Spiegel, a talented professional actuary (pictured in fig. 5.6 with his wife, Barbara, at his 2003 wedding), succeeded Roloff.

Irene Yuan

In 2002 Irene Yuan received her Bachelor of Fine Arts degree from the Art Center College of Design in Pasadena, California, one of the foremost institutions for art and design education. She currently designs

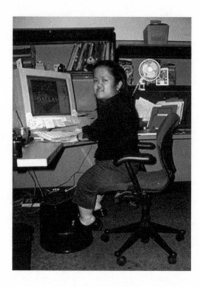

Fig. 5.12. Irene Yuan, graphic designer. Photograph courtesy of Irene Yuan.

for *City and Travel Magazine*, where she is also acquiring experience in lifestyle and fashion projects (fig. 5.12). Coordinator of the LPA Dwarf Artists' Coalition, she has set up a Web site for the group.

The outspoken Yuan is active in the Young Democrats group in Sacramento, California; she joined them in a lobbying effort against Jeffrey Sutton, candidate for a federal judgeship, whose record indicated that he would vigorously attempt to weaken disability laws. Yuan has alerted LPs to a good many other significant issues, making cogent arguments and enlisting their support. An activist in dwarfism-related matters and national issues, she opposed preemptive military action in Iraq.

Yuan's decision to become a graphic artist resembles that of other talented LPs who continue to pursue fine arts while using their abilities commercially to support themselves. The advent of computers has increased their chances for employment; many are employed in Web site design and behind-the-scenes work in film. Australian LP Nancy Adams, for example, worked on digital technology for *Lord of the Rings.*

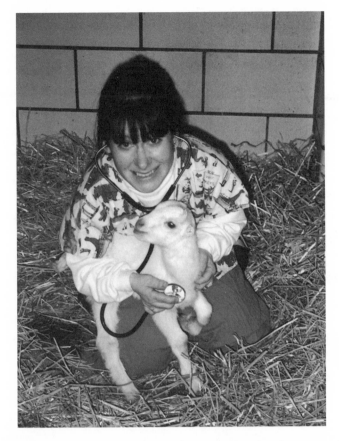

Fig. 5.13. Melinda Keel North, veterinary technologist. Photograph courtesy of Katherine Pudelek.

Melinda Keel North

Melinda Keel North, married to financial analyst Jonathan North, grew up with many animals in her house and even raised a pair of raccoons and a baby squirrel in her basement.[71] Majoring in the sciences, she received a Bachelor of Science degree and went on to work in a laboratory doing DNA fingerprinting. After volunteering at the National Zoo, however, she rediscovered her passion for animals (fig. 5.13). She returned to school to become a veterinary technologist, a position similar to physician's associate or nurse.

Many persons question how a person of North's stature could function in such a physically demanding job. She explains that she works with a team; although she can do restraint, animal handlers do a great deal. The veterinarian and technologist perform the skilled procedures, such as inserting an intravenous catheter or inducing anesthesia. North assists with surgery, does physical exams, administers vaccinations and medications, and does dental cleanings and extractions; she also deals with radiology and diagnostics.

Although there is a two-year technician degree, she took the four-year program and became a technologist. The field is competitive, and by maximizing her qualifications and proving herself during two internships, she found rewarding work in veterinary offices in New York, and later at the Chicago Zoo. North's story raises an issue that often arises when dwarfs make unusual job choices. Their families or professionals in the field sometimes discourage short-statured persons from entering physically demanding occupations. Although occupations such as hairstylist, nurse, or surgeon are uncommon choices, persons enthusiastic about their work often devise ways to manage.

Grady Horndt

Grady Horndt is one of a minority of dwarfs who work at various physically demanding jobs (fig. 5.14). Among the crafts positions others hold are automobile mechanic, cabinetmaker, electrician, machinist, and boilermaker; two individuals are employed by the forest service and four are farmers; there are ten hairstylists and a barber, several cooks and a chef.

Horndt first became interested in welding in 1967 when he learned about it in a high school shop class. A friend of the family offered him employment in a welding shop, and Grady worked for him for two years. Subsequently, he went to trade school in Houston and then returned to welding, working with pipes of all sizes for Brown and Root,

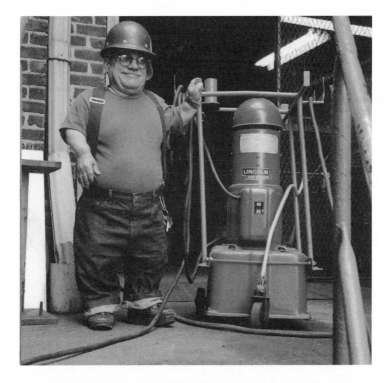

Fig. 5.14. Grady Horndt, pipe welder. Photograph courtesy of Grady Horndt.

a large and respected national firm. Although the work was physically demanding and required lifting, walking, and climbing, he worked for the firm for 15 years. Subsequently, he was employed as an aircraft welder for seven years; at present, he works as a pipe welder in construction in Farmington, Connecticut.

Horndt has pseudoachondroplasia, a condition accompanied by arthritic, deteriorating joints, and his type of work did take its toll. He required hip replacements in 1989 and again in 2003, and although he made good recoveries, his recent experience has given him pause. He has acquired considerable skill and loves the work, but he may seek employment in an easier aspect of it, bench work, something he has also done before.

Horndt remains devoted to his two children, Christal and Christopher, young adults, now living on their own in other states. He was fortunate during his surgery and convalescence to have the support of his fiancée, Alice Higgins, a science technician for a pharmaceutical company and former president of the Mid-Hudson chapter of LPA. Now, after having married in October 2004, and feeling restored to better health, he is looking forward to the next stage of life.

Anna Adelson

Anna Adelson is a confirmed Brooklynite, at home in the lively Park Slope neighborhood where she resides and enjoys lifelong friend-

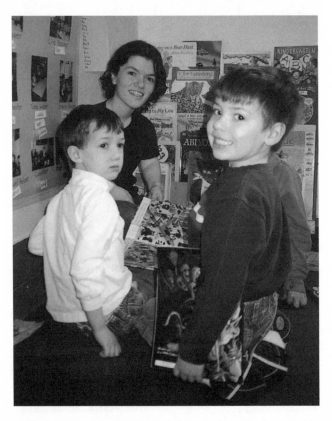

Fig. 5.15. Anna Adelson, nursery school teacher. Photograph courtesy of Karen Bacal.

ships. The community has afforded her continuity in a variety of ways, including her present employment. At age four in 1978 she attended a local nursery school; now she is teaching another generation of four-year-olds in that same preschool program (fig. 5.15).

After two years at Skidmore College, Adelson was employed as an administrative assistant in a couple of nonprofit settings, including the grassroots Brooklyn Bridge Park Coalition. Although the work made good use of her organizational, computer, graphic, and people skills, she sought adventure and the opportunity to travel, and joined a Pokemon children's theater tour that took her to Great Britain, Portugal, and Belgium; she also worked in Chicago as part of the Radio City Christmas road show.

When she returned, she was offered a position as co-teacher of the four-year-old group at the center where she had previously supervised counselors in the after-school program. She has been praised for how well she relates to the children—planning activities, tuning in to their personalities and moods, and allowing them to learn and connect with each other at their own pace.

At first, some children inquired about why their teacher was not much taller than they were. At this age, especially aware of size because of their desire to grow bigger themselves, children can be perplexed by a surprising discrepancy between age and size. Anna explained that she was a short grown-up, and the issue soon disappeared without threat to her authority. Once the relationship with a class is established, Anna, like other LPs, finds that she is simply accepted for who she is. She enjoys the school's atmosphere and appreciates the enthusiasm and sense of wonder in these young, unfolding personalities.

Other significant interests include ceramics and LPA. Having been introduced to the group in childhood, she had left it as a teenager. At the Portland convention in 1999 she rediscovered her dwarfism, and since then she has felt equally comfortable in the short and average-statured worlds.

The Influence of Dr. Steven Kopits

One thing the next three individuals have in common is their view of their relationship with Dr. Steven Kopits as a vital aspect of their professional success. Each had been his patient from childhood well into adulthood. Like Julie Rotta, graphics editor of this book, they spoke about his having initiated a discussion of careers with them while they were still adolescents. His belief in them became a central part of their own self-confidence.

In his eulogy for Dr. Kopits, actor Danny Woodburn related that even when he was a boy, Kopits had spoken to him as an equal—patiently explaining every detail of his syndrome, SED congenita—while lightheartedly joking. Recognizing how his physician had loved each of his patients, Woodburn expressed his return of that love. He concluded, "I thank him for my life," noting that without this "Michelangelo of the bones" he would not have had the chance to graduate from college, pursue his successful career, or marry his beloved wife. (He married actress/playwright Amy Buchwald in 1998.)

Pediatrician Dr. Jennifer Arnold also remembers Dr. Kopits asking her about career plans. His enthusiastic response when she talked of becoming a doctor helped confirm her decision. Like Woodburn, Arnold considered Kopits a friend and another father. She had chosen medicine in the hope that perhaps one day she might be as important in her patients' lives as he was.[72]

Julie Williams, a clinical psychologist specializing in neuropsychology, recalled an incident in which Dr. Kopits had calmed *her* when she was a young adult scheduled for surgery. Julie had announced to the whole staff that she would not submit to yet another surgery; she was feeling somewhat panicky, and after all these years was just fed up. Dr. Kopits had arrived after others' attempts to persuade her had failed. "My good friend," he said warmly, "how wonderful it is to see you!" Williams' anxiety and anger immediately melted, doctor and patient spent some easy moments together, and the operation went forward.

Many years later, she had an adolescent patient whose mother could be heard raging outside her office. All at once, Dr. Kopits's strategem leapt into mind: "Hello, my friend," Williams said warmly, "I'm glad you're here. I've been looking forward to meeting with you." The mother's anger was quickly defused, and client and doctor had a productive discussion.

These remarks are included not only to pay homage to Dr. Kopits, but also to emphasize that medicine, as it is practiced by the best physicians, is a profound, existential human encounter.

Julie Williams

Julie Williams, a clinical psychologist, is an example of someone whose vocational direction developed over time. She majored in rehabilitation at college and then took a routine administrative job with the State of Ohio Bureau of Disability. She yearned for more challenge, and so three years later she enrolled for her doctorate in psychology. For the next five years, while working as a clinician with adolescents with physical and emotional disabilities, she became increasingly interested in adolescents with brain injuries; she began to work exclusively with that group while continuing doctoral studies.

Growing up in Dayton, Ohio, Williams had yearned to experience big city life on the East or West coast. Now confident about her abilities, she got her chance when she was accepted for an internship in neuropsychology at Mt. Sinai School of Medicine in New York in 2002–03. Her success in that position led to a postdoctoral post. Despite significant mobility limitations, she has been able to navigate the hospital with two kinds of scooters, as well as the New York City bus system, which has lifting devices.

Jennifer Arnold

Dr. Jennifer Arnold, a pediatrician, is recognized as a role model both within and outside dwarfism circles (fig. 5.16). She is increasingly

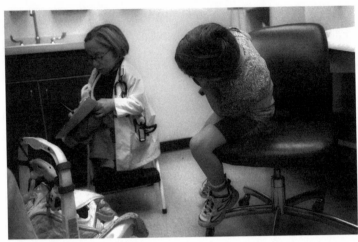

Fig. 5.16. Jennifer Arnold, M.D., pediatrician. Photograph by Annie O'Neill. Copyright, Pittsburgh Post-Gazette 2004

sought out by the media: she has been featured on a number of documentaries and talk shows, and in newspaper articles.[73] Now in her late twenties, she has completed her residency at Children's Hospital in Pittsburgh. Arnold has received high praise both from doctors and patients' families. Dr. Dena Hofkosh, pediatric residency program director, commented, "She's got this very lovely ability to connect with the kids and with parents. They trust her. If she were just a Little Person it would be a novelty. The fact is, she's a fabulous doctor."[74] One of Arnold's favorite stories involves a young patient who announced, "When I grow up, I want to be a little doctor like you!" Arnold laughingly replied, "You can't—but you can be a big doctor!"

Despite having had more than twenty orthopedic surgeries, some of them "tune-ups" performed to prevent her bones from bending and deforming as she grew and gained weight, she continued to experience distress and in 2001 had a hip replacement. Helped by what seems like a constitutionally cheerful personality, she has overcome the painful experiences that have often interrupted progress and the difficulties that medical school presents: "Academics didn't come easy to me; after studying for hours I was often stressed, and of course there were the physical obstacles. There were great days and difficult days; I was often tired and frustrated. Fortunately, there were enough good days to counteract the bad days."

Her parents were supportive, but they hadn't necessarily wanted her to do something so demanding. She had to love what she did to make it worthwhile. Arnold would like to find a niche with fewer physical obstacles, but she finds also herself attracted to neonatology and pediatric emergency intensive care, giving extremely sick kids a chance at life they might not otherwise have.

Danny Woodburn

A graduate of Temple University, talented actor Danny Woodburn has appeared in comedy clubs, theater, and film, but he is noted most of all for his television performances. He first achieved fame for his portrayal of Mickey Abbot, Kramer's volatile but lovable friend on *Seinfeld.* The role was an enormous breakthrough, in that a dwarf was playing a character like any other in the sitcom—outrageous and funny just as they were. Woodburn also made repeated appearances on *Baywatch, Tracy Takes On* (with Tracy Ullman), and *Murder She Wrote.*

He has also been cast in dramatic roles, receiving high praise for his performance in the made-for-TV movie "Things You Can Tell Just By Looking at Her." In that film he plays Albert, an accountant who becomes involved with an average-statured woman; dwarf actors are almost never seen in romantic roles. He has spoken out about the images of dwarfs in television and film, commenting at a Little People's Research Fund benefit in 1998: "Little people are often seen as freaks, as evil, dirty-minded, diabolical men with devious minds and lecherous hearts. On the other side of the coin they are seen as pathetic, pitiful, sad, and lonely, unwanted members of society. Or else they are presented as jokes, mistakes, clowns to be laughed at and dehumanized, instead of laughed with."

Woodburn has turned down roles of this kind and rewritten others; even when he has played fantasy characters, as in *Conan the Bar-*

barian and *Special Unit 2,* he has felt that the roles were well drawn. Woodburn also registered that he could never have played any of these active, demanding parts without the reconstructive surgery he had undergone.

As a stand-up comedian, he expresses his views about little people and society's perception of them. Unlike earlier dwarf performers, who submitted to being made ridiculous, and even major actors who never accepted themselves as dwarfs, Woodburn takes pride in his place in his profession, and, when he can, tries to influence the theater world and society.

Cara Egan

When Cara Egan was still in her twenties, she wrote an article for *Newsweek* entitled "The Seven Dwarfs and Me," expressing her indignation at the treatment she had sometimes experienced, and the portrayal of dwarfs in the media. Later, she chose a profession (public health administration) that allowed her to make a difference, for her group and others with disabilities.

After her stint as manager of communications at Holy Cross Hospital in Silver Spring, Maryland, she was hired as Special Projects Administrator for the American College of Physicians in Philadelphia, her current position (fig. 5.17). Her master's thesis, written for her degree at the School of Hygiene and Public Health at Johns Hopkins University, is entitled "LPA, Inc.: Coming of Age in the Policy Arena." It traces the organization's progress from social group to advocacy.

Egan served LPA for several years as vice president for public relations and advocacy; in that capacity she responded to countless provocations in the media, contacting media representatives when ridicule or distorted accounts appeared, consulting with producers or advertising executives about whether a given portrayal might be considered offensive. She also offered praise when it was due.

These days, she is LPA senior vice president, helping to revitalize local chapters, while continuing to promote political action for issues impacting the dwarf community, including health and disability. LPA

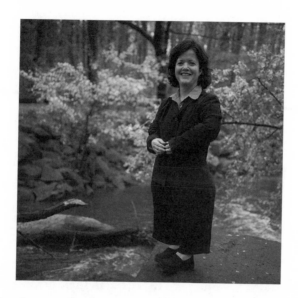

Fig. 5.17. Cara Egan, special projects administrator, American College of Physicians. Photograph courtesy of the Philadelphia Enquirer.

joined with the National Organization of Rare Diseases (NORD) to lobby for the Rare Diseases Act and the Rare Diseases Orphan Product Development Act. Despite the Bush administration's cutting of most social programs, these two bills passed and became law in October 2002.

Egan empathizes with the struggles of support groups and ethnic groups as well. She knows that there is a hard road ahead, given the health care rationing that has increasingly marked the managed care era. But she is glad to have acquired the expertise that allows her, both in her professional life and in LPA, to join the battle for patient rights and care. Her bountiful life, in a family that includes seven sisters and a brother, has become even richer: in 2004, she married Gibson Reynolds, rare-book dealer and long-time member of LPA.

Paul Miller

President Clinton appointed attorney Paul Miller as commissioner at the Economic Employment Opportunity Commission in 1994 (fig.

5.18). Miller achieved a distinguished record during his two terms, re-signing in 2004.[75] In 1997 his career success had been capped by the joy he felt on marrying Jennifer Mechem (a disability policy coordinator in the Education Department) and several years later by the birth of their daughter Naomi.

His path had not always been easy. Although he had graduated from the University of Pennsylvania and Harvard Law School, he had been shocked and dismayed when law firms that had actively pursued him denied him employment because of his stature. He received forty-five rejection letters. Miller commented on the experience: "I didn't begin to understand until I was told by one law firm that even though they personally did not have a problem with my size, they feared their clients would think that they were running . . . 'a circus freak show' if their clients were to see me in their firm."[76]

After a friend from Harvard helped him obtain a job with a prominent California law firm, Miller went on to demonstrate his excellence in several positions: he was director of litigation for the Western Law Center for Disability Rights and also taught at several law schools. This background helped prepare him for his role at the EEOC, where

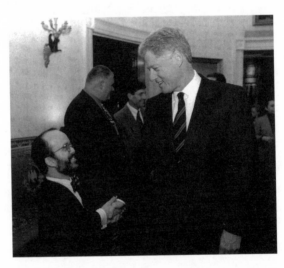

Fig. 5.18. Paul Steven Miller, commissioner, U.S. E.E.O.C., with President Bill Clinton. Photograph courtesy of the White House Photographers and the Clinton Presidential Library.

he aided others—women, persons with disabilities, and various minorities—in their battles against the very bigotry that he had encountered; he also actively defended the privacy of genetic records.

When Miller was asked what had made the difference for him, he
said, "My parents gave me the kind of confidence in myself that I
needed in order not just to assimilate and have the same dreams, the
same goals, but also to recognize that I *was* different, there is a difference—and to have the understanding, no matter how different or imperfect it was then, that this was something to be developed." A member of LPA since childhood, he feels that children who are told, "You're
no different—you don't need to be in LPA"—are left empty and confused, missing something important; on the other hand, he believes
that one also needs what the rest of the world has to offer, including
supportive teachers and friends outside the dwarf community, and
some lucky breaks along the way.

Miller's efforts to protect marginalized groups from discrimination gained him recognition both in the United States and abroad. In
2002, he was invited to Israel to participate in a conference aimed at
integrating the Arab citizens of Israel in the workplace.[77] In 2004,
having noted how few persons with disabilities were members of law
faculties, he accepted a position as Professor at the University of
Washington School of Law in Seattle (where his wife's family lives),
with the expectation that his new post would offer him a platform for
translating his legal expertise in the area of disability into the achievements of the next generation.

REMAINING PROBLEMS

Reading about such persons' careers, or perusing the list of more than
160 individuals and their diverse occupations and avocations that
Fred Short compiled in 2003, it is easy to feel sanguine about the future of all dwarf individuals.[78] However, everyone in the community
knows some who have not thrived. There are those who have not addressed their health issues adequately or have simply been unlucky—

beset by overwhelming medical complications. Some were born into dysfunctional families who did not help them gain self-esteem. Still others, like one man in his forties who telephoned me after seeing a television documentary on dwarfs, feel trapped in an impoverished, unwelcoming neighborhood, unable to change their situations.

This man described how he had felt beaten down not only by his medical and economic problems, but also by the steady onslaught of mockery he experienced in his community. The hopeful dwarfism documentary had brought him to tears; he longed to attend a meeting, but could not bring himself to do so. Repeatedly, many of us are confronted with the problem of finding the considerable time and effort needed to engage with newcomers who have multiple problems and so clearly need our help.

Some young people express feeling at a disadvantage when they see others their age marrying and having babies and do not anticipate that these things will happen for them. Still struggling with their bodies and their lives, they wonder at the positive, optimistic statements they hear all around them. Even when life goes well, the mature individual acknowledges that it is not easy. Here is an excerpt from an eloquent posting, written by a 37-year-old LP from the Netherlands to the mother of an 8-year-old, who wondered about how to reply to her daughter who was finding it hard to accept being small:

> Of course it is important to explain to her that she is a valuable person, and that being a dwarf doesn't mean she can't have any dreams or hopes, and that there are various dwarfs in the world who made it "big" . . . but despite all the positive messages there is still a huge downside to being a dwarf which she didn't choose and neither did you. Being a dwarf means you are different (and as a child being "normal" is extremely important), you have physical limitations, maybe even physical pain, a lot of things you want to do have to be carefully planned whereas other people can do them without thinking, things like friendship and love. . . . And believe me, all of this is no fun! You can learn to take it into stride, with empathy and humor, you can de-

velop your own style in handling all the problems and pain and discomfort, but it isn't as if you have a choice! Some days the world gets on your case worse than others, but on your case it is.[79]

The writer continues that the child needs to be given the opportunity to express her anger and frustration at being a little person. Although she herself feels very fortunate in her love life and career, there are still days when she is upset with the world for not taking her special needs into account, and just sad and tired of having to struggle. Despite all that is good in her life, she speculates that if offered medicine that could make her average statured overnight, she would take it.

Others, feeling they have benefited tremendously from the understanding that their struggles have conferred, state that they would not for all the world give up being a dwarf: "It's who I am!" However, even these individuals can rail against some aspects of their conditions, like the joint degeneration that increases with age. Maria Perez, an assistant director of media/technology at a university, looks at the honeymoon pictures of a young Harvard student and doesn't long so much for the companionship aspect, as for the European tour she will never have. She writes:

> (And I finally have the money and the time!) It's not about men and dating. . . . It is about the fact that there is so much of Europe that is inaccessible from a scooter. (*sighs*) Yes, I realize that I can go to tour but not unencumbered as I would like it, and being a loner it is important for me to experience some things without interruption and distraction. Perhaps this is because I had another life before body rot, and still struggle accepting the accommodations and frustrations. Heck, these days even Puerto Rico is becoming too much of a problem. . . .
>
> Although I don't have a motherly bone in my entire body . . . this is not my main reason for not reproducing, in all fairness I couldn't pass on my medical problems to another human being and not take responsibility for their pain. Wouldn't it be wonderful to know that if I did reproduce that although there was a possibility of that child having the same genetic mutation, they could have lived without the phys-

ical pain associated with it? Yes, it is most likely that I am who I am because of what I am, but would gladly trade some of who I am for someone in less pain. [80]

Along with the pain and accessibility problems are the seemingly endless observations of strangers. LPs often exchange amusing and not so amusing stories of what it is like to have "an LP day"—one in which there has been some sort of negative experience in a supermarket, or someone has patted them on the head, or has offered them $20 for permission to touch them "for good luck." One must decide whether to seize an educational opportunity, or simply move on.

In *Against Tall Odds*, Matt Roloff addresses the issue of how to respond to stares, questions, and comments.[81] When possible, he tries to live by his father's dictum that it is not worth the energy it takes to get angry when people look at you. Originally, his father, exasperated, confronted people he caught staring at his children, and let them know that they were real children with feelings and not a sideshow. Later, he used the opportunities to help people understand why Matt and his brother looked the way they did and what it was like to live with their condition. Roloff often extends himself and takes the initiative when he encounters shock or discomfort in others.

Dwarf Tossing

Dwarf tossing is an activity that has engendered significant opposition. This "sport" originated in 1985 when bouncers at an Australian night club decided it would be entertaining for customers to compete by seeing who could throw a dwarf the farthest. In the ensuing decade, the activity spread to many other countries. In the United States, some, like Chicago mayor Harold Washington, called it "degrading and mean-spirited, repugnant to everyone truly committed to eliminating prejudice against any group."[82] Others, such as philosophy Professor Peter Suber, defended it as akin to riding a motorcycle without a helmet, and that society was exercising needless paternalism when it attempted to "protect people from themselves."[83]

The practice was banned in Florida and New York as a result of active lobbying campaigns by LPA—in Florida led by Nancy Mayheux and Beth Tatman and in New York by Angela Van Etten. They felt that it was particularly dangerous to dwarfs because of their vulnerable spines and that it had led to people picking up little people in the streets and swinging them around, as well as to a hostile, mocking atmosphere in the workplace. There was an undercurrent of feeling that at its core dwarf tossing was an affront to the dignity of dwarfs. Why were dwarfs chosen for tossing, rather than women or children of the same weight? The dwarf seemed to have been placed in a category distinct from humanity—somewhat human, but not quite. Although there are occasional recurrences of the practice, at least in some states bar owners can be threatened with losing their licenses. In September 2002 the U.N. Human Rights Committee affirmed a French ban on dwarf tossing, calling it "necessary in order to protect public order, including considerations of human dignity."[84]

Dwarfs in the Media

Legal decisions are one thing; personal decision making is more complex. A good portion of the dwarf community is upset when their fellows engage in activities that they see as personally demeaning, reminiscent of jesters and sideshows of former days. In this era of self-affirmation and advocacy, there is increased sensitivity to "dwarf dignity," and ongoing controversy about television and film performances and appearances at private parties. Some LPs, unfazed, declare that all persons have the right to make a living as they see fit.

Dwarfs in outlandish costumes still abound in MTV videos, creating "atmosphere," and they are reputed to be in great demand in the pornography industry. There seems to be no dearth of terrible parts in terrible movies for dwarfs. Do members of minority groups have a responsibility to the entire community not to accept positions that may open that group to criticism or ridicule, or recall a past history of discrimination and oppression? It is not always easy to agree about which jobs inspire innocent laughter and which have the power to make a laughingstock of the whole dwarf community.

An aphorism that recalls the era of court and exhibiting dwarfs comes to mind: "Andeme yo caliente y riase la gente:" "I don't care if people laugh at me, as long as I keep warm."[85] One constituency believes that today's little people, who have more choices, should choose more dignified ways to support themselves. Others respond, "Average-sized people do some pretty stupid things for money, too."[86] The fear that the retrograde actions of a few individuals will necessarily tar the image of the rest has beset every vulnerable minority group.

A signal event occurred in 2003 when *The Station Agent* appeared, in which consummate actor Peter Dinklage offered one of the first emotionally authentic depictions of a dwarf protagonist. Audiences responded enthusiastically, enjoying its humor, and its portrayal of the nuances of loneliness and the growing friendships among the film's three central characters. Both the distinctive characteristics of Fin, the singular dwarf that Dinklage plays, and the human commonalities among all the characters are highlighted.

The many documentaries that have been produced in the past two decades have proven to be honest inquiries, rather than either sensationalistic potboilers or unrelieved positive propaganda. By 2006, for the first time, a documentary by an American dwarf filmmaker will have appeared: Steve Delano will have released *No Bigger than a Minute,* in which his own perspective is imprinted on the experiences of persons with dwarfism whom he includes. Memoirs, and the first fiction by dwarf authors with dwarf characters, are now being written. The LPA database is being reconfigured so that LPs can extract information that might be of value to projects they choose. They look forward to studying themselves, not being studied exclusively by others. "Nothing about us without us"—the maxim of the disability movement—is finally resonating within the dwarf community.

The current situation affords many contrasts. A significant number of individuals have become successful, many assuming leadership positions in their workplaces, their churches, their communities, and in politics—some with important roles as disability activists. Far more individuals, however, especially in less affluent nations but in the United States as well, still feel limited and discouraged, unable to forge meaningful, enjoyable lives.

The factors that make the difference are not hard to discern. In the vignettes offered in this volume, one can observe that those persons who have been blessed with exceptional talents and temperaments, who are fortunate enough to have been born into loving and determined families, who have access to expert medical care, and who live in a society that provides both economic opportunity and social acceptance, these are most likely to flourish. Just having a few such advantages can be sufficient.

The fact that, even in a selected group of persons with achondroplasia (Gollust et al.), 31 percent now make $50,000 or more a year is an amazing statistic. These individuals turn out to be the same ones who have a positive self-concept and enjoy the highest quality of life. Correlations do not always reveal causality; variables like these tend to interact and influence each other. But what becomes increasingly clear, as studies of disability have demonstrated for decades, is that persons who are poor—from low-income families in "bad" neighborhoods—are at the greatest risk. They also have the least access to good health care, which scandalously is unavailable to a significant proportion of persons in the United States. Family income may be the single factor that best predicts to quality of life; especially when there is a person in the family with a disability, the possibility of adapting one's living quarters, traveling to get good medical care and attend meetings and conventions, and have something left over for personal comforts and recreation is crucial.

Of course, progress brings with it higher expectations. Despite obvious improvement, it is hard not to be impatient for much more. In a world where poverty is the rule rather than the exception, where the

United Nations are far from united, and no matter how many candles are lit in vigils held to ward it off, war seems to be as inevitable as forest fires, it is not surprising that the needs of this relatively small group of individuals often go unmet. They still confront formidable economic problems, inadequate medical care, and stigma. However, those of us who are familiar with what life was like in past eras for most persons with dwarfism can nevertheless find ourselves grateful for having been born during this hopeful and sometimes exhilarating era.

Appendix 1 ∼

DWARFISM
Conditions and Descriptions

The most common currently accepted definition of dwarfism is short stature of 4′10″ or under that has resulted from a medical condition. Although persons may be also be this short as a result of ethnic or family origins (constitutional short stature), these persons most often tend not to consider themselves dwarfs or be focused on in most of the literature. Because several hundred types of dwarfism exist, persons should supplement the brief descriptions below by consulting the Web sites of Little People of America and other dwarfism groups to find specialized material that will ensure a fuller understanding. LPA Online is particularly useful because it now contains a medical resource site that offers alternative accounts and links to articles about each condition.

I. Disorders of Bone and Cartilage (also called skeletal dysplasia or chondrodystrophy)
   A. Short-limbed dwarfism
      1. *Achondroplasia:* This is the most common form of dwarfism, representing approximately half of all cases of profound short stature. Achondroplastic dwarfism is characterized by an average-sized trunk, short arms and legs, and a slightly enlarged head and prominent forehead. Other distinctive features include a relatively low or flat nasal bridge, swayback, and prominent buttocks and abdomen. Most achondroplastic dwarfs are born to average-sized parents and account for approximately 1 in 25,000 births.
         Babies should routinely be evaluated for potential problems in the foramen magnum and cervical spine areas be-

cause untreated these can cause difficulties like muscle weakness, apnea, or, in extreme cases, sudden infant death syndrome. Other potential concerns are hydrocephalus and ear infections. Beginning with the toddler years, bowlegs may present a problem. In later decades spinal stenosis necessitates careful assessment, and sometimes requires surgery.

2. *Hypochondroplasia:* Although hypochondroplasia can appear simply to be a milder form of achondroplasia, it is actually a different genetic condition entirely. Children are often not diagnosed until they are two to four years old. Hypochondroplasia manifests itself in a similar way to achondroplasia as short-limbed dwarfism; affected individuals are somewhat taller than those with achondroplasia and have fewer medical problems.

3. *Diastrophic Dysplasia:* A relatively common form of dwarfism (about 1 in 100,000 births) first differentiated in 1960; before that, diastrophic dysplasia had been thought to be a different form of achondroplasia. The condition is characterized by short-limbed dwarfism and, in some cases, cleft palate, clubfeet, "hitchhiker's thumb," and ears with a cauliflower appearance. Respiratory problems are sometimes present in infancy, but life span is normal. Serious orthopedic problems often require numerous surgical procedures and should be performed in a timely fashion by experts familiar with the limited research about techniques.

4. *Pseudoachondroplasia:* As the name implies, pseudoachondroplasia, like hypochondroplasia, was once thought to be closely related to achondroplasia. However, geneticists have since learned otherwise. Growth retardation is usually not apparent until the child is 1 year old, often not until 2 or 3 years old, when delayed walking or an abnormal gait is evident. Pseudoachondroplastic dwarfs average about four feet tall, but there is great variability in range, with adult heights ranging from 36 inches to 61 inches. Head growth and facial features are normal. Pseudoachondroplasia is associated with

osteoarthritis and other orthopedic problems that often require surgery.

5. *Cartilage-Hair Hypoplasia (CHH)*, also referred to as metaphyseal chondrodysplasia, McKusick type: This is a rare form of dwarfism except among certain ethnic groups, in particular, the Amish and Finns. CHH is characterized by short-limb dwarfism, fine, sparse, and light-colored hair, and hyperextendability of the fingers and wrists. Because of risk and susceptibility to chicken pox, children should be treated with antiviral medication and gamma globulin when exposed. About 10 percent of individuals may have Hirschsprung disease (intestinal malabsorption).

6. *Ellis–van Creveld (EVC) Syndrome*, also known as chondroectodermal dysplasia: This rare genetic disorder is characterized by short-limb dwarfism, additional fingers and/or toes, abnormal development of fingernails and teeth, and, in more than half of the cases, congenital heart defects. As with CHH, EVC syndrome disproportionately affects the Amish.

7. *Multiple Epiphyseal Dysplasia (MED)*, also known as Fairbank disease: This rare genetic condition that is present at birth but does not usually manifest itself till between 5 and 10 years old, when the child affected begins to notice unexplained pain in the hips, knees, and/or ankles. The shortening of the limbs is variable, and the trunk is normal; the hands, especially the thumbs, may appear short and stubby. Severe degenerative arthritis of the hips often develops in older patients, although some affected persons remain asymptomatic. The short stature associated with MED is not severe.

8. *Acromesomelic Dysplasia:* This extremely rare genetic condition is characterized by short arms, legs, and fingers and a slightly enlarged head. These are disorders in which there is disproportionate shortening of the middle segments (forearms and forelegs) and distal segments (hands and feet). Types include Hunter-Thompson, Maroteaux, and Grebe syndromes.

9. *Pycnodystososis or Pyknodystostosis:* The major signs of this condition are failure to thrive with resultant short stature in childhood and the persistence of an open anterior fontanel into adulthood. The head is large in relation to the body, and the face is small in proportion to the cranium, with a sharp nose, receding chin, and dental abnormalities. Arm span is less than normal. Because of increased bone density, trauma—even tooth extraction—can cause fractures. Fractures of the long bones may occur, with subsequent deformities and short stature common as a result of malunion. Kyphosis, scoliosis, and lumbar lordosis may also occur.

10. *Campomelic Dysplasia:* This is a rare, more serious form of short-limbed dwarfism. People with campomelic dysplasia often have severely bowed lower legs and complications that involve the cardiac, respiratory, urinary tract, and central nervous system. Stillbirths or significant problems in the early months are common, but with early intervention more children survive into young adulthood.

11. *Rhizomelic Chondrodysplasia Punctata (RCP):* Occurring once in 100,000 births, RCP is a severe condition marked by profound delays in developmental and physical growth, and a shortened life span. Babies have shortening of the upper arms and face and characteristic facial features. RCP is a peroxisomal disorder, a condition in which cell structures cannot break down chemicals the body needs. An excellent pamphlet about this disorder is available from the Midwest Bone Dysplasia Clinic.

B. Short-Trunk Dwarfism

1. *Hypochondrogenesis:* Children born with hypochondrogenesis have both a short trunk and short limbs, a large, oval-shaped head, and, in many cases, a cleft palate and small chin. Because of respiratory distress caused by a small rib cage, many babies die shortly after birth. Those who survive are generally reclassified as having spondyloepiphyseal dysplasia.

2. *Spondyloepiphyseal Dysplasia Congenita* (SEDC or SEDc): More commonly known as SEDC, or simply as SED, these bone disorders represent a group of skeletal alterations characterized by progressive abnormalities of the epiphyses (growing ends of the long or short tubular-shaped bones) and "spondylo" or spine changes. SEDC is the best known of several varieties of these dysplasias. Adult height may vary from slightly under three feet to slightly over four feet, although some adults are much taller. Other characteristics can include clubfeet, a cleft palate, and barrel-chested appearance.

   SED is associated with a variety of medical problems, mainly orthopedic, but about half of affected individuals have a cleft palate, and there is some increased risk for retinal detachment or myopia (nearsightedness). Ligaments tend to be loose and joint mobility is increased. The cervical spine should be carefully monitored for abnormality of motion. Various surgeries are often indicated. SED occurs approximately once in every 100,000 births, making it, along with achondroplasia and diastrophic dwarfism, one of the most common forms of dwarfism.

3. *Spondyloepimetaphyseal Dysplasia, Strudwick:* Although this condition, known as SEMD (or SMD), has a unique genetic cause, its characteristics are virtually indistinguishable in most respects from those of spondyloepiphyseal dysplasia.

4. *Spondyloepiphyseal Dysplasia Tarda:* Yet another variation of SED, also called SEDT. Because it is linked to the X chromosome, this condition affects only males. Short stature is mild, with adult height ranging from 4′10″ to 5′6″.

5. *Metatropic Dysplasia:* This rare type of skeletal dysplasia is sometimes confused with Kniest syndrome, which is why Kniest is often referred to as metatropic dysplasia, type II.

6. *Kniest Syndrome or Kniest Dysplasia,* also known as Metatropic Dysplasia type II: This condition shares many similarities with spondyloepiphyseal dysplasia congenita (SEDc) and spondyloepimetaphyseal dysplasia, Strudwick (SEMD).

7. *Osteogenesis Imperfecta* (OI): There are five major types of osteogenesis imperfecta, a condition characterized by unusually fragile bones that fracture easily. OI is a genetic disorder of collagen 1, the major building block of bone and other connective tissues. There are different degrees of severity: people with the mildest form of OI are average statured, with few fractures and the least bone deformity. In a great many instances, however, in addition to brittle bones, the condition is accompanied by short stature, skeletal deformities, brittle teeth, hearing loss, or respiratory difficulties. An estimated 30,000 people in the United States have OI. Although a cure has not yet been found, common treatments include placement of casts or splints on fractured bones, braces, and a surgical procedure called rodding. Physical exercise and dietary measures are also recommended, and several promising medications and treatments are currently being explored.

II. Endocrine Disorders: Hormone Failure
About 15 percent of serious growth retardation is caused by failures in the endocrine system.
A. Growth Hormone Deficiency: Hypopituitarism
Growth hormone is a protein produced by the pituitary gland that is vital for normal growth. Growth hormone deficiency exists when this hormone is absent or produced in inadequate amounts. Panhypopituitarism is due to a deficit of all of the anterior pituitary hormones; it accounts for approximately two-thirds of pituitary dwzarfism cases and results in lack of sexual maturity. *Hypopituitarism* or *pituitary dwarfism* due to an isolated deficiency of growth hormone accounts for approximately one third of cases, and persons with this condition may reproduce. Other variants of the condition exist, including a hereditary inability to form an insulin-like growth factor; African pygmies are an example of that situation.
It is estimated that 10,000 to 15,000 children in the United States have growth failure due to growth hormone deficiency;

this number is being reduced as more families seek treatment for their children. Early diagnosis and treatment with synthetic growth hormone over a period of several years, given by injection, may result in achieving average stature.

Further information about other hormones affecting growth, such as thyroid-stimulating hormone (THS), adrenocorticotropic hormone (ACTH), luteinizing hormone, and follicle-stimulating hormone (FSH), may be found on the Human Growth Foundation and Magic Foundation Web sites.

B. Hypothyroidism

Any problem of the thyroid gland can interfere with growth. It may be congenital or acquired. Symptoms may include growth retardation, sluggish behavior, puffy face and skin, and neurological problems and mental retardation. These days in most Western nations screening is done at birth and necessary supplementation is provided, but damage to the thyroid gland or acquired autoimmune thyroiditis may occur later and require treatment. Early diagnosis and treatment with thyroid replacement is very important. In nations without iodized salt, iodine deficiency has led to cretinism (now more commonly called IDD, a condition that includes short stature and retardation).

III. Dwarfism Caused by Absent or Abnormal Chromosomes

A. Turner Syndrome

Turner syndrome is a chromosomal condition that exclusively affects girls and women. It occurs when one of the two X chromosomes normally found in females is missing or incomplete. It results in short stature in almost 100 percent of those with this disorder and infertility and ovarian dysfunction in about 95 percent. The physical features that accompany the condition are webbed neck, arms that turn out slightly at the elbow, and a low hairline in back of the head. Some, but by no means all, individuals may be affected by cardiovascular, kidney, and thyroid problems, skeletal disorders such as scoliosis or dislocated hips, and hearing and ear disturbances. Intelligence is normal, although some difficulties occur in learning spatial relations, which can be helped through tutoring.

Turner syndrome occurs in about 1 of every 2,500 live female births; approximately 50,000 girls and women are affected in the United States. Treatment with androgen and estrogen are used to bring about sexual development and growth; treatment with synthetic growth hormone is now common, causing an average height gain of two to four inches in patients who were treated with growth hormone early, whereas estrogen treatment is started after age 14 years.

B. Down Syndrome

This is a genetic disorder characterized by an anomaly in cell development that results in 47 instead of the usual 46 chromosomes in every cell of the body, interfering with aspects of body and brain development. The condition is marked by a distinct physical appearance that includes slanting eyes with folds at the inner corners and short broad hands and feet.

At least one-fourth of individuals with Down syndrome are short statured. They have poor muscle tone, delayed motor skills, and some degree of mental retardation. Approximately one-third of babies have heart defects and many have gastrointestinal defects, most of which can now be surgically corrected. Weight gain is an ongoing problem that has an impact on health, longevity, and social functioning and may be helped by a diet and exercise program. Down Syndrome is one of the most common dwarfing conditions, occurring about once in every 800 to 1,000 births. Now, a vast literature and many groups offer information and support to affected families.

IV. Mucopolysaccharidoses (MPS) and Mucolipidoses (ML): Lysosomal Storage Disorders

Mucopolysaccharidoses and mucolipidoses are rare genetically determined conditions caused by the body's inability to produce certain enzymes, resulting in an abnormal deposit of complex sugars in tissues and cells. The process causes progressive damage that can range in severity from strictly bone and joint involvement to massive complications in all organ systems, causing early death.

A. MPS Disorders

These include Hurler syndrome, Scheie syndrome, Hurler-Scheie syndrome, Hunter syndrome (mild and severe), San Filippo (A, B, C, and D), Morquio (A and B), Maroteaux-Lamy (classic severe, intermediate, and mild), and Sly syndrome.

Persons with Morquio syndrome have a better prognosis than persons with some of the other disorders, although a somewhat shorter than average life span. Occurring in about 1 in 100,000 births, Morquio syndrome is characterized by skeletal, respiratory, cardiac, and hearing problems. Surgical intervention for Morquio syndrome has improved. A good number of individuals with this condition are in LPA, and a Morquio Web site and links may be found on LPA Online.

B. ML Disorders

I-cell disorder and pseudo-Hurler polydystrophy. There is no cure available at present, but promising research is being conducted in several areas, most notably in enzyme replacement therapy and, to a lesser degree, in gene replacement therapy.

V. Intrauterine or In Utero Growth Disorders (IUGDs)

Some disorders originate while the infant is still in the mother's womb, resulting in full-term babies whose height and weight may be as much as two standard deviations below the mean, or less than the third percentile compared with other newborns. Etiology is variable and often not identifiable, but sometimes involves complicated interactions of causes. There may be defects relating to the placenta, blood supply, or heart, or environmental factors, such as medication, drugs, or alcohol taken by the mother. Even living in a high altitude may be a contributor. It is important to have an expert medical evaluation to determine whether the correct diagnosis is IUGR (intrauterine growth retardation), SGA (small for gestational age, below the 10th percentile on growth chart), or prematurity. Most cases of IUGD do not catch up completely, but finding the cause is essential in determining treatment. The terms IUGR and SGA are sometimes used under a more generic label, primordial short stature or dwarfism. Recently, growth hormone has proved helpful in some instances.

A. Russell-Silver Syndrome

While the many complicated (named and unnamed) IUGR conditions cannot be identified here, Russell-Silver syndrome, also known as Silver-Russell syndrome, Silver syndrome, and Russell syndrome, is one of the most fully explored. It is characterized by short stature, a small, triangular face, low-set ears, and an incurved fifth finger. It is marked by low birth weight, and appetite is often poor for the first few years of life. A full account of the syndrome is available from the Magic Foundation.

VI. Chronic Systemic Disease or Iatrogenic Dwarfism

Many diseases and infections, such as renal, cardiac, hepatic, and gastrointestinal, can interfere with children's achieving their full growth potential. Recently, growth hormone has shown some promise in treating Crohn disease, a gastrointestinal disorder. Among the other diseases that sometimes result in dwarfism are rheumatoid arthritis in childhood and tuberculosis, which can cause Pott disease. Iatrogenic dwarfism results when therapy for a condition (e.g., the treatment of colitis, nephritic disease, or asthma with excessive cortisone) causes growth failure.

VII. Dwarfism Caused by Emotional Deprivation

Among the many names for this condition are psychosocial failure to thrive (PFTT), psychosocial dwarfism, deprivation dwarfism, and Kasper Hauser syndrome. When children are abused or neglected emotionally, their growth may be seriously compromised. When they are transferred to more salubrious conditions, growth tends to resume. Sometimes, when the child is not "rescued" and instead experiences prolonged emotional deprivation, dwarfism may result. These individuals rarely join dwarfism groups, and little is known about their functioning in adulthood.

VIII. Dwarfism caused by Nutritional Deprivation

Chronic malnutrition remains a major cause of growth failure in much of the world. Overall protein deprivation is a primary factor, but historically, lack of nutritional vitamin D and lack of sunlight has been identified as the cause of rickety dwarfism, and iodine deficiency (IDD) as the cause of the condition formerly known as cretinism.

Appendix 2 ~

RESOURCES
Medical and Support Groups

DWARFISM ORGANIZATIONS

Little People of America, the largest organization, is listed first. Other major organizations and small support groups are listed alphabetically.

- **Little People of America**
  5289 NE Elam Young Parkway, Suite F-700
  Hillsboro, OR 97124
  phone: (1-888) LPA-2001 (English and Spanish)
  or (1-503) 846-1562   fax: (1-503) 846-1590
  www.lpaonline.org
  ~ LPA consists of persons who are 4'10" and under because of various medical disorders, as well as family members and related professionals. Its extensive Web site offers links to other groups, and to its medical advisory board, personal sites, discussion groups and chat rooms, and recent news of interest to dwarf individuals. Persons with skeletal dysplasias constitute the largest percentage of LPA's membership, but many other diagnostic categories are also represented.
      A good way to obtain assistance is to consult the members of LPA medical advisory board or physicians associated with organizations listed below. These individuals, after evaluating the special needs of the persons who contact them, may be able to suggest appropriate referrals in their geographical area.

- **Association for Children with Russell-Silver Syndrome, Inc.**
  22 Hoyt Street
  Madison, NJ 07940
  phone: (1-201) 377-4531 or (1-313) 242-2219

- **Camp Little People**
  150 Mill Street
  Benton, PA 17814
  http://pages.prodigy.net/ritzycat/d2/camplp.htm
  ∽ Summer vacation experience for children and adults with dwarfism.

- **Camp Little People II**
  phone: (1-303) 773-9112
  ∽ Summer vacation experience for children and adults with dwarfism.

- **Ellis–Van Creveld Syndrome Support Group**
  540 South Forest Street, 4-203
  Denver, CO 80246
  http://ouray.cudenver.edu/~dsurek/index.htm

- **Human Growth Foundation**
  997 Glen Cove Avenue
  Glen Head, NY 11545
  phone: (1-800) 451-6434
  www.hgfound.org
  ∽ This is a support group that publishes educational materials, offers small research grants, and offers services for persons with various short-stature disorders, but with special emphasis on conditions such as growth hormone deficiency and allied conditions.

- **The MAGIC Foundation**
  1327 North Harlem Avenue
  Oak Park, IL 60302
  phone: (1-708) 383-0808   fax: (1-708) 383-0899
  www.magicfoundation.org
  ∽ The MAGIC (Major Aspects of Growth in Children) Foundation emphasizes various short-stature conditions that lend themselves to treatment, such as human growth hormone deficiency, offering published materials and providing a network of 100 types of growth disorders, with eleven divisions.

- **National Mucopolysaccharidosis (MPS) Society**
  45 Packard Drive
  Bangor, ME 04401
  www.mppsociety.org
  ∼ The MPS Society is devoted to finding a cure for the mucopolysaccharidoses and mucolipidoses syndromes, genetic lymosomal storage
  disorders. The society supports families, publishes educational materials, finances research, and offers a family assistance program.

- **The Osteogenesis Imperfecta Foundation**
  804 West Diamond Avenue, Suite 210
  Gaithersburg, MD 20878
  phone: (1-801) 981-2663 or (1-301) 947-0083
  fax: (1-301) 947-0456
  www.oif.org
  ∼ The foundation's mission is to improve quality of life for persons
  with "brittle bone" disorders, genetic conditions characterized by bones
  that break easily. The organization supports research, education, and
  public awareness and provides mutual support.

- **Restricted Growth Association**
  P.O. Box 4744
  Dorchester, Dorset
  England DT2 9FA
  phone: 01-308-898445
  www.rgaonline.org.uk
  ∼ This is the British organization for persons with dwarfism.

- **Rhizomelic Chondrodysplasia Punctata (RCP)**
  Support Group
  137 25th Avenue
  Monroe, WI 53566
  phone: (1-608) 325-2717
  ∼ RCP is a rare, severe type of dwarfism. Children are seriously delayed, both developmentally and physically.

- **Turner Syndrome Society of the United States**
  14450 TC Jester, Suite 269
  Houston, TX 77014
  phone: (1-832) 249-9988   fax: (1-612) 379-3619
  http://turner-syndrome-us.org
  ∼ Provides research, awareness and support for persons affected by Turner syndrome.

- **Turner's Syndrome Society of Canada**
  21 Blackthorn Avenue
  Toronto, ON,
  Canada M6N 3H4
  phone: (1-800) 465-6744 or (1-416) 781-2086
  fax: (1-416) 660-7450
  www.turnersyndrome.ca

MEDICAL CENTERS WITH EXPERTISE IN DWARFISM

These are only a few of the recognized centers that have specialists with experience in the treatment of dwarfing conditions. Additional appropriate referral sources may be found by contacting LPA medical advisory board members. LPA is currently assembling a list of knowledgeable clinics and physicians.

- **Alfred I. duPont Skeletal Dysplasia Clinic**
  P.O. Box 269. Wilmington, DE 19899
  phone: (1-302) 651-5916   fax: (1-302) 651-5033

- **Greenberg Center for Skeletal Dysplasia**
  Johns Hopkins Hospital-Blalock 1012-C
  600 North Wolfe Street
  Baltimore, MD 21287
  phone: (1-410) 614-0977   fax: (1-410) 614-2522

- **Skeletal Dysplasia Clinic at the Medical Genetics Birth Defects Center**
  Cedars-Sinai Medical Center
  8700 Beverly Boulevard, North Tower, Fourth Floor
  Los Angeles, CA 90048
  phone: (1-800) CEDARS-2 or (1-310) 233-2771
  fax: (1-310) 423-1402
  www.csmc.edu/medgenetics/3086.asp

- **Center for Skeletal Dysplasias**
  Hospital for Special Surgery
  535 East 70th Street
  New York, NY 10021
  phone: (1-212) 774-7332   fax: (1-212) 774-7827
  e-mail: csd@hss.edu

- **Midwest Regional Bone Dysplasia Clinic**
  Clinical Genetics Center
  University of Wisconsin–Madison
  1500 Highland Avenue
  Madison, WI 53705
  phone: (1-608) 262-9722   fax: (1-608) 263-3496
  http://waisman.wisc.edu

- **Northern California Regional Skeletal Dysplasia Clinic**
  〜 The Northern California Regional Skeletal Dysplasia Clinic is a
  collaboration between Kaiser Permanente and Children's Hospital, Oakland. At the Web site, click on "Our Services," then "Specialty Clinics," then "Skeletal Dysplasia."

1. **Kaiser Permanente Skeletal Dysplasia**
   Department of Genetics
   280 West MacArthur Boulevard
   Oakland, CA 94611-5693
   phone: (1-510) 752-6367
   www.dor.kaiser.org

2. Children's Hospital Oakland
Department of Medical Genetics
747 Fifty-Second Street
Oakland, CA 94609-1809
phone: (1-510) 428-355
www.childrenshospitaloakland.org

- **Regional Skeletal Dysplasia Center**
Akron Children's Hospital
One Perkins Square
Akron, OH 44308
phone: (1-330) 535-6633
www.akronchildren's.org/depts-services/skil_dysplasia

- **Vermont Regional Genetics Center**
1 Mill Street, Box B-10
Burlington, VT 05401
phone: (1-802) 658-4310

UMBRELLA GROUPS AND OTHER SOURCES
OF USEFUL PUBLICATIONS

In addition to informational material obtainable from the groups listed above, useful information and publications may be obtained from the following sources.

Umbrella Groups

1. Genetic Alliance
430 Connecticut Avenue NW, Suite 404
Washington, DC 20008-2304
phone: (1-800) 336-4363 or (1-202) 966-5557
fax: (1-202) 966-8553
www.geneticalliance.org

~ The Genetic Alliance is an international coalition composed of millions of individuals with genetic conditions and more than 600 advocacy, research, and health care organizations. One of its major goals is to translate genetic advances into quality health care. It offers a genetics helpline and has a great many valuable publications.

2. National Organization of Rare Disorders
www.rarediseases.org

~ NORD is a federation of voluntary health organizations dedicated to helping people with rare "orphan" diseases and assisting the organizations that serve them. It has programs for education, advocacy, research, and service. Descriptions of a great number of dwarfing disorders are available at NORD's Web site where visitors may read abstracts of reports on more than 1,120 conditions free of charge or purchase full-text reports for $7.50 each. It also has published The NORD Guide to Rare Disorders, a 900-page medical text for physicians and other health care professionals.

Valuable Publications

Several organizations or centers listed above have particularly valuable publications. In addition to each specialized organization's brochures about the condition(s) it represents, the following are notable:

1. The Human Growth Foundation has brochures on achondroplasia, growth hormone deficiency, adult growth hormone deficiency, intrauterine growth retardation, septo-optic dysplasia, Turner syndrome, and readiness for school.
2. LPA Medical Resource Center has links to varied articles about specific conditions and their complications, and information about other medical issues: (www.lpa-medical.org).
3. The Midwestern Regional Skeletal Dysplasia Clinic has superb booklets and fact sheets. Booklets are available for rhizomelic chondroplasia punctata, for understanding developmental differences in young children with achondroplasia, and for entering school. Fact sheets are available for achondroplasia,

diastrophic dysplasia, pseudoachondroplasia, and spondyloepiphyseal dysplasia, congenita. Medical histories are available for
achondroplasia, campomelic dysplasia, diastrophic dysplasia,
Ellis–Van Creveld syndrome, hypochondroplasia, Kniest dysplasia, and multiple epiphyseal dysplasia congenita.

4. The Restricted Growth Association offers excellent brochures,
   including several on skeletal dysplasias and Turner syndrome, as
   well as other "lifestyle" publications on babies, going to school,
   the teen years, having a baby, limb lengthening, adoption, the
   mature years, etc. A list of publications and an order form are
   available via e-mail at rga1@talk21.com

ESSENTIAL SCIENTIFIC RESOURCES FOR MEDICAL PROFESSIONALS

- **American Society for Matrix Biology**
  Hospital for Special Surgery
  535 East 70th Street
  New York, NY 10021
  phone: 212-774-7598
  ∽ This interdisciplinary group consists of medical professionals and
  other scientists who conduct research and disseminate information
  about investigations involving the extracellular matrix, intracellular signaling and gene expression, and related factors influencing growth and
  development.

- **Coalition for Heritable Disorders of Connective Tissue**
  4301 Connecticut Avenue, N.W.
  Washington, DC 20008
  www.chdct.org/
  ∽ This group encourages awareness of connective tissue disorders
  among medical professionals and the public. Its goals are to encourage
  teaching about these conditions in medical schools, to train health care
  practitioners to diagnose and treat them, and to foster research.

- **International Skeletal Dysplasia Registry**
  Cedars-Sinai Medical Center
  444 South San Vicente Boulevard, Suite 1001
  Los Angeles, CA 90048
  phone: (1-301) 423-9915
  fax: (1-310) 423-9946
  www.cedars-sinai.edu/3805.html
  ∿ The ISDR at Cedars-Sinai serves as the core facility for a National
  Institutes of Health (NIH) project. The registry provides a unique service for professional researchers and physicians, and individuals with
  various conditions worldwide. The ISDR and the associated clinic are a
  major resource for clinical, radiographic, morphological, and biochemical materials. The registry collects materials on patients with rare skeletal dysplasias and provides investigators throughout the world with diagnostic and research assistance, illuminating the natural history and
  treatment of skeletal dysplasias.

- **Lawson Wilkins Pediatric Endocrine Society**
  http://lwpes.org/AboutUs.aspx
  ∿ The mission of this professional organization of pediatric endocrinologists is to promote the acquisition and dissemination of knowledge
  about endocrine and metabolic disorders from conception through
  adolescence.

- **Little People's Research Fund, Inc.**
  phone: (1-800) 232-5773 or (1-410) 494-0055
  fax: (1-410) 494-0062
  http://lprf.org
  ∿ This is the foundation associated with the work of orthopedist
  Dr. Steven E. Kopits. It is currently engaged in producing articles about
  his research findings and editing videos demonstrating his surgical techniques. Interested professionals may contact the office for further information as publications become available.

- **Medline: PubMed**
  www.pubmed.net
  ∿ This is the National Library of Medicine's comprehensive Internet
  database, offering references and synopses of journal articles written

during the past several decades. Most are directed to medical professionals, but many may prove of interest to the intelligent lay reader.

- **National Institute of Arthritis and Musculoskeletal and Skin Diseases**
NIAMS Information Clearinghouse
National Institutes of Health
1 AMS Circle
Bethesda, MD 20892-3675
phone: (1-301) 495-4484   fax: (1-301) 718-6366
TTY: (1-301) 565-2966
http://niams.nih.gov/
~ NIAMS is a part of the NIH. Its mission is to support research into
the causes, treatment, and prevention of the diseases noted above. It offers grants, trains basic and clinical researchers, and publishes many
useful pamphlets. Because skeletal dysplasias are often accompanied by
arthritis, this group is valuable both for research and information.

- **Online Mendelian Inheritance in Man (OMIM)**
www.ncbi.nlm.nih.gov
~ This is the updated online version of *Mendelian Inheritance in
Man*, the "bible of genetics," by Victor A. McKusick. The online version
is regularly updated by Dr. McKusick and his colleagues at Johns Hopkins and elsewhere. Textual information, pictures, and links to Medline
articles are provided. Despite their specialized scientific terminology,
entries may provide the general reader with an overview of the history
of the condition's discovery and major relevant research areas.

- **Relevant Social Science Databases**
~ For further information about psychosocial aspects, several databases may prove of value, among them PsycInfo, PsycArticles (APA),
and ASSIA (Applied Social Science Index and Abstracts.)

- **Sources of General Information about Dwarfs, Dwarfism, and Short Stature**
~ Two additional popular Web sites are Centralized Dwarfism
Resources, www.dwarfism.org, and Short Persons Support,

www.shortsupport.org. Although these are "works in progress" and not always updated, they contain useful references to books, articles, videos, and other links. For general history, biography, and information about dwarfs in the arts, as well as further bibliographical references, see Betty M. Adelson, *The Lives of Dwarfs: Their Journey from Public Curiosity toward Social Liberation* (Piscataway, NJ: Rutgers University Press, 2005).

Notes ⌒

PREFACE

1. Betty M. Adelson, *The Lives of Dwarfs: Their Journey from Public Curiosity toward Social Liberation* (New Brunswick, NJ: Rutgers University Press, 2005).
2. "Developmental Diseases of the Skeleton," in *Mercer's Orthopedic Surgery*, ed. Robert B. Deithee, 8th ed. (Baltimore: George Keightley, 1983), 207. First published by Edward Arnold, Ltd., London, 1932.

INTRODUCTION

1. See Yi-Fu Tuan, *Dominance and Affection: The Making of Pets* (New Haven, CT: Yale University Press, 1984), for a searching analysis of the relationship of the treatment of dwarfs to that of other minorities.
2. Monique Coneley, "Dwarfism and Me," *UMW Post*, 29 January 2003, 13, 21.
3. Tad Friend, "What's So Funny," *New Yorker*, 11 November 2002, 90.

CHAPTER 1. MEDICAL ASPECTS

1. J. M. Tanner, *A History of the Study of Human Growth* (Cambridge: Cambridge University Press, 1981).
2. M. le Dr. Godin, "Observation d'une Naine," *Société d'Anthropologie de Paris Bulletins et Mémoires* 9, ser. 4 (1898): 531–35.
3. G. O. Jacobson, "A Family of Dwarfs," *Lancet* 1 (1891): 1040.
4. A. Bloch, "Observations sur Les Nains du Jardin d'Acclimation," *Société d'Anthropologie de Paris Bulletins et Mémoires* 10, ser. 5 (1909): 533–74.
5. A. Poncet and R. Leriche, "Nains d'aujourd'hui et nain de autre fois," *Revue Scientifique (Paris)* 20, ser. 4 (1903): 587–93. Poncet and Leriche were influential scientists at the turn of the century who believed that persons with dwarfism were descended from an ancient dwarf race mentioned by Homer.
6. M. Howard, *Victorian Grotesque: An Illustrated Excursion into Medical Curiosities, Freaks and Abnormalities, Principally of the Victorian Age* (London: Jupiter Books, 1977), 103.
7. Victor A. McKusick, interview with the author, early 1990s.
8. J. G. Gamble, "Charles Dickens: His Quaint Little 'Person of the House' and the English Disease," *Pharos* 59, no. 4 (1996): 24–28.
9. H. Burgi, Z. Supersaxo, and B. Selz, "Iodine Deficiency Disease in Switzerland One Hundred Years after Theodor Kocher's Survey: A Historical Review with Some New Goiter Prevalence Data," *Acta Endocrinologica* 123, no. 6 (1990): 577–90.
10. See, for example, A. Marie, "Nano-infantilisme et Folie," *Société d'Anthropologie de Paris Bulletins et Mémoires* 5, ser. 10 (1909): 101–17.

11. H. Rischbieth and A. Barrington, "Achondroplasia," in *Treasury of Human Inheritance* (London: University of London, Francis Galton Laboratory for Human Eugenics, 1912), 1:364.

12. M. Jansen, *Achondroplasia: Its Nature and Its Cause* (Leiden: Brill, 1912).

13. T. Parvin, "The Influence of Maternal Impression upon the Foetus," *International Medical Magazine* 1 (1893): 487–93.

14. J. Warkany, *Congenital Malformations* (Chicago: Yearbook Medical Publishers, 1971), 12–14.

15. G. M. Gould and W. L. Pyle, *Anomalies and Curiosities of Medicine* (1896; repr., New York: Bell Publishing Company, a division of Crown Publishers, Inc., 1956), 337–38.

16. J. M. Warren, "An Account of Two Remarkable Indian Dwarfs Exhibited in Boston under the Name of Aztec Children," *American Journal of the Medical Sciences* 42 (1851): 286–93.

17. "The Marriage of Dwarfs," *Hospital Gazette*, in *Archives of Clinical Surgery* 4, no. 5 (1878): 81–82.

18. "Transactions of the Obstetrical Society of Philadelphia," *American Journal of Obstetrics* (October 1879): 766–70.

19. W. Bodin and B. Hershey, *It's a Small World: All about Midgets* (New York: Coward-McCann, Inc., 1934), 41.

20. A. Hamilton, "If You Were a Midget," *Science Digest* 55 (1964): 33.

21. L. Fiedler, *Freaks: Myths and Images of the Secret Self* (New York: Simon and Schuster, 1978), 52.

22. "Developmental Diseases of the Skeleton," in *Mercer's Orthopedic Surgery*, 8th ed., ed. R. B. Deithee, 207 (Baltimore: George Keightley, 1983). First published by Edward Arnold, Ltd., London, 1932.

23. "Dwarfism," an *Encarta Encyclopedia Article*. http://encarta.msn.com/index/conciseindex/0A/00AFC000.htm?z=1&pg=2&br=1.

24. This presentation follows the organization used in B. Linder and F. Cassorla, "Short Stature: Etiology, Diagnosis and Treatment" (Grand Rounds of the National Institute of Health) *JAMA* 260, no. 21 (1988): 3171–75. Wording and details have been altered.

25. *Criteria for Determining Disability in Infants and Children: Short Stature.* Summary, Evidence Report / Technology Assessment: no. 33, AHRQ Publication no. 03-E025, 2003. Agency for Healthcare Research and Quality, Rockville, MD, www.ahrq.gov/clinic/epcsums/shortsum/htm. Free copies available by calling (1–800) 358-9295.

26. P. Beighton, "Osteochondrodysplasias in South Africa," *American Journal of Medical Genetics* 63 (1996): 7–11. I. M. Orioli, E. E. Castilla, and J. G. Barbosa-Neto, "The Birth Prevalence Rates for the Skeletal Dysplasias," *Journal of Medical Genetics* 23, no. 4 (1986): 328–32, discuss Latin America. An excellent Australian population study of achondroplastic dwarfs in Australia, finding an incidence of 1 in 26,000 is F. Oberklaid, D. M. Danks, F. Jensen, L. Stace, and S. Rosshandler, "Achondroplasia and Hypochondroplasia: Comments on Frequency, Mutation Rate and Radiological Features in Skull and Spine," *Journal of Medical Genetics* 16, no. 2 (1979): 140–46.

27. J. Ablon, *Little People in America: The Social Dimensions of Dwarfism* (New York: Praeger, 1984), 4.

28. Spiegel completed his evaluation of the Departments of Motor Vehicles in Spring 2003 and kindly forwarded the results to me in August 2003.

29. Clair A. Francomano, interview with the author, 23 June 2000.

30. See V. A. McKusick, R. Eldridge, J. A. Hostetler, U. Ruanguit, and J. A. Egeland, "Dwarfism in the Amish, I. The Ellis–van Creveld Syndrome," *Bulletin of Johns Hopkins Hospital* 115 (1964): 306–36; R. Eldridge. J. A. Hostetler, O. Ruanguit, and J. A. Egeland, "Dwarfism in the Amish, II. Cartilage-Hair Hypoplasia," *Bulletin of Johns Hopkins Hospital* 116 (1965): 285–326; V. A. McKusick, "The Amish," *Endeavor* 4 (1980): 52–57. V. A. McKusick, *Medical Genetic Studies of the Amish* (Baltimore: Johns Hopkins University Press, 1978); V. A. McKusick, "Ellis-van Creveld Syndrome and the Amish," *Nature Genetics* 24, no. 3 (2000): 203–4.

31. O. Makitie, "Cartilage-Hair Hypoplasia in Finland: Epidemiological and Genetic Aspects of 107 Patients," *Journal of Medical Genetics* 29, no. 9 (1992): 652–55.

32. V. A. McKusick, *Heritable Disorders of Connective Tissue* (St. Louis: C. V. Mosby, 1972).

33. J. Spranger, "Pattern Recognition in Bone Dysplasias," *Progress in Clinical and Biological Research* 200 (1985): 315–42.

34. J. W. Spranger, P. W. Brill, and A. Poznanski, *Bone Dysplasias: An Atlas of Genetic Disorders of Skeletal Development* (New York: Oxford University Press, 2002); J. W. Spranger, L. O. Langer, and H. R. Wiedmann, *Bone Dysplasias: An Atlas of Genetic Disorders of Skeletal Development* (Philadelphia: W. B. Saunders, 1974).

35. Spranger, Brill, and Poznanski, *Bone Dysplasias*, vi.

36. S. E. Kopits, "Orthopedic Complications of Dwarfism," *Clinical Orthopaedics and Related Research* 114 (1976): 153–79.

37. Ekman's original article has been published as "The Classic Congenital Osteomalacia" in *Clinical Orthopaedics and Related Research* 159 (1981): 2–5, along with an editorial comment and introduction. See also K. S. Seedorf, *Osteogenesis Imperfecta* (Copenhagen: Munksgaard, 1949).

38. W. A. Horton, "Evolution of the Bone Dysplasia Family," *American Journal of Medical Genetics* 63, no. 1 (1996): 4–6.

39. Among the important historic surveys describing hereditary disorders of the skeleton are these: C. I. Scott, Jr., "The Genetics of Short Stature," in *Progress in Medical Genetics*, ed. A. Steinberg and A. Bearn (New York: Grune & Stratton, 1972), 8:243–99; D. L. Rimoin, "The Chondrodystrophies," Chap. 1 in *Human Genetics*, ed. H. Harris and K. Hirschhorn (New York: Plenum Press, 1970), vol. 5; P. Maroteaux, *Bone Diseases of Children*, trans. from the French and adapted by H. J. Kaufmann (Philadelphia: J.B. Lippincott, 1979).

40. V. A. McKusick, *Heritable Disorders of Connective Tissue*, 4th ed. (St. Louis: C. V. Mosby, 1972); V. A. McKusick, *Mendelian Inheritance in Man*, 13th ed. (Baltimore: Johns Hopkins University Press, 1998). This database has been on a computer since 1964; since 1998 it has been available online as OMIM, and on CD-ROM.

41. "International Nomenclature of Constitutional Disorders of Bone," www.csmc.edu/genetics/skeldys/nomen.1.html.

42. C. M. Hall, "International Nosology and Classification of Constitutional Disorders of Bone (2001)," *American Journal of Medical Genetics* 113 (2002): 65–77.

43. A. Superti-Furga, "Molecular Pathology of Skeletal Development," www.cloettastiftung.ch/superti_ref.pdf. A. Superti-Furga, L. Bonafe, and D. L. Rimoin, "Molecular-Pathogenetic Classification of Genetic Disorders of the Skeleton," *American Journal of Medical Genetics* 106, no. 4 (2001): 282–93. J. F. Crow, "There's Something Curious about Paternal-Age Effects," *Science* 301 (2003): 606–607.

44. C. S. Pandav and K. Anand, "Toward the Elimination of Iodine Deficiency Disorders in India," *Indian Journal of Pediatrics* 62, no. 5 (1995): 545–55.

45. "Screening for Congenital Hypothyroidism" in *Guide to Clinical Preventive Services*, 2nd ed. (Washington, D.C.: U.S. Department of Health and Human Services, Office of Disease Prevention and Health Promotion, 1996). American Academy of Pediatrics, "Newborn Screening for Congenital Hypothyroidism: Recommended Guidelines," *Pediatrics* 91, no. 6 (1993): 1203–09.

46. M. M. Grumbach, B. S. Bin-Abbas, and S. L. Kaplan, "The Growth Hormone Cascade: Progress and Long-Term Results of Growth Hormone Treatment in Growth Hormone Deficiency," *Hormone Research* 49, suppl. 2 (1998): 41–57.

47. F. Huet, J. C. Carel, J. L. Nivelon, and J. L. Chaussain, "Long-Term Results of GH Therapy in GH-Deficient Children Treated before One Year of Age," *European Journal of Endocrinology* 140 (1999): 29–34.

48. M. Vanderschueren-Lodeweyckx, "Who Is Treated with Growth Hormone Today? The Executive Scientific Committee of the Kabi International Growth Study," *Acta Paediatrica Scandinavica Supplement* 370 (1990): 107–13.

49. See, for example, M. Dattani and M. Preece, "Growth Hormone Deficiency and Related Disorders: Insights into Causation, Diagnosis, and Treatment," *Lancet* 363 (2004): 1977–87. G. Rosenfeld and V. Hwa, "Toward a Molecular Basis for Ideopathic Short Stature," *Journal of Clinical Endocrinology and Metabolism* 89, no. 3 (2004): 1066–67; R. G. Rosenfeld, "Insulin-like Growth Factors and the Basis of Growth," *New England Journal of Medicine* 349, no. 23 (2003): 2184–86; R. G. Rosenfeld, "Transition from Pediatric to Adult Care for Growth Hormone Deficiency," *Journal of Pediatric Endocrinology and Metabolism*, Suppl. no. 3 (2003): 645–69. For an excellent comprehensive work that includes some chapters relevant to short stature, see M. E. Sperling, *Pediatric Endocrinology*, 2nd Ed. (Philadelphia: W. B. Saunders, 2002).

50. L. L. Key, Jr., and A. J. Gross, "Response to Growth Hormone in Children with Chondrodysplasia," pt. 2, *Journal of Pediatrics* 5 (1996): S14–S17.

51. "Growth Hormone for Short Kids, " *Pediatrics Blog Archives*, http:pediatrics. about.com/b/a/2003_07_26.htm.

52. G. Stock, "Stamping Out Short People," www.wired.com/wired/archive/11.11/ view.html?pg=2. L. M. Fisher, "A Clinical Trial of Growth Drug Shows Promise," *New York Times*, 17 June 2004, C1.

53. Z. Hochberg and Z. Zadik, "Final Height in Young Women with Turner Syndrome after GH Therapy: An Open Controlled Study," *European Journal of Endocrinology* 141, no. 3 (1999): 218–24. This study reports a final height gain of 4.4 cm, or corrected mean gained height of 5.3 above the control group, with shorter girls showing a better response than taller girls.

54. L. Hanton, L. Axelrod, Y. Bakalov, and C. A. Bondy, "The Importance of Estrogen Replacement in Young Women with Turner Syndrome," *Journal of Women's Health*, 12, no. 10 2003): 971–77. (See Turner Syndrome Society Web site for updates.

55. P. J. Hilts, "Fetus to Fetus Transplant Blocks Deadly Genetic Defect, Researchers Say," *New York Times*, 21 November 1991, B14. This encouraging report later ended in the patient's death.

56. E. D. Kakkis, J. Muenzer, G. E. Tiller, et al, "Enzyme-Replacement Therapy in Mucopolysaccaridosis I," *New England Journal of Medicine* 344, no. 3 (2001): 182–88; S. Tomatsu, "Toward Development of Treatment for Morquio Patients." www.aguaforte.com/morquio/letter2.html.

57. G. S. Bassett, "Neck Disorders in Little People," www.lpa.on.ca/NECKDISOR DERS.HTM.

58. R. M. Pauli, V. K. Horton, L. P. Glinski, et al., "Prospective Assessments of Risks for Cervicomedullary-Junction Compression in Infants with Achondroplasia, *American Journal of Medical Genetics* 56, no. 3 (1995): 732–44.

59. J. Money, *The Kaspar Hauser Syndrome of "Psychosocial Dwarfism": Deficient Statural, Intellectual and Social Growth Induced by Child Abuse* (Buffalo, NY: Prometheus Books, 1994). This influential volume discusses Kaspar Hauser, a foundling abandoned in Nuremberg in 1828 and research by Money and associates at Johns Hopkins. Since Money's reputation was damaged by disclosures about improperly authorizing sex reversal surgery on sexually ambiguous children and misreporting results, this formerly respected researcher has come under a cloud. Nevertheless, *Kaspar Hauser* provides an interesting introduction to psychosocial dwarfism. Important contributions in this field were made by Drs. Robert Blizzard, Dagfinn Aarskog, Gerald Powell, Salvatore Raiti, and others.

60. L. Gardner, "Deprivation Dwarfism," *Scientific American,* 227, no. 1 (1972): 76–82; R. M. Blizzard and A. Bulatovic, "Syndromes of Psychosocial Short Stature," in *Pediatric Endocrinology,* 3rd ed. (New York: Marcel Dekker, 1996).

61. D. Skuse and J. Gilmour, "Psychosocial Short Stature: Follow-up to Adolescence and Adulthood," in *Growth, Stature, and Psychosocial Well-Being,* ed. U. Eiholzer, F. Haverkamp, and L. Voss, 179–92 (Seattle, WA: Hogrefe & Huber Publishers, 1999); J. Gilmour and D. Skuse, "A Case Comparison Study of the Characteristics of Children with a Short Stature Syndrome Induced by Stress (Hyperphagic Short Stature) and a Consecutive Series of Unaffected Stressed Children," *Journal of Child Psychology and Psychiatry* 40, no. 6 (1999): 969–78.

62. D. Burgin, "Psychosocial Failure to Thrive," in *Growth, Stature, and Psychosocial Well-Being,* ed. U. Eiholzer, F. Haverkamp and L. Voss, 193–201 (Seattle, WA: Hogrefe & Huber Publishers, 1999).

63. H. McCarthy, "Failure to Thrive: Sergei, Mighty Mite," *Eastern European Adoption Coalition,* 31 August 1998, www.eeadopt.org/home/parenting/development/failureto thrive/. Although this article is no longer posted, the Eastern European Adoption Coalition Web site provides valuable information and support.

64. A. G. Hunter, A. Bankier, J. G. Rogers, D. Sillence, and C. I. Scott, Jr., "Medical Complications of Achondroplasia: A Multicentre Patient Review," *Journal of Medical Genetics* 35, no. 9 (1998), 705–12; A. G. Hunter, "Perceptions of the Outcome of Orthopedic Surgery in Patients with Chondrodysplasia," *Clinical Genetics* 56, no. 6 (1999): 343–40.

65. N. N. Mahomed, M. Spellmann, and M. J. Goldberg, "Functional Health Status of Adults with Achondroplasia," *Am J Med Genet* 78, no. 1 (1998): 30–35.

66. R. M. Pauli, C. I. Scott, Jr., E. R. Wassman, et al., "Apnea and Sudden Unexpected Death in Infants with Achondroplasia," *Journal of Pediatrics* 104, no. 3 (1984): 342–48.

67. J. G. Hall, "Results of the survey of medical complications in classical achondroplasia," photocopy, 1974–75.

68. E. Owen, K. Smalley, D. D'Allessio, et al., "Resting Metabolic Rate and Body Composition of Achondroplastic Dwarfs," *Medicine* (Baltimore) 69 (1990): 56–67.

69. A. G. Hunter, J. T. Hecht, and C. I. Scott, Jr., "Standard Weight for Height Curves in Achondroplasia," *American Journal of Medical Genetics* 62 (1996): 255–61; J. G. Hall, "Nutrition and the Little Person," *LPA Online,* www.lpa.on.ca/NUTRITION.HTM.

70. L. Munk, "A Conversation with Victor A. McKusick, MD," www.aabb.org/ Professionals/Professional_Development/Annual_Mee . . . /56amsunmck.ht

71. L. Hook Porter, "Invitation," in *The Marfan Writer's Anthology* (Jersey City, NJ: Publ. by Angela Hebert and Julie Kurnitz, 1999), 47.

72. V. A. McKusick, "Forty Years of Medical Genetics," *JAMA* 261, no. 21 (1989): 3155–58.

73. Lasker Living Library: "Victor McKusick Interview," www/laskerfoundation.org/ library/mckusick/interview-main.htm.

74. V. A. McKusick, *Heritable Disorders of Connective Tissue* (St. Louis: C. V. Mosby Co., 1956).

75. "First Genetic Trust and the Johns Hopkins University's McKusick-Nathans Institute for Genetic Medicine," *First Genetic Trust*, www.firstgenetic.net/about_partners .html.

76. "Victor McKusick and Al Sommer: Medical Researchers, Baltimoreans of the Year," *Baltimore Online*, www.baltimoremag.com/main/archives/98–01/boty2.html.

77. For information about the background of the creation of HUGO (the Human Genome Organization) and other aspects of the gene-mapping movement, see V. A. McKusick, "Mapping and Sequencing the Human Genome," *New England Journal of Medicine* 320, no. 14 (1989): 910–15.

78. K. Ledger, "And So to Maine," *Hopkins Medical News*, Summer 1999. http:// hopkins.med.jhu.edu/ReadingRoom/jhmn/S99/annals.html.

79. Kathryn (Kay) Smith, telephone interview with the author, 31 July 2000. For the account of the Greenberg Center, I am also grateful to Kay Smith.

80. Clair A. Francomano, interview with the author, 23 June 2000.

81. Here are a few of her notable publications: Z. Vajo, C. A. Francomano, and D. J. Wilkin, "The Molecular and Genetic Basis of Fibroblast Growth Factor Receptor 3 Disorders: The Achondroplasia Family of Skeletal Dysplasias, Muenke Craniosynostosis and Crouzon Syndrome with Acanthosis Nigricans," *Endocrine Reviews* 21, no. 1 (2000): 23– 39; L. P. Fried, C. A. Francomano, S. M. McDonald, et al., "Career Development for Women in Academic Medicine: Multiple Interventions in a Department of Medicine," *JAMA* 276, no. 11 (1996): 898–905; V. A. McKusick, J. S. Amberger, and C. A. Francomano, "Progress in Medical Genetics: Map-Based Gene Discovery and the Molecular Pathology of Skeletal Dysplasias," *American Journal of Medical Genetics* 63, no. 1 (1996): 98–105; C. A. Francomano, "The Genetic Basis of Dwarfism," *New England Journal of Medicine* 332, no. 1 (1995): 58–59; T. Sulisalo, C. A. Francomano, P. Sistonen, et al., "High Resolution Genetic Mapping of the Cartilage-Hair Hypoplasia (CHH) Gene in Amish and Finnish Families," *Genomics* 20, no. 3 (1994): 347–53.

82. C. A. Francomano, "Division of Intramural Research, investigators and advisors." www.nhgri.nih.gov/Intramural_research/People/francoman.html.

83. R. Henderson and M. Centofanti, "Life as a Little Person," *Hopkins Medical News*, Spring-Summer 1995. Available on LPA Online.

84. Vajo, Francomano, and Wilkin, "The Molecular and Genetic Basis of FGFR3 Disorders," 21: 23–39.

85. N. Wade, "Now the Hard Part: Putting the Genome to Work," Science Times, *New York Times* F1, 27 June 2000, 1–8.

86. H. C. Gooding, K. Boehm, R. E. Thompson, D. Hadley, C. A. Francomano, and B. B. Biesecker, "Issues Surrounding Prenatal Genetic Testing for Achondroplasia," *Prenatal Diagnosis* 10 (2002): 933–40.

87. Clair Francomano, e-mail message to author, 4 November 2002.

88. Ibid., 16 March 2004.

89. D. L. Rimoin and R. N. Schimke, *Genetic Disorders of the Endocrine Glands* (St. Louis: C. V. Mosby, 1971; later editions in 1977, 1983, 1992).

90. "Shriners Hospital for Children, Intermountain Shrine Telemedicine Initiative," www.shrinershq.org/WhatsNewArch/Archives99/telemedicine10–99.html.

91. Further information about contacting the International Skeletal Dysplasia Registry may be obtained at their Web site, www.csmc.edu/3992.html.

92. L. Jaroff, "Keys to the Kingdom: An Autism Genetics Tutorial," *Time,* Special Medical Issue, Fall 1996, 24–26, 28–29.

93. Summary of APHMG 1997 Workshop, www.faseb.org/genetics/aphmg/aphmg8d.htm.

94. Rimoin co-chaired the Strategic Planning Task Force on genetics and biology for the National Institute of Child Health and Human Development, NIH agency. "NICHD Strategic Plan," www.nichd.nih.gov/strategicplan/cells/strategicplan.pdf.

95. C. S. Reid, "Management of Major Craniofacial Anomalies: A Pediatric Perspective," *The Cleft Palate-Craniofacial Journal* 29, no. 6 (1992): 570, 575–77.

96. C. S. Reid, "Respiratory Studies in Achondroplasia during Childhood," *LPA Today,* March–July 1992, 6–7.

97. H. Wang, A. E. Rosenbaum, C. S. Reid, et al., "Pediatric Patients with Achondroplasia: CT Evaluation of the Craniocervical Junction," *Radiology* 164, no. 2 (1987): 515–19; C. S. Reid, R. E. Pyeritz, S. E. Kopits, et al., "Cervicomedullary Compression in Young Patients with Achondroplasia: Value of Comprehensive Neurologic and Respiratory Evaluation," *Journal of Pediatrics* 110, no. 4 (1987): 522–30.

98. A. G. Hunter, C. S. Reid, R. M. Pauli, and C. I. Scott, Jr., "Standard Curves of Chest Circumference in Achondroplasia and the Relationship of Chest Circumference to Respiratory Problems," *American Journal of Medical Genetics* 62, no. 1 (1996): 91–97.

99. Michael Wright, quoted in M. Hendricks, "Aiming High," *Johns Hopkins Magazine,* April 1999, 9; www.lpaonline.org/resources_library.html.

100. E. A. Sisk, D. G. Heatley, B. J. Borowski, G. E. Leverson, and R. M. Pauli, "Obstructive Sleep Apnea in Children with Achondroplasia: Surgical and Anesthetic Considerations," *Otolaryngology and Head and Neck Surgery* 120, no. 2 (1999): 248–54; R. C. Tasker, I. Dundas, A. Laverty, et al., "Distinct Patterns of Respiratory Difficulty in Young Children with Achondroplasia: A Clinical, Sleep, and Lung Function Study," *Archives of Disease in Childhood* 79, no. 2 (1998): 99–108.

101. M. Bachstein, "Clinics," in *Toward Solomon's Mountain: The Experience of Disability in Poetry,* ed. J. Baird and D. S. Workman, 38 (Philadelphia: Temple University Press, 1986).

102. G. Kobren and E. J. Malashuk, "God's Gift to the Little People," *Sun Magazine,* 20 September 1981, 6–16.

103. B. Lemley, "The Big Man of Little People," *Washington Post Magazine,* 9 December 1984, n.p.

104. J. Phillips, "A New Way to Run," available from the Little People's Research Fund.

105. M. Segal, "In Their Own Words," *Pierre House Happenings: Biannual Newsletter of the Little People's Research Fund,* Fall-Winter 1999–2000, 2.

106. C. Brown III, "In Their Own Words," *Pierre House Happenings: Biannual Newsletter of the Little People's Research Fund,* Fall-Winter 1999–2000, 2.

107. Ibid.

108. G. Kobrun and E. J. Malashuk, "God's Gift to the Little People," *Sun Magazine*, 20 September 1981, 1.

109. Ibid.

110. G. P. Matysek, Jr., "St. Joseph's Doctor Saves the Lives of Two 'Little People,'" *Catholic Review*, 7 October 1999; repr. in *Diastrophic Dynamics*, www.pixelscapes.com/ddnewsletter/kopits-juliana.html.

111. Charles McElwee (executive director of the Little People's Research Fund), in telephone interview with the author, 9 August 2000.

112. Vita Gagne, e-mail to author, 19 September 2000.

113. Letter from Steven Kopits, then at Johns Hopkins, 20 November 1980.

114. Charles McElwee, in telephone conversation with the author, 29 August 2000.

115. Melissa Hendricks, "Aiming High," *Johns Hopkins Magazine*, April 1999.

116. J. Bor, "Profile: Dr. Ain." *Baltimore Sun*, 6 September 1998, www.dwarfism.org/library/index.php.

117. Ibid.

118. Michael Ain, in telephone interview with the author, 26 September 2000.

119. B. Ziegler Rothenhausier and C. P. Scott, "Michael Ain, MD: Dedicated to Enhancing Lives," *Orthopedic Technology Review* 3, no. 6 (2001): 26. www.orthopedictech review.com/issues/novdec01/pg26.htm.

120. M. C. Ain, I. Elmaci, O. Hurko, R. E. Clatterbuck, R. R. Lee, and D. Rigamonti, "Reoperation for Spinal Restenosis in Achondroplasia," *Journal of Spinal Disorders* 13, no. 2 (2000): 168–73; M. C. Ain, B. M. Andres, D. S. Somel et al., "Total Hip Arthroplasty in Skeletal Dysplasia: Patient Selection, Preoperative Planning and Operative Techniques," *Journal of Arthroplasty* 19, no. 1 (2004): 1–7; M. C. Ain and E. D. Shirley, "Spinal Fusion for Kyphosis in Achondroplasia," *Journal of Pediatric Orthopedics* 24, no.5 (2004): 542–45.

121. B. Carson and C. Murphey, *Gifted Hands: The Ben Carson Story* (Grand Rapids, MI: Zondervan Publishing House, 1992); B. Carson and C. Murphey, *Think Big: Understanding Your Potential for Excellence* (Grand Rapids, MI: Zonderveer Publishing House, 1992).

122. Hendricks, "Aiming High," 7–8.

123. Rothenhausier and Scott, "Michael Ain," 3:26.

124. "A Distinction of the Highest Order," *Canadian Paediatric Society News* (March/April 1999), www.cps.ca/english/publications/cpsnews/1999/March/DistinctionHighest Order.htm.

125. Judith G. Hall and Lynn T. Staheler, Medical Advisors, "What it is and How it is Treated" *AVENUES*, A Publication of the National Support Group for Arthrogryposis Multiplex Congenita, http://sonnet1.sonnet.com/avenues/publications/pamphlet.htm.

126. American Academy of Pediatrics, "Health Supervision for Children with Achondroplasia," *Pediatrics* 95, no. 3 (1995): 443–51.

127. News and Analysis, *Canadian Medical Association Journal* 160, no. 1 (1999): 15.

128. R. E. Stevenson, R. Goodman, and J. G. Hall, *Human Malformations and Related Anomalies* (New York: Oxford University Press, 1993).

129. L. T. Staheli, J. G. Hall, and K. M. Jaffee, *Arthrogryposis* (Cambridge: Cambridge University Press, 1998).

130. J. G. Hall, U. G. Froster-Iskenius, and J. E. Allanson, *Handbook of Normal Physical Measurements* (New York: Oxford University Press, 1990).

131. D. A. Applegarth, J. E. Dimmick, and J. G. Hall, *Organelle Diseases* (London: Chapman & Hall Medical, 1999).

132. "Profile of Dr. Judith Hall, " British Columbia Research Institute for Children's and Women's Health, www.bcricwh.bc.ca/profiles/hall.html.

133. S. B. Cassidy and J. Allanson, eds., *The Management of Genetic Syndromes*, 2nd ed. (New York: Wiley, 2004)

134. "Mendel Might Get Dizzy," *Canadian Medical Association Journal* 157, no. 12 (1997): 1669–70.

135. J. G. Hall, "The Value of the Study of Natural History in Genetic Disorders and Congenital Anomaly Syndromes," *Journal of Medical Genetics* 25, no. 7 (1988): 434–44.

136. "Revolution in Genetics Just Beginning Predicts Malcolm Brown Lecturer," *Info Spec,* official newspaper of the Annual Meeting of the Royal College of Physicians and Surgeons of Canada, 1999 issue. http://www.mednet.ca/InfoSpec1999p14.htm.

137. J. G. Hall, "Folic Acid: The Opportunity That Still Exists," *Canadian Medical Association Journal* 162, no. 11 (2000): 1571–2.

138. News and Analysis, *Canadian Medical Association Journal* 160, no. 1 (1999): 15.

139. C. I. Scott, Jr., "Dwarfism," *CIBA-GEIGY Clinical Symposia* 40, no. 1 (1988); C. I. Scott, Jr., "Medical and Social Adaptation in Dwarfing Conditions," *Birth Defects: Original Articles Series* 13 (3C): 29–43 (March of Dimes Birth Defects Foundation, 1977).

140. C. I Scott, Jr., N. Mayeux, R. Crandall, J. O. Weiss, *Dwarfism: The Family and Professional Guide,* eds. R. Crandall and T. Crosson (Irvine, CA: Short Stature Foundation & Information Center, Inc., 1994).

141. J. O. Weiss and J. S. Machta, *Starting and Sustaining Genetic Support Groups* (Baltimore: Johns Hopkins University Press, 1996).

142. E. V. Lapham, C. Kozma, and J. O. Weiss, "Genetic Discrimination: Perspectives of Consumers," *Science* 274, no. 5287 (1996): 621–24.

143. See the several studies that cast light on this question in E. Eiholzer, F. Haverkamp, and L. Voss, eds., *Growth, Stature and Psychosocial Well-Being* (Seattle, WA: Hofgrefe & Huber Publishers, 1999).

144. M. M. Grumbach, B. S. Bin-Abbas, and S. L. Kaplan, "The Growth Hormone Cascade: Progress and Long-Term Results of Growth Hormone Treatment in Growth Hormone Deficiency," *Hormone Research* 49, suppl. no. 2 (1998): 41–57.

145. J. Monson, ed., *Challenges in Growth Hormone Therapy* (Oxford: Blackwell Science, 1999).

146. M. Winerip, "Our Towns: Enduring Agony, A Boy's Made Taller," *New York Times,* 30 December 1986, B1.

147. R. Samghabadi, "In New Jersey a Boy Grows Towering Tall," *Time,* 22 August 1988, 12–13.

148. John Herzenberg, telephone interview with the author, 24 April 2004.

149. This description is adapted from *Limb Surgery,* n.p., published by the British Restricted Growth Association; this booklet describes the procedure and considerations in decision making.

150. The information that follows is drawn largely from two sources: "Historical Review," *ASAMI (Association for the Study and Application of the Method of Ilizarov)* http://62.94.230.179:8081/asami_story/default.asp; S. Green, "How the Ilizarov Method Came to North America," *Distraction* 4, no. 1 (1996), www.asaminorthamerica.org/main/archive/1996nov.pdf.

151. R. Gross, "Leg-Lengthening," adapted from *Lancet* 354 (1999): 1574–75. www
.findarticles.com/cf_0/m)/m0833/9190_354/57820884/print.jhtml. This is an excellent
review of the history of limb lengthening; see also S. Green, "Ilizarov Method," 2.

152. A. D. Aaron and R. E. Eilert, "Results of the Wagner and Ilizarov Methods of
Limb-Lengthening," *Journal of Bone and Joint Surgery. American Volume* 78, no. 1 (1996):
20–29.

153. R. Aldegheri, "Distraction Osteogenisis for Lengthening of the Tibia in Patients
Who Have Limb-Length Discrepancy or Short Stature," *Journal of Bone and Joint Surgery.
American Volume* 81, no. 5 (1999): 624–34.

154. S. E. Kopits, B. Nicoletti, et al., *Human Achondroplasia: A Multidisciplinary Approach*, Basic Life Sciences (New York: Plenum, 1989), vol. 48.

155. Steven E. Kopits, lecture at LPA Conference in Baltimore, Summer 1989.

156. J. G. Hall, "Summary of the First International Conference on Human Achondroplasia, 26 November 1986, *LPA District 2 Newsletter*, Spring 1987; S. E. Kopits, B.
Nicoletti, et al., *Human Achondroplasia: A Multidisciplinary Approach*, Basic Life Sciences
(New York: Plenum, 1989), vol. 48.

157. "Little People of America: Position Statement on Extended Limb Lengthening
(ELL), November 1988." www.dwarfism.org/library/ell.php.

158. J. Correll, "Surgical Correction of Short Stature in Skeletal Dysplasias," *Acta Paediatrica Scandinavica Supplement* 377 (1991): 143–48.

159. M. T. Dahl, B. Gulli, and T. Berg, "Complications of Limb-Lengthening: A Learning Curve," *Clinical Orthopaedics and Related Research* 301 (1994): 10–18.

160. "Device Allows Noninvasive Monitoring of Nerve Function," *Academy News,
The Annual Meeting Edition of the AAOS Bulletin* (American Academy of Orthopaedic
Surgeons), 5 February 1999. www.aaos.org/wordhtml/99news/nerve1.htm.

161. J. E. Herzenberg and D. Paley, "Methods and Strategies in Limb Lengthening and
Realignment for Skeletal Dysplasia" in *Limb Lengtheninng: For Whom, When and How?"*
ed. Z. Laron, S. Matragostino, and C. Romano (London: Freund Publishing House, 1995),
181–99.

162. John Herzenberg, in a telephone interview with the author, 25 April 2004.

163. Papers on these subjects and others by Drs. Paley and Herzenberg on bilateral
tibial and humeral lengthening were forwarded to me by the International Center for
Limb Lengthening and Reconstruction (ICLLR).

164. A. Ganel and H. Horoszowski, "Limb Lengthening in Children with Achondroplasia. Difference Based on Gender," *Clinical Orthopaedics and Related Research* 332
(1996): 179–83.

165. R. Aldegheri and C. Dall'Oca, "Limb Lengthening in Short Stature Patients,"
Journal of Pediatric Orthopaedics Part B 10, no. 3 (2001): 238–47.

166. John Herzenberg, telephone conversation with author, 25 April 2004: discussed
the several levels of difficulty—problems (e.g., infections); obstacles (premature fusing
that requires returning to the operating room); and complications (very serious, permanent sequelae). The first two are relatively common; the last, quite rare.

167. G. Mueller, "Extended Limb-Lengthening: Setting the Record Straight," 2000.
www.dwarfism.org/library/index.php.

168. D. Rimoin, "Extended Leg Lengthening," *LPA Today* (January-February 1991):
7–8; J. M.Villerubias, I. Ginebreda, and E. Jimeno, "Lengthening of the Lower Limbs
and Correction of Lumbar Hyperlordosis in Achondroplasia," *Clinical Orthopaedics and
Related Research* 250 (1990): 143–49.

169. P. Bregani, G. Weber, A. Cucchiani, et al., "Emotional Implications of Limb Lengthening in Adolescents and Young Adults with Achondroplasia," *Life Span and Disability,* July/December 1998. www.lifespan.it/vol1n2/uk/pag6.htm.

170. Mary and Anthony Tarabocchia, telephone conversation with the author, 18 April 2004.

171. David Rimoin, e-mail message to the author, 20 April 2004.

172. "Stats and Facts of Shriners Hospitals," www.pixi.com/~shriners/stats.html.

173. Thanks to Cheryl Reid for offering this information.

174. "Gene Therapy: What and Why," *March of Dimes* Research Annual Report, 1997–98. www.modimes.org.

175. My thanks to Priscilla Ciccariello, former chair of the Marfan Foundation and former president of the Coalition of Heritable Disorders of Connective Tissue. She quotes Reed Pyeritz as calling the matrix "the glue that holds the body together."

176. W. Bodin and B. Hershey, *It's a Small World: All about Midgets* (New York: Coward-McCann, Inc., 1934), 302.

177. "Shriners Hospital Researchers Discover Dwarfism Gene: Discovery May Lead to Better Ways to Treat Bone, Joint Disorders," www.shriners.com/WhatsNewArch/Archives96/dwarf8-96.html.

178. *LPA Today,* July–October 1998, 38.

179. William Horton, e-mail message to the author, 16 March 2004. See also W. A. Horton, S. Garofolo, and G. P. Lunstrum, "FGFR3 Signaling in Achondroplasia: A Review," *Cells and Materials* 8 (1998): 83–87; D. Aviezer, M. Golumbo, and A. Yayon, "Fibroblast Growth Factor Receptor-3 as a Therapeutic Target for Achondroplasia: Genetic Short Limbed Dwarfism," *Current Drug Targets* (2003):353–65; A. Yasoda, Y. Komatsu, H. Chusho, et al., "Overexpression of CNP in Chondrocytes Rescues Achondroplasia through a MAPK-dependent Pathway," *Nature Medicine* 10, no. 1 (2004): 80–86.

180. M. Jones, "The Genetic Report Card That Will Tell You if Your Embryo Will Get Prostate Cancer," *New York Times Magazine,* 11 June 2000.

181. NORD Orphan Disease Update, Summer 2000, 3.

182. P. Modaff, V. K. Horton, and R. M. Pauli, "Errors in the Prenatal Diagnosis of Children with Achondroplasia," *Prenatal Diagnosis* 16, no. 6 (1996): 525–30.

183. C. Stoll, P. Manini, J. Bloch, and M. P. Roth, "Prenatal Diagnosis of Hypochondroplasia," *Prenatal Diagnosis* 5, no. 6 (1985): 423–26. Marginal note made by Dr. Rimoin when he kindly reviewed the chapter for accuracy in November 2000.

184. Christina Dunigan, "Doctors: Don't Want No Short People 'Round Here," *Real Choice* 5 July 2000. www.shortsupport.org/cgt/news_list.cgi.

185. G. Hayden, "Late Pregnancy Termination for Dwarfism Provokes Controversy," *AccessLife.com.* http://www.accesslife.com/scripts/saisapi.dll/catalog.class/life/20000811-ETH-dwarfabortion.html.

186. Ibid., 2.

187. J. Gillott, "The Spectre of Eugenics," *LM Archives.* Reproduced from *Living Marxism,* January 1996, 1–5, www.prochoiceforum.org.uk/and3.asp.

188. H. C. Gooding, K. Boehm, R. E. Thompson, D. Hadley, C. A. Francomano, and B. B. Biesecker, "Issues Surrounding Prenatal Genetic Testing for Achondroplasia," *Prenatal Diagnosis* 10 (2002): 933–40.

189. S. Mawer, *Mendel's Dwarf* (New York: Harmony Books, a division of Crown Publishers, 1998), 238–39.

190. International Center for Bioethics, Culture, and Disability, www.bioethicsand disability.org.

191. See, for example, D. C. Wertz, "Society and the Not-So-New-Genetics: What Are We Afraid Of? Some Future Predictions from a Social Scientist," www.umassmed.edu/shriver/research/socialscience/staff/wertz/lawjrl.cfm.

192. "The Regulation of Pre-implantation Genetic Diagnosis: Response to the HFEA/ACGT Consultation from the Campaign Against Human Genetic Engineering," www.users.globalnet.co.uk/~cahge/pgd.htm.

193. British Council of Disabled People, "The New Genetics and Disabled People: A Discussion Document," www.bcodp.org.uk/general/genetics.html.

194. "Frequently Asked Questions," 4. LPA Online, www.lpaonline.org/resources_faq.html.

195. R. E. Ricker, "Do We Really Want This: Little People of America Inc. Comes to Terms with Genetic Testing," LPA Online, July 1995, http://home.earthlink.net/~dkennedy56/dwarfism_genetics.html

196. T. Shakespeare, "RGA Genetics Survey Report," October 2000. Discrepant attitudes about aborting a fetus with restricted growth may result from greater awareness in short-statured respondents of potential double-dominance problems.

197. G. Kolata, "In Late Abortions Decisions Are Painful and Options Few," *New York Times*, 5 January 1992, A1. The Letter to the Editor appeared on 5 February 1992. Its position was supported in an article by J. G. Hall and D. Gilchrist in *Current Issues in Pediatric and Adolescent Endocrinology*. They note that intelligence is average or above average in persons with Turner syndrome.

198. Simi Linton, Columbia University Disability Studies Seminar, 30 March 2004.

199. L. P. Sawisch, "Psychosocial Aspects of Short Stature: The Day to Day Context," in *Slow Grows the Child: Psychosocial Aspects of Growth Delay,* ed. B. Stabler and L. E. Underwood (Mahwah, NJ: Lawrence Erlbaum Associates, 1986), 47.

200. Richard Pauli, e-mail message to the author, 25 November 2002.

CHAPTER 2. PSYCHOSOCIAL ASPECTS

1. Joan Ablon, *Little People in America* (New York: Praeger, 1984).

2. Rainer Maria Rilke, "The Dwarf's Song," *Selected Poems of Rainer Maria Rilke*. Translation and commentary by Robert Bly (New York: Harper & Row, Perennial, 1981), 126–27. The translation here is by Betty Adelson.

3. For an analysis of the dwarf in painting and literature, see Betty Adelson, *The Lives of Dwarfs: Their Journey from Public Curiosity toward Social Liberation* (Piscataway, NJ: Rutgers University Press, 2005).

4. See *Criteria for Determining Disability in Infants and Children: Short Stature,* Evidence Report/Technology Assessment no. 73, U.S. Department of Health and Human Services, www.ahrq.gov/clinic/epcsums/shortsum, htm. Full report available by calling (1-800) 358-9295. This report contains charts and bibliographies that include the physiological and psychological aspects of dwarfing conditions.

5. Joan Ablon, *Living with Difference* (New York: Praeger, 1988). See summary, Appendix C.

6. Brian Stabler and Louis E. Underwood, eds., *Slow Grows the Child: Psychosocial As-*

pects of Growth Delay (Hillsdale, NJ: Lawrence Erlbaum Associates, 1986); Urs Eiholzer, Fritz Haverkamp, and Linda Voss, eds., *Growth, Stature and Psychosocial Well-Being* (Seattle, WA: Hogrefe & Huber Publishers, 1999); Leslie F. Martel and Henry B. Biller, *Stature and Stigma: The Biopsychosocial Development of Short Males* (Lexington, MA: DC Heath and Company, 1987).

7. B. Stabler, R. R. Clopper, P. T. Siegel, "Academic Achievement and Psychological Adjustment in Short Children," *Developmental and Behavioral Pediatrics* 15, no, 1 (1994): 1–6; B. Stabler, R. R. Clopper, P. T. Siegel, et al, "Links between Growth Hormone Deficiency, Adaptation, and Social Phobia," *Hormone Research* 45 (1996): 30–33; B. Stabler, P. T. Siegel, R. R. Clopper, et al, "Behavior Change after Growth Hormone Treatment of Children with Short Stature," *Journal of Pediatrics* 133 (1998): 336–73; L. Stace and D. M. Danks, "A Social Study of Dwarfing Conditions," *Australian Paediatric Journal* 17 (1981): 167–82; A.G. Hunter, "Some Psychosocial Aspects of Nonlethal Achondroplasias," *Journal of Medical Genetics* 78, no.1 (1998): 1–29; J. Ablon, "Personality and Stereotype in Osteogenesis Imperfecta: Behavioral Phenotype or response to Life's Hard Challenges," *American Journal of Medical Genetics* 122A, no. 3 (2003): 201–14; S.E. Gollust, R.E. Thompson, H.C. Gooding, B.B. Biesecker, "Living with Achondroplasia in an Average-Sized World: An Assessment of Quality of Life," *American Journal of Medical Genetics* 120A, no.4 (2003): 447–58.

8. K. Y. Lai, D. Skuse, R. Stanhope, and P. Hindmarsh, "Cognitive Abilities Associated with the Silver-Russell Syndrome," *Archives of Disease in Childhood* 71, no. 6 (1994): 490–96.

9. P. Chatelain, "Children Born with Intra-uterine Growth Retardation (IUGR) Small for Gestational Age (SGA): Long Term Growth and Metabolic Consequences," *Endocrine Regulations* 35, no. 1 (2000): 33–36.

10. C. S. Holmes, R. G. Thompson, and J. T. Hayford, "Factors Related to Grade Retention in Children with Short Stature," *Child: Care, Health and Development* 10, no. 4 (1984): 199–210.

11. P. Drash, N. E. Greenberg, and J. Money, "Intelligence and Personality in Four Syndromes of Dwarfism," in *Human Growth: Body Composition, Cell Growth*, ed. D. B. Cheek, *Energy and Intelligence* (Philadelphia: Lea & Febinger, 1968), 568–81.

12. J. G. Rogers, M. A. Perry, and L. A. Rosenberg, "IQ Measurement in Children with Skeletal Dysplasias," *Pediatrics* 63, no. 2 (1979): 894–97.

13. L. J. Low, M. J. Knudson, and C. Sherrill, "New Interest Area for Adapted Physical Activity," *Adapted Physical Activity Quarterly* 13, no. 1 (1996): 1–15.

14. L. O. Langer, R. K. Beals, I. L. Solomon, et al., "Acromesomelic Dwarfism: Manifestations in Childhood," *American Journal of Medical Genetics* 1, no. 1 (1977): 87–100.

15. R. Wynne-Davies and M. A. Patton, "The Frequency of Mental Retardation in Hypochondroplasia," *Journal of Medical Genetics* 28, no. 9 (1991): 644. This article cites separate previous studies by Langer and Spranger from which the conclusions about mental retardation were drawn.

16. This information from a statement by Dr. Bellus about a study done by Bellus, Art Aylworth, Thad Kelly, and Susan Blanton was sent by Dee Miller, coordinator of the Greenberg Center, to Dan Kennedy and posted by him on the Dwarfism List on 3 December 2003.

17. G. Brinkmann, H. Schlitt, P. Zorowka, and J. Spranger, "Cognitive Skills in Achondroplasia," *American Journal of Medical Genetics* 47, no. 5 (1993): 800–4.

18. J. T. Hecht, N. M. Thompson, T. Weir, L. Patchell, and W. A. Horton, "Cognitive and Motor Skills in Achondroplastic Infants: Neurologic and Respiratory Correlates," *American Journal of Medical Genetics* 41, no. 2 (1991): 208–11.

19. N. M. Thompson, J. T. Hecht, T. P. Bohan, et al., "Neuroanatomic and Neuropsychological Outcome in School Age Children with Achondroplasia," *American Journal of Medical Genetics* 88, no. 2 (1999): 145–53.

20. E. Pollitt and J. Money, "Studies in the Psychology of Dwarfism, I. Intelligence Quotient and School Achievement," *Journal of Pediatrics* 64 (1964): 415–421; P. Drash, N. E. Greenberg, and J. Money, "Intelligence and Personality in Four Syndromes of Dwarfism," in *Human Growth*, ed. D. B. Cheek (Philadelphia: Lea and Febiger, 1968): 568–81; F. Cacciaguerra, "Research in Some Aspects of Mental Levels and Their Developmental Process in Chondrodystrophic and Hypopituitary Dwarfism," *Acta Medica Auxologica* 10, no. 2 (1978): 103–11; H. Steinhausen, "Psychoendocrinological Studies of Dwarfism in Childhood and Adolescence," *Zeitschr fur kinder und jugend psychiatrie* 5, no. 4 (1977): 346–59.

21. A. Sartorio, A. Conti, E. Molinari, et al., "Growth, Growth Hormone, and Cognitive Functions," *Hormone Research* 45, no. 1–2 (1996): 23–29.

22. P. T. Siegel and N. Hopwood, "The Relationship of Academic Achievement and the Intellectual Functioning and Affective Conditions of Hypopituitary Children," in Stabler and Underwood, 57–72.

23. See B. Stabler et al., "Academic Achievement and Psychological Adjustment in Short Children," *Developmental and Behavioral Pediatrics* 15, no. 1 (1994): 1–6, for discussion of lag in achievement.

24. D. Abbott, D. Rotnem, M. Genem, and D. J. Cohen, "Cognitive and Emotional functioning in Hypopituitary Short-Statured Children," *Schizophrenia Bulletin* 8 , no. 2 (1982): 310–19

25. Holmes, Thompson, and Hayford, 1984.

26. H. Steinhausen and J. Smith, "Cognitive Development in Turner Syndrome," in Stabler and Underwood, 111–22; J. Downey, E. J. Elkin, A. A. Ehrhardt, H. F. Meyer-Bahlburg, et al., "Cognitive Ability and Everyday Functioning in Women with Turner Syndrome, "*Journal of Learning Disabilities* 24, no. 1 (1991): 32–39.

27. R. A. Richman, M. Gordon, P. Tegtmayer, et al., "Academic and Emotional Difficulties Associated with Constitutional Short Stature," in Stabler and Underwood, 13–26; M. Gordon, E. M. Post, C. Crouthamel, and R. A Richman, "Do Children with Constitutional Delay Really Have More Learning Problems?" *Journal of Learning Disabilities* 17(1984): 291–93.

28. D. M. Wilson, L. D. Hammer, P. Duncan, et al., "Growth and Intellectual Development," *Journal of Pediatrics* 78, no. 4 (1985): 646–50.

29. M. N. Peck and O. Lundberg, "Short Stature as an Effect of Economic and Social Conditions in Childhood," *Social Science and Medicine* 41, no. 5 (1995): 733–38.

30. D. Burgin, "Psychosocial Failure to Thrive," in Eiholzer, Haverkamp, and Voss, eds., 193–200.

31. G. F. Powell, J. A. Brasel, S. Raiti, and R. M. Blizzard, "Emotional Deprivation and Growth Retardation Simulating Idiopathic Hypopituitarism," *New England Journal of Medicine* 276 (1967): 1279–83.

32. J. Money, C. Annecillo, and J. F. Kelley, "Growth of Intelligence: Failure and Catchup Associated Respectively with Abuse and Rescue in the Syndrome of Abuse Dwarfism," *Psychoneuroendocrinology* 8, no. 3 (1983): 309–19.

33. W. H. Green, M. Campbell, and R. David, "Psychosocial Dwarfism: A Critical Review of the Evidence," *Journal of the American Academy of Child Psychiatry* 23, no. 1 (1984): 39–48.

34. D. Skuse and J. Gilmour, "Psychosocial Short Stature: Follow-up to Adolescence and Adulthood," in Eiholzer, Haverkamp, and Voss, eds., 179–92.

35. Steven J. Gould, *The Mismeasure of Man* (New York: W.W. Norton & Co., 1981), 155. Many other writers since have detailed the quest for defining and measuring intelligence, but this work presents a good overview of the process and the important figures, such as Spearman, Goddard, Burt, Terman, and Yerkes, involved in its accomplishments and failures.

36. Erica Good, "His Goal: Making Intelligence Tests Smarter," *New York Times*, 3 April 2001, F1, 7.

37. F. Haverkamp and M. Noeker, "Short Stature in Children—A Questionnaire for Parents: A New Instrument for Growth Disorder-specific Psychosocial Adaptation in Children," *Quality of Life Research: An International Journal of Quality of Life Aspects of Treatment, Care and Rehabilitation* 7, no. 5 (1998): 47–55; S. E. Gollust, R. E. Thompson, H. C. Gooding, and B. B. Biesecker, "Living with Achondroplasia in an Average-Sized World: An Assessment of Quality of Life." *American Journal of Medical Genetics* 120A, no. 4 (2003): 447–58.

38. Drash, Greenberg, and Money, "Intelligence and Personality," 568–81.

39. J. S. Brust, C. V Ford, and D. R Rimoin, "Psychiatric Aspects of Dwarfism," *American Journal of Psychiatry* 133 (1976): 160–64.

40. S. E. Folstein, J. O. Weiss, F. Mittleman, and D. Ross, "Impairment, Psychiatric Symptoms, and Handicap in Dwarfs," *Johns Hopkins Medical Journal* 148 (1981): 273–77.

41. Ablon, *Little People*, 13–30, 184–89.

42. M. Kusalic and C. Fortin, "Growth Hormone Treatment in Hypopituitary Dwarfs: Longitudinal Psychological Effects," *Canadian Psychiatric Association Journal* 20 (1975): 325–31.

43. J. Money and E. Pollitt, "Studies in the Psychology of Dwarfism II: Personality Maturation and Response to Growth Hormone Treatment in Hypopituitary Dwarfs," *Journal of Pediatrics* 68 (1966): 381–90.

44. H. C. Steinhausen and N. Stahnke, "Negative Impact of Growth-Hormone Deficiency on Psychological Functioning in Dwarfed Children and Adolescents," *European Journal of Pediatrics* 126, no. 4 (1977): 263–70; D. Drotar, R. Owens, and J. Gotthold, "Personal Adjustment of Children and Adolescents with Hypopituitarism," *Annual Progress in Child Psychiatry and Child Development* 11(1981): 306–14.

45. B. Stabler, J. K. Whitt, D. M. Moreault, et al., "Social Judgments by Children of Short Stature," *Psychological Reports* 46 (1980): 743–46; B. Stabler, J. R. Turner, S. S. Girdler, et al. "Reactivity to Stress and Psychological Adjustment in Adults with Pituitary Insufficiency," *Clinical Endocrinology* 36, no. 5 (1992): 467–73; B. Stabler, M. E. Tancer, J. Ranc, and L. E. Underwood, "Evidence for Social Phobia in Adults Who Were Growth Hormone Deficient in Childhood," *Anxiety* 2, no. 2 (1996): 86–89.

46. D. M. Eminson, R. P. Powell, and S. Hollis, "Cognitive Behavioral Interventions with Short-statured Boys: A Pilot Study," in *Growth, Stature, and Adaptation,* ed. Brian Stabler and Louis Underwood (Chapel Hill, NC: University of North Carolina Press, 1994).

47. A. Sartori, G. Peri, E. Molinari, et al., "Psychosocial Outcomes of Adults with GH

Deficiency," *Acta Medica Auxologica* 18 (1986): 123–28; H. D. Dean, T. L. McTaggart, D. G. Fish, and H. G. Friesen, "Long-term Social Follow-up of Growth Hormone Deficient Adults Treated with Growth Hormone during Childhood," in Stabler and Underwood (1986); B. Stabler, J. R. Turner, S. S. Girdler, et al., "Reactivity to Stress and Psychological Adjustment in Adults with Pituitary Insufficiency, *Clinical Endocrinology* 36, no. 5 (1992): 467–73; B. Stabler, R. R. Clopper, P. T. Siegel, et al., "Links between Growth Hormone Deficiency, Adaptation and Social Phobia," *Hormone Research* 45, no. 1–2 (1996): 30–33; L. M. Nicholas, M. E. Tancer, S. G. Silva, et al., "Short Stature, Growth Hormone Deficiency and Social Anxiety," *Psychosomatic Medicine* 59, no. 4 (1997): 372–75.

48. A. Glatzer, O. Aran, N. Beit-Halachmi, et al., "The Impact of Long-term Therapy by a Multidisciplinary Team on the Education, Occupation and Marital Status of Growth Hormone Deficient Patients after Termination of Therapy," *Clinical Endocrinology* 27(1987): 191–96.

49. Stabler, Turner, Girdler, Light, and Underwood, 1992.

50. G. McGauley, R. Cuneo, F. Salomon, and P. Sonksen, "Growth Hormone Deficiency and Quality of Life," *Hormone Research* 45 (1996): 34–37.

51. "Adults Who Live with Growth Hormone Deficiency (GHD)," The Magic Foundation, www.magicfoundation.org/adultlwghdp.html.

52. E. McCauley, J. Ito, and T. Kay, "Psychosocial Functioning in Girls with Turner Syndrome and Short Stature: Social Skills, Behavior Problems, and Self-concept," *Journal of the American Academy of Child Psychiatry* 25, no. 1 (1986): 105–12; E. McCauley, T. Kay, and R. Treder, "The Turner Syndrome, Cognitive Deficits, Affective Discrimination, and Behavior Problems," *Child Development* 58 (1987): 64–73.

53. J. Downey, A. A. Ehrhardt, R. Gruen, A. Morishima, and J. Bell, "Turner Syndrome vs. Constitutional Short Stature: Psychopathology and Reaction to Height," in Stabler and Underwood, 1986; J. Downey, A A. Ehrhardt, R. Gruen, et al., "Psychopathology and Social Functioning in Women with Turner Syndrome," The *Journal of Nervous and Mental Disease* 177, no. 4 (1989): 191–201.

54. E. McCauley, V. P. Sybert, and A. A. Ehrhardt, "Psychosocial Adjustment of Adult Women with Turner Syndrome," *Clinical Genetics* 29, no. 4 (1986): 284–90.

55. K. Pavlidis, E. McCauley, and V. P. Sybert, "Psychosocial and Sexual Functioning in Women with Turner Syndrome," *Clinical Genetics* 47, no. 2 (1995): 85–89.

56. J. Ross, A. Zinn, and E. McCauley, "Neurodevelopmental and Psychosocial Aspects of Turner Syndrome," *Mental Retardation and Developmental Disabilities Research Review* 6, no. 2 (2000): 135–41.

57. J. E. Toublanc, F. Thibaud, and C. Lecointre, "Psychosocial and Sexual Outcome in Women with Turner Syndrome," *Contraception Fertilite Sexualite (Paris)* 25, no. 7–8 (1997): 633–38.

58. G. Calo, G. Guzzaloni, D. Moro, et al., "Social Integration in Adulthood in a Group of Subjects with Turner Syndrome," *Minerva Pediatrica* 45, no. 6 (1993) 247–51.

59. L. Sylven, C. Magnusson, K. Hagenfeldt, and B. Van Schoultz, "Life with Turner's Syndrome: A Psychosocial Report from 22 Middle-aged Women," *Acta Endocrinologica* 129, no. 3 (1993): 201–6.

60. L. L. Mullins, J. Lynch, J. Orten, and L. K. Youll, "Developing a Program to Assist Turner's Syndrome Patients and Their Families," *Social Work Health Care* 16, no. 2 (1991): 69–79; P. T. Siegel, R. Clopper, and B. Stabler, "The Psychological Consequences of Turner Syndrome and Review of the National Cooperative Growth Study Psychological Substudy," *Pediatrics* 102, no. 2, Pt. 3 (1998): 488–91.

61. D. Dorholt, M. Noeker, M. Ranke, and F. Haverkamp, "Body Height, Body Image and General Well-being in Adult Women with Turner's Syndrome," in Eiholzer, Haverkamp, and Voss, 95–103.

62. See Shirley Poirier, "Autobiographical Reminiscences and Journal," www.cnwl.igs .net/~poirier/page3.html.

63. Drash, Greenberg, and Money (1968): 574.

64. Ibid., 577.

65. J. Brust , C. Ford, and D. Rimoin, "Psychiatric Aspects of Dwarfism," 161.

66. Ablon, Little People.

67. Ibid., 60.

68. M. S. Weinberg, "The Problems of Midgets and Dwarfs and Organizational Remedies: A Study of the Little People of America," Journal of Health and Social Behavior 9 (1968): 65–71; W. Ricker, "Problems of Parents with Children of Short Stature" (unpublished paper distributed by LPA and HGF; n.d.); Sonny Kleinfeld, "Our Smallest Minority: Dwarfs," Atlantic, September 1975, 65; C. I. Scott, "Medical and Social Adaptation in Dwarfing Conditions," Birth Defects Original Articles Series 13, no. 3C (1977): 29–43; J. O. Weiss, "Social Development of Dwarfs," in Proceedings of a Conference on Genetic Disorders: Social Service Intervention, ed. W. T. Hall and C. L. Young (Pittsburgh: University of Pittsburgh Graduate School of Public Health, 1977), 56–61.

69. J. O. Weiss, "Social Development of Dwarfs," 56–61.

70. Folstein, Weiss, Mittleman, and Ross, "Impairment and Psychiatric Symptoms in Dwarfs," 1981.

71. L. Stace and D. M. Danks, "A Social Study of Dwarfing Conditions," Australian Paediatric Journal 17(1981): 167–82.

72. A. G. Hunter, "Some Psychosocial Aspects of Nonlethal Chondrodysplasias," American Journal of Medical Genetics 78, no. 1 (1998): 1–29.

73. Alasdair Hunter, e-mail message to the author, 30 March 2001.

74. Gina Zingaro, "A Study of the Impact of Organizational Membership and Parental Attitudes on the Development of Self-esteem of the Adolescent Dwarf Individual," Senior Thesis in Sociology, Goucher College, 1981.

75. C. Sherrill, M. Hinson, B. Gench, S. O. Kennedy, and L. Low, "Self-concepts of Disabled Youth Athletes," Perceptual and Motor Skills 70, no. 3 pt. 2 (1990): 1093–8.

76. M. Mulberg, "The Relationship between Negative Body Image and Depressive Symptomatology in Dwarf-Statured Individuals" (Ph.D. dissertation, New York University, 1985).

77. R. Griggs, "A Comparison of the Self Concept of Short-statured versus Average-statured Individuals and Their Perception of Each Other" (master's thesis, Abilene Christian University, 1988).

78. J. Moneymaker, "The Social Significance of Short Stature: A Study of the Problems of Dwarfs and Midgets," Loss, Grief, and Care 3, no. 3–4 (1989), 183–89.

79. N. Roizen, E. Ekwo, and C. Gosselink, "Comparison of Education and Occupation of Adults with Achondroplasia with Same-sex Sibs," American Journal of Medical Genetics 35(1990): 257–60.

80. S. A. Frankel, "Psychological Complications of Short Stature in Childhood: Some Implications of the Role of Visual Comparisons in Normal and Pathological Development," Psychoanalytic Study of the Child 51 (1996): 455–74.

81. L. Ancona, "The Psychodynamics of Achondroplasia," in Human Achondroplasia: An Interdisciplinary Approach, ed. N. Benedetto and S. E. Kopits, Proceedings of the First

International Symposium in Rome, Italy, 19–21 November 1986, Basic Life Sciences (New York: Plenum, 1989), 48:447–51.

82. W. G. Shakespeare, "Social Implications of Achondroplasia: A Public Health View," in *Human Achondroplasia: An Interdisciplinary Approach*, 453–55.

83. D. Skuse, "The Psychological Consequences of Being Small," *Journal of Child Psychology and Allied Disciplines* 28, no. 5 (1987): 641–50; D. E. Sandberg, W. M. Bukowski, C. M. Fung, and R. B. Noll, "Height and Social Adjustment: Are Extremes a Cause for Concern and Action?" *Pediatrics* 114, no. 3 (2004): 744–50; J. L. Ross, D. E. Sandberg, and S. R. Rose, "Psychological Adaptation in Children with Idiopathic Short Stature Treated with Growth Hormone or Placebo," *Journal of Clinical Metabolism* 89, no. 10 (2004): 4873–78.

84. Leslie F. Martel and Henry B. Biller, *Stature and Stigma: The Biopsychosocial Development of Short Males* (Lexington, MA: DC Heath and Company, 1987). Quotes are from pp. 14 and 86.

85. Eiholzer, Haverkamp, and Voss, *Stature and Well-being*.

86. M. Noeker and F. Haverkamp, "Can Clinical and Empirical Evidence regarding Adjustment to Short Stature Be Reconciled," in Eiholzer, Haverkamp, and Voss, 107–20.

87. Ibid, 117.

88. M. Noeker, D. Dorholt, M. Ranke, and F. Haverkamp, "Stress, Resources and Social Adaptation to Short Stature in Childhood: A Study in Pathological Growth Disorders," in Eiholzer, Haverkamp, and Voss, 59–72.

89. J. Ablon, "Personality and Stereotype in Osteogenesis Imperfecta," *American Journal of Medical Genetics* 122A (2003): 201–14. Quotations by OI subjects appear on pp. 203, 209, and 210. For a study indicating high adaptability and resiliency in diastrophic patients, see P. Vaara, H. Sintonen, J. Peltonen, et al., "Health-Related Quality of Life in Patients with Diastrophic Dysplasia," *Scandinavian Journal of Public Health* 27, no. 1 (1999): 38–42.

90. M. Reite, K. Davis, C. C. Solomons, and J. Ott, "Osteogenesis Imperfecta: Psychological Function," *The American Journal of Psychology* 128, no, 12 (1972): 1540–45.

91. Joan Ablon, e-mail message to the author, 25 February 2004.

92. S. E. Gollust, R. E. Thompson, H. C. Gooding, B. B. Biesecker, "Living with Achondroplasia in an Average-sized World".

93. Andrew Solomon, *The Noonday Demon: An Atlas of Depression* (New York: Simon and Schuster, 2001).

94. Leslye Sneider, "Thoughts on the Untimely Death of a Longtime Friend," unpublished article, August 2003.

95. Bonnie Rothman Morris, "Two Types of Brain Problems Are Found to Cause Dyslexia," *New York Times*, 8 July 2003, F5.

96. J. L. Tringo, "The Hierarchy of Preference toward Disability Groups," *Journal of Special Education* 4 (1970): 295–306.

CHAPTER 3. THE BIRTH OF A CHILD

1. Robert and Suzanne Massie, *Journey* (New York: Alfred E, Knopf, 1973); Helen Featherstone, *A Difference in the Family* (New York: Basic Books, 1980).

2. Dan Kennedy, *Little People: Looking at the World through My Daughter's Eyes*

(Emmaus, PA: Rodále Press, 1993); Joan Ablon, "Ambiguity and Difference: Families with Dwarf Children," *Social Science and Medicine* 30, no. 8 (1990); Joan Ablon, *Living with Difference* (New York: Praeger, 1988).

3. Ablon, "Ambiguity and Difference," 880.

4. V. Hill, M. Sahhar, M. Aitkin, et al., "Experience at the Time of Diagnosis of Parents Who Have a Child with a Bone Dysplasia Resulting in Short Stature," *American Journal of Medical Genetics* 122A, no. 2 (2003): 100–7.

5. Ablon, *Living with Difference*, 14.

6. Ibid., 14–15.

7. Bill Loman, "Standing Tall: Chesterfield Teacher's Spirit 'Defies Words,'" www.timesdispatch.com/flair/MGBQTGVLPLC.html.

8. Sue Thurman, letter to the author, Fall 1980.

9. See American Academy of Pediatrics, "Health Supervision for Children with Achondroplasia," *Pediatrics* 95, no. 3 (1995): 443–51.

10. Ablon, *Living with Difference*, 27.

11. R. M. Pauli, P. Modaff, E. Fowler, and C. A. Reiser, *To Celebrate: Understanding Developmental Differences in Young Children with Achondroplasia* (Madison: University of Wisconsin, Midwestern Bone Dysplasia Clinic, 1997), n.p.

12. Vita Gagne, e-mail message to the author, 12 October 2001.

13. "The Individual with Dwarfism as Parent: A Position Statement by Little People of America Inc.," www.lpaonline.org/library-dwarfasparent.html.

14. Ellen Highland Fernandez, *The Challenges Facing Dwarf Parents* (Tamarac, FL: Distinctive Publishing Group, 1990).

CHAPTER 4. ORGANIZATIONS

1. Edward J. Wood, *Giants and Dwarfs* (London: Edward Bentley, 1868), 315–16.

2. Billy Barty, telephone interview with the author, 19 December 1998.

3. Joan Ablon, *Little People in America* (New York: Praeger Publishers, 1984), and *Living with Difference* (New York: Praeger Publishers, 1988), 101.

4. Martin S. Weinberg, "The Problems of Midgets and Dwarfs and Organizational Remedies: A Study of Little People of America," *Journal of Health and Social Behavior* 9 (1968): 65–72.

5. Weinberg, "Problems of Midgets and Dwarfs," 68.

6. *LPA Today*, January–February 1998, 21–23.

7. Nancy Rockwood, telephone interview with the author, 26 January 1999.

8. National MPS Society, Inc., www.mpssociety.org/mps-factsheet.html.

9. Marie Capobianco, telephone interview with the author, January 1999; Linda Shine, telephone interview with the author, 28 January 1999.

10. Philip J. Hilts, "Fetus to Fetus Transplant Blocks Deadly Genetic Defect, Researchers Say," *New York Times*, 21 November 1991, B14.

11. "Clinical Trials, MPS I: FDA Panel Backs Efficacy, Safety of Aldurazyme for MPS I," National MPS Society Web site, www.mpssociety.org/news-clinical.html.

12. Sally Motomuro, interview with the author, 24 March 2004.

13. A grant for research on genetic defects and storage disorders, including Fabry and Hunters, was announced by NORD on 11 October 2001. See "The NORD/Roscoe Brady

328   NOTES TO PAGES 201–213

Lysosomal Storage Diseases Fellowship," for information about awards granted in 2001, 2002, and 2003. www.rarediseases.org/research/roscoe.

14. See Web sites of Brian Daugherty, Danette Baker, and Shawn Brush at www. LPAOnline.org.

15. *Turner Syndrome and Short Stature: QA—Answers to commonly asked questions,* a publication of the Turner Syndrome Society.

16. L. G. Tesch, "Turner Syndrome: A Personal Perspective," *Adolescent and Pediatric Gynecology* 2 (1989): 186–88.

17. *Fast Facts on Osteogenesis Imperfecta* is a superb pamphlet developed by Michael Whyte, chair of the OI Foundation Medical Advisory Committee. It discusses medical, management, and psychosocial issues and is available from the Osteogenesis Imperfecta Foundation.

18. Ellen Dollar, public relations director of Osteogenesis Imperfecta Society, telephone conversation with the author, 25 January 1999.

19. One such account is Osteogenesis Imperfecta Type I: Jojos Story," www.ptialaska .net/~sturm/OI_JoJo.html.

20. F. H. Glorieux, N. J. Bishop, H. Plotkin, et al., "Cyclic Administration of Pamidronate in Children with Severe Osteogenesis Imperfecta," *New England Journal of Medicine* 339 (1998): 947–52; "Montreal Shriners Hospital Study Advances Potential Drug Treatment for Children with OI," in *OIF Breakthrough* November/December 1998, 1.

21. See "New Research Strategies in Osteogenesis Imperfecta," www.oif.org/site/ PageServer?pagename=03ResStratMtg; S. Adami, D. Gatti, F. Colapietro, et al, "Intravenous Neridronate in Adults with Osteogenesis Imperfecta," *Journal of Bone and Mineral Research* 18, no.1 (2003): 126–30; R. Sakkers, D. Kok, R. Engelbert, et al, "Skeletal Effects and Functional Outcome with Olpadronate in Children with Osteogenesis Imperfecta," *Lancet* 363 (2004): 1427–31; N. P. Camacho, C. L. Raggio, S. B. Doty, et al, "A Controlled Study of the Effects of Alendronate in a Growing Mouse Model of Osteogenesis Imperfecta," *Calcified Tissue International* 69, no.2 (2001): 94–101; "Bisphosphonates, An Information Update from the OI Foundation's Medical Advisory Council," *OIF Breakthrough,* Summer 2004.

22. See discussion in Psychology chapter of J. Ablon, "Personality and Stereotype in Osteogenesis Imperfecta," *American Journal of Medical Genetics* 122A (2003): 201–14.

23. C. I. Scott, N. Mayeux, R. Crandall, and J. O. Weiss, *Dwarfism: The Family and Professional Guide* (Short Stature Foundation Pr., 1994). Available through LPA.

24. Dan Kennedy, "Not alone anymore." www.salon.com/sept97/mothers/alone970917 .html. This article also discusses the experiences and Web sites of other disability groups.

25. Dan Kennedy, personal communication, 23 November 2001.

26. Kennedy, "Not Alone Anymore," 8–9.

CHAPTER 5. LIVES TODAY

1. For a full account of the history of advocacy among persons with disabilities, see Doris Zames Fleischer and Frieda Zames, *The Disability Rights Movement* (Philadelphia: Temple University Press, 1999).

2. This legal process is described in greater detail by Cara Egan, "LPA, Inc.: Coming

of Age in the Policy Arena" (master's thesis, School of Hygiene and Public Health, Department of Health Policy and Management, Johns Hopkins University, 2001). It provides an essential background to the growth of advocacy among the disabled, especially dwarfs.

3. C. Angela Van Etten, "Little People and Disability from a Personal and Legal Perspective," *LPA Today,* May–September 1999, 50, http://gate.net/~vanetten/ergochair.htm. See also the Americans with Disabilities Act (Civil Rights Division, U.S. Department of Justice, Washington, D.C. 201 514-0301). New York Lawyers for the Public Interest, Inc., facilitates complaints.

4. Angel and Eileen Shields, telephone interview with the author, 27 October 2000.

5. "Survey: Disabled are Disadvantaged Too," www.dwarfism.org/library/survey.phtml.

6. Bethany Jewett, "Watson Final Report," 1988, 20 pages, photocopy.

7. Bethany Jewett Stark, telephone interview with the author, 12 March 2000.

8. Jewett, 11.

9. *Careers, Employment and Education* (Restricted Growth Association, P.O. Box 8, Countesthorpe, Leicestershire, LE8 5ZS, n.p).

10. Ibid.

11. Van Etten, "Little People and Disability from a Personal and Legal Perspective."

12. Egan, "LPA, Inc.: Coming of Age in the Policy Arena."

13. Jenny Clark, "Battling Your HMO: Your Second Job." *LPA Today,* Conference Wrap-Up 2001, 1, 10.

14. Honor Rawlings, e-mail message to the author, 21 January 2000.

15. Martin Monestier, *Les Nains* (Paris: J.C. Simeon, 1977), 183.

16. George Sofkin, e-mail messages to the author, 12 February, 2000; 26 August 2004.

17. Luke Oyawiri, "Dwarfs Lament Prejudice against Them," THISDAY online, www.thisdayonline.com/archive/2003/05/19/20030519da02.html.

18. Monestier, *Les Nains,* 177.

19. Lee Kitchens, former LPA vice president, e-mail message to the author, 22 November 2001.

20. Duncan Hewitt, "Asia-Pacific Short Chinese Walk Tall," *LPA Today,* May–September 1999, 17. Originally appeared on BBC Online Network (http://news.bbc.co.uk/), 10 April 1999.

21. Hanna Beech, "High Hopes," *Time asia,* 17 December 2001. TIMEasia.com, www.time.com/time/asia/news/magazine/0,9754,187654,00.html, 1–3.

22. Elisabeth Rosenthal, "College Entrance in China: 'No' to the Handicapped," *New York Times,* 23 May 2001, A3.

23. "A Handicapped Man Accuses His Mother," *Beijing Daily News,* 7 April 1989, translated from Chinese by Professor Tao Jie.

24. Professor Tao Jie, letter to the author, 10 August 1989.

25. Nicholas D Kristof, "Outcast Status Worsens Pain of Japan's Disabled," *New York Times,* 7 April 1996, Sect. l, 3.

26. Ibid.

27. Stephanie Strom, "Social Warming: Japan's Disabled Gain New Status," *New York Times,* 7 July 2001, B7.

28. Etsuko Enami Nomachi, e-mail message to the author, 13 December 2001.

29. Susan Orlean, "Fertile Ground," *The New Yorker,* 7 June 1999, 64.

30. Helene Whitaker, Dwarfism List posting, 2002 (exact date unavailable).

31. *The Teenage Years*, Restricted Growth Association, PO Box 8, Countesthorpe, Leicestershire, LE8 5ZS United Kingdom).

32. Ibid.

33. Nicola Persico, Andrew Postlewaite, and Dan Silverman, "The Effect of Adolescent Experience on Labor Market Outcomes: The Case of Height," mimeo, University of Pennsylvania, 2002. Quoted online in "Shorter Men Earn Less Money in Careers," *Science News*, 19 April 2002. www.cosmiverse.com/news/science04190206.html.

34. Steven Landsburg, "Short Changed: Why Do Tall People Make More Money?" *Slate*, 25 March 2002. http://slate.msn.com/?id=2063439

35. E. T. Mörch, *Chondrodystrophic Dwarfs in Denmark* (Copenhagen: Einar Munksgaard, 1941).

36. Judith Hall, "Results of the Survey of Medical Complications in Classical Achondroplasia," photocopy, 1974–75.

37. S. E. Folstein, J. O. Weiss, F. Mittleman, and D. J. Ross, "Impairment, Psychiatric Symptoms, and Handicap in Dwarfs," *Johns Hopkins Medical Journal* 148 (1981): 273–77.

38. Ken Wolf, "Big World, Little People," *Newsday*, 20 April 1989, 8–17.

39. John H. Richardson, "Dwarfs: A Love Story," *Esquire*, February 1998, 74–121.

40. John Wolin, "Dwarf Like Me," *Miami Herald Tropic*, 24 January 1993, 12–21. Wolin became increasingly disabled as a result of spinal compression and died on 30 August 2004 after spinal surgery. See Greg Cote, "Epitaph for John Wolin: Nobody Cared More," *Miami Herald*. Wolin's article, "Walking Tall": also appears on the Web site of the Society of Professional Journalists, spjsofla.net.

41. John Richardson, *In the Little World: A True Story of Dwarfs, Love, and Trouble* (New York: HarperCollins, 2001).

42. Dan Kennedy, *Little People: Through My Dwarf Daughter's Eyes* (Emmaus, PA: Rodale Press, 2003).

43. Wolin, quoting Tatman, 18.

44. Ibid.

45. Wolin, describing his own experience.

46. Ibid.

47. Walter Bodin and Burnett Hershey, *It's a Small World: All about Midgets* (New York: Coward-McCann, Inc., 1934), 29.

48. Elsa Davidson, "Size Matters," is a freelance writer and graduate student in cultural anthropology in New York City. Her article was previously at www.feedmag.com/deepread/dr261.html (site now discontinued; check lpaonline.org for possible reappearance.)

49. Marcello Truzzi, "Lilliputians in Gulliver's Land," in *Sociology and Everyday Life*, ed. Marcello Truzzi (Englewood Cliffs, NJ: Prentice Hall, 1968), 208.

50. Monestier, *Les Nains*, 166.

51. *Scots Magazine* for August 1751, quoted in Wood, 357.

52. A. G. Hunter, "Some Psychosocial Aspects of Nonlethal Chondrodysplasias: IV. Dyadic Scale of Marital Adjustment, "*American Journal of Medical Genetics* 78, no.1 (1998): 17–21.

53. Leslie Fiedler, *Freaks: Myths and Images of the Secret Self* (New York: Simon and Schuster, 1977), 53.

54. Van Etten, *Dwarfs*, 185.

55. Christopher Smart, "The Author Apologizes to a Lady for His Being a Little Man,"

The Collected Poems of Christopher Smart, ed. Norman Callan (Cambridge, MA: Harvard University Press, 1950), 1:112–13.

56. Matt Roloff with Tracey Sumner: *Against Tall Odds: Being a Goliath in a David World.* Sisters (Sisters, OR: Multnomah Publishers, Inc.), 1999.

57. Van Etten, *Dwarfs,* 215, Sawitch and McDonald quotations.

58. Mark Andrew Berseth, "When an O.I.'er begets an O.I.'er." *Signal,* publication of the Osteogenesis Imperfecta Foundation, Spring 1989, 1.

59. Simon Minty, e-mail message to the author, 23 February 2002.

60. Ruth Ricker, "Retirement Project," *LPA Today,* January–February 1998, 8.

61. Kim Silarski, "Little People Bridge Two Worlds," *Detroit News,* 20 December 2001. http://detnews.com/2001/homelife/0112/20/c01-371098.htm.

62. Fred and Linda Short, "My Garden," *Carryongardening,* 24 September 2002. www.carryongardening.org.uk/mygarden.asp.

63. Bodin and Hershey, *Small World,* 89–90.

64. Truzzi, "Lilliputians in Gulliver's Land."

65. Ernst Trier Mörch, *Chondrodystrophic Dwarfs in Denmark* (Copenhagen: Einar Munksgaard, 1941).

66. Dave Elsila, "Solidarity: Little People with Big Jobs," October 1997, www.uaw.org/solidarity/9707/06_1.html.

67. C. I. Scott, Jr., "Medical and Social Adaptation in Dwarfing Conditions," *Birth Defects Original Article Series* 13, no. 3C, 29–43 (The National Foundation, 1977), 34.

68. J. E. Gollust, R. E. Thompson, H. C. Gooding, and B. B. Biesecker, "Living with Achondroplasia in an Average-Sized World: An Assessment of Quality of Life," *American Journal of Medical Genetics* 120A (2003): 447–58.

69. I obtained the assistance of Berna Miller Torr, demographer at Brown University, in finding online sites and approaching data analysis. However, because she did not oversee the process, or check the results, I alone am responsible for any inadequacies. Nevertheless, I am confident that this summary represents a reasonably accurate picture of the vocational pattern of the group.

70. Matt Roloff, with Tracy Sumner, *Against Tall Odds* (Sisters, OR: Multnomah Publishers, 1999).

71. "An Interview with Melinda North," *LPA Today,* Winter 2002, 8.

72. Jennifer Arnold, telephone conversation with the author, 2 March 2003.

73. See, for example, the documentary *Dwarfs: Little People, Big Steps* and Anita Srikameswaran, "Meet Dr. Arnold," *Pittsburgh Post Gazette,* 7 August 2001. www.postgazette.com/healthscience/20010807hlittledoc.3.asp, 1–4.

74. Dena Hofkosh quotation, "She's got this very lovely ability . . . ," Srikameswaren, 1; "Academics don't come easy . . . ," Jennifer Arnold, telephone conversation with the author, March 2003.

75. Quotations of Miller's views are drawn from an interview with the author on 7 January 2002. Miller is featured at greater length in Betty M. Adelson, *The Lives of Dwarfs: Their Journey from Public Curiosity toward Social Liberation* (Piscataway, NJ: Rutgers University Press, 2005).

76. Paul Steven Miller, "The Changing Face of Civil Rights," *LPA Today,* July–October 1998, 48.

77. Uriya Shavit, "The Times That Really Matter," *Ha'aretz Magazine,* 22 February 2002.

78. Fred Short, "Occupations and Avocations," www.lpaonline.org/library_fredslist.html.

79. Cisca Pijpers, author of works on disability, Dwarfism List posting, 31 August 2001.

80. Maria Perez, former senior vice president of LPA, Dwarfism List posting, 4 January 2003.

81. Roloff, *Against Tall Odds*, 124.

82. Angela Van Etten, *Dwarfs Don't Live in Doll Houses* (Rochester, NY: Adaptive Living, 1988), 237.

83. Peter Suber, "Paternalism," *Philosophy of Law: An Encyclopedia, ed. Christopher Grey* (New York: Garland Publishing Co., 1999), vol. 2, 632–35. Also www.earlham.edu/-perers/writingpaternal.htm.

84. "U. N. backs dwarf-tossing ban," www.cnn.com/2002/WORLD/europe/09/27/dwarf.throwing/.

85. Sheila Ackerlind, *Patterns of Conflict: The Individual and Society in Spanish Literature to 1700* (New York: Peter Lang, 1988).

86. Roloff, *Against Tall Odds*, 125.

Index 〰